# CONTENTS

# KEY TOPICS IN
# PSYCHIATRY

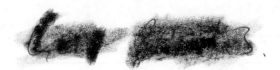

# The KEY TOPICS Series

**Advisors:**

**T.M. Craft** *Department of Anaesthesia and Intensive Care, Royal United Hospital, Bath, UK*
**C.S. Garrard** *Intensive Therapy Unit, John Radcliffe Hospital, Oxford, UK*
**P.M. Upton** *Department of Anaesthetics, Treliske Hospital, Truro, UK*

---

**Anaesthesia, Second Edition**

**Obstetrics and Gynaecology**

**Accident and Emergency Medicine**

**Paediatrics**

**Orthopaedic Surgery**

**Otolaryngology and Head and Neck Surgery**

**Ophthalmology**

**Psychiatry**

Forthcoming titles include:

**General Surgery**

**Oncology**

**Oral Surgery**

**Renal Medicine**

# KEY TOPICS IN
# PSYCHIATRY

## C.E. SMITH
MA, BMBCh, MRCPsych
*Clinical Lecturer, Oxford University Department of Psychiatry*
*Honorary Senior Registrar, Warneford Hospital, Oxford, UK*

## L. SELL
MA, MBBS, MRCP, MRCPsych
*The Maudsley Hospital, London, UK*

## P. SUDBURY
MA, BMBCh, MRCPsych
*Consultant Psychiatrist, Wexham Park Hospital, Slough, UK*

**Consultant Editor**

## C. BASS
MA, MD, FRCPsych
*Consultant in Liaison Psychiatry, John Radcliffe Hospital, Oxford, UK*

βIOS
SCIENTIFIC
PUBLISHERS

© BIOS Scientific Publishers Limited, 1996

First published 1996

A CIP catalogue record for this book is available from the British Library.

ISBN 1 872748 17 1

BIOS Scientific Publishers Ltd
9 Newtec Place, Magdalen Road, Oxford OX4 1RE, UK
Tel. +44 (0)1865 726286. Fax. +44 (0)1865 246823

DISTRIBUTORS

*Australia and New Zealand*
    DA Information Services
    648 Whitehorse Road, Mitcham
    Victoria 3132

*India*
    Viva Books Private Limited
    4325/3 Ansari Road, Daryaganj
    New Delhi 110002

*Singapore and South East Asia*
    Toppan Company (S) PTE Ltd
    38 Liu Fang Road, Jurong
    Singapore 2262

*USA and Canada*
    Books International Inc.
    PO Box 605, Herndon VA 22070

Typeset by Chandos Electronic Publishing, Stanton Harcourt, UK.
Printed by Redwood Books, Trowbridge, UK.

**Front cover:** *adapted from an illustration on p. 226 of* Practical Problems in Clinical Psychiatry, *edited by K. Hawton and P. Cowen, with permission from M. Sharpe and Oxford University Press.*

[a] Contributed by K.A. Smith ( MRCPsych), Wellcome Training Fellow and Honorary Senior Registrar, Littlemore Hospital, Oxford, UK

[b] Contributed by C. Bass (MA, MD, FRCPsych), Consultant in Liaison Psychiatry, John Radcliffe Hospital, Oxford, UK

[c] Contributed by D. Gill (MRC), Health Services Research Fellow, Institute of Health Sciences, Oxford, UK

[d] Contributed by D. Rowe (BMedSci, BM, BS, MRCPsych), Senior Registrar in Psychiatry of Learning Disability, The Slade Hospital, Oxford, UK

# ABBREVIATIONS

| | |
|---|---|
| ACh | acetylcholine |
| ACTH | adrenocorticotrophic hormone |
| AD | Alzheimer's disease |
| ADH | anti-diuretic hormone |
| AIDS | acquired immune deficiency syndrome |
| AN | anorexia nervosa |
| ANa | autonomic nervous system |
| APP | amyloid precusor proteins |
| ASP | antisocial personality disorder |
| ASW | approved social worker |
| BNF | British National Formulary |
| BP | bipolar |
| BPD | borderline personality disorder |
| BS | behavioural syndrome |
| BT | behaviour therapy |
| BN | bulimia nervosa |
| C and R | control and restraint |
| CBT | cognitive behaviour therapy |
| CCF | congestive cardiac failure |
| CCK | cholecystokinin |
| ChAT | choline acetyl transferase |
| CIS | Clinical Interview Schedule |
| CJD | Creutzfeld-Jacob disease |
| CLAT | choline acetyltransferase |
| CNS | central nervous system |
| COAs | children of alcoholics |
| CPK | creatine phosphokinase |
| CRF | corticotrophin releasing factor |
| CSA | child sex abuse |
| CT | computerized tomography |
| CTC | clinical trials certificate |
| CTX | clinical trials exemption certificate |
| CVA | cerebrovascular accident |
| DA | dopamine |
| DD | dissociate (conversion) disorder |
| DIS | Diagnostic Interview Schedule |
| DSH | deliberate self-harm |
| DVT | deep vein thrombosis |
| DZ | dizygotic |
| ECA | epidemiological catchment area |
| ECT | electroconvulsive therapy |
| EE | expressed emotion |

| | |
|---|---|
| EEG | electroencephalogram |
| EP | evoked potentials |
| EPQ | Eysenck Personality Questionnaire |
| EPSE | extrapyramidal side effect |
| ESR | erythrocyte sedimentation rate |
| FBC | full blood count |
| FSH | follicle stimulating hormone |
| GABA | gamma-aminobutyric acid |
| GAD | generalized anxiety disorder |
| GFR | glomerular filtration rate |
| GH | growth hormone |
| GI | gastrointestinal |
| GMS | geriatric mental state |
| GnRH | gonadotrophin releasing hormone |
| HD | Huntington's disease |
| HGPRT | hypoxanthineguanine phosphoribosyl transferase |
| 5-HIAA | 5-hydroxyindoleacetic acid |
| HIV | human immunodeficiency virus |
| HLA | human leucocyte antigen |
| HPA | hypo–pituitary–adrenal axis |
| HR | heart rate |
| 5-HT | 5-hydroxytryptamine |
| HVA | homovallinic acid |
| ICD | International Classification of Diseases |
| IPT | interpersonal therapy |
| LH | luteinizing hormone |
| LNANs | large neutral amino acids |
| LTM | long-term memory |
| MAOI | monoamine-oxidase inhibitor |
| MARI | monoamine reuptake inhibitor |
| MDMA | methoxydesmethyl amphetamine (ecstasy) |
| ME | myalgic encephalomyelitis |
| MHA | Mental Health Act |
| MHPG | 3-methoxy-4-hydroxyphenylethylene gycol |
| MHRT | Mental Health Tribunal |
| MHV | Mill Hill Vocabulary Test |
| MID | multi-infarct dementia |
| MMSE | mini-mental state examination |
| MRI | magnetic resonance imaging |
| MZ | monozygotic |
| NA | noradrenaline |
| NART | National Adult Reading Test |
| NMDA | $N$-methyl D-aspartate |
| NMR | nuclear magnetic resonance imaging |
| NMS | neuroleptic malignant syndrome |

| | |
|---|---|
| NPY | neuropeptide Y |
| OCD | obsessive-compulsive disorder |
| PCP | phencyclidine |
| PD | Parkinson's disease |
| PET | positron electron tomography |
| PHF-tau | paired helical filament-tau |
| PMS | post marketing surveillance |
| PRL | prolactin |
| PSE | Present State Examination |
| PTA | post-traumatic amnesia |
| PTSD | post-traumatic stress disorder |
| RAS | reticular activating system |
| RBD | recurrent brief depression |
| RCBF | regional cerebral blood flow |
| RDC | Research Diagnostic Criteria |
| REM | rapid eye movement |
| RFLP | restriction fragment length polymorphisms |
| RPM | Ravens Progressive Matrices |
| SAD | seasonal affective disorder |
| SD | somatization disorder |
| SDAT | senile dementia of the Alzheimer type |
| SDLT | senile dementia of Lewy body type |
| SEC | socioeconomic class |
| SLPE | schizophrenia-like psychosis of epilepsy |
| SPECT | single photon emission tomography |
| SSRIs | selective serotonin reuptake inhibitors |
| STM | short-term memory |
| STS | short-term store |
| SWS | slow wave sleep |
| TD | tardive dyskinesia |
| TENS | transcutaneous electrical nerve stimulation |
| THC | tetrahydrocannabinol |
| TRH | thyroid releasing hormone |
| TRP | tryptophan |
| TSH | thyroid stimulating hormone |
| UP | unipolar |
| VIP | vasoactive intestinal peptide |
| WAIS | Wechsler Adult Intelligence Scale |
| WHO | World Health Organization |

# PREFACE

Psychiatry continues to undergo rapid development and changes. This applies as much to training and the examination for the membership of the Royal College of Phsychiatrists as it does for clinical practice. This book aims to provide the reader with a framework of information about a number of key topics. Basic information is contained in some topics (e.g. conditioning, learning, rating scales), and a symptom-oriented approach is used in others (e.g. the intoxicated patient, stuporose patient, hyperventilation and dangerousness). Topics on specific commonly seen disorders (e.g. anxiety and panic, schizophrenia, chronic fatigue syndrome) are also included. Other material which does not lend itself to this format has been included in the relevant topics, and in particular we have attempted to cover 'topical' subjects such as the Care Programme Approach, supervision registers, services for patients with deliberate self harm, suicide prevention and treatment of chronic fatigue syndrome.

Although this book is aimed predominantely at psychiatrists in training, particularly those who are studying for their membership examinations, it should also be an ideal introduction to the speciality for medical students. General practioners, especially those on vocational training schemes in psychiatry, should also find the book a valuable and accessible reference.

Throughout the book we have attempted to use a multi-axial classification of psychiatric disorder, and have been guided by the clinical descriptions and diagnostic guidelines contained in the International Classifications of Diseases Classification of Mental and Behavioural Disorders (10th edition, 1992). Wherever possible, however, we have also made reference to the North American classification (Diagnostic and Statistical Manual, 4th Edn, 1994).

During the preparation of the book, there have been important recent changes in the subjects covered. We have attempted to include these, and the reader is encouraged to fill out the information further by referring to those topics of related interest and by consulting the references cited at the end of each topic. A short index is provided to help locate certain key areas within the book.

We would like to thank Dr Jonathan Ray and Jane Campbell at BIOS for their patience and support.

*C. Smith*
*L. Sell*
*P. Sudbury*

# ADDICTION – AETIOLOGY

The aetiology of addictive behaviour is complex, and only a brief overview can be attempted here. We can divide factors into societal / subcultural, familial and individual.

**Societal/subcultural influences**

*1. Price.* The prime determinant of consumption of drugs, or any other goods, across a society, is the relative price thereof. Per capita alcohol consumption of alcohol or cigarettes is correlated, both within and across countries, with price relative to the standard of living. There is no evidence that legality or otherwise makes any difference to this economic law. In Vietnam, where opiates were cheap and plentiful, 40% of US servicemen at some point experienced physical dependence (Robins, 1993). Interesting questions arise about the 'elasticity' of demand; that is the degree to which consumption is sensitive to price. With cigarettes, a 15% increase in price leads to a 7% reduction in consumption (in economic terms, these goods are described as 'inelastic'). It is possible with some drugs that the elasticity varies, with many casual users dropping out of the market as prices begin to rise, leaving a 'hard core' much more resistant to price increases, who may only be affected if prices rise considerably more (Wagstaff, 1989).

*2. Socialization.* The manner in which drugs are taken is influenced by social norms. Violence in association with alcohol consumption is rare in France, but common in Britain, despite the fact that far more alcohol is consumed in France (the relative price is much lower), and rate of alcoholic cirrhosis is much higher there.

*3. Subculture.* The epidemic nature of drug use in inner cities in many countries suggests that subcultural factors may operate. Drugs go through phases when they are popular with different groups: cocaine in the early 1980s was a yuppie recreational drug; in the form of 'crack' in the 1990s, it is a 'scourge of inner cities' (and note the change of perception depending on which social class it is used by!). In inner-city Liverpool, the only people who are busy are the drug users, and the 'drug scene' can provide a sense of 'belonging' for those otherwise marginalized by society (Preble, 1969).

*4. Secular trends.* Alcoholism is progressively more common in western countries with later birth cohorts. In the

USA, lifetime prevalence was double in the 1955–65 birth cohort, compared to the 1935–45 cohort (Dinwiddie and Reich, 1991). The age of onset is also decreasing in later birth cohorts. These changes are more pronounced in women, resulting in a narrowing of the gender difference in age of onset and prevalence. Changes seem to be concentrated in those at risk of familial alcoholism (i.e. those with alcoholic relatives), with the result that the heritability of alcoholism is higher in later birth cohorts (Reich *et al.*, 1988).

**Familial influences**

The influence of family of origin on addiction is difficult to study, as most families consist of biologically related individuals, who share the same genetic as well as environmental influences. What evidence there is from adoption or twin studies suggests that family of origin is more important than family of upbringing; that is, genes are more important than environment (Cloninger *et al.*, 1981). This is perhaps hardly surprising, given that alcohol is environmentally ubiquitous, and it might be expected that the same will be shown to be true of drugs, given the increasing ease of their availability to all sections of society. The inheritance of addiction is probably polygenic, although genetics is not the whole story but Reich *et al.* (1988) conclude that their data strongly suggest additional non-genetic familial transmission. One of the major inherited mediating factors in addiction is probably temperament. Extremes of temperamental factors in childhood, particularly harm avoidance and novelty seeking, have been shown to be highly predictive of adult alcohol problems. Work on children of alcoholics (COAs) is generally fraught with methodological difficulties, but there are relatively robust findings of differences in sensitivity to alcohol in COAs (Sher, 1991). They may be more sensitive to the reinforcing effects, particularly associated with increasing blood levels, and less sensitive to the punishing effects, particularly associated with decreasing blood levels. COAs also seem to have more positive expectancies for the effect of alcohol. There are also fairly consistent findings of psychophysiological abnormalities, particularly relating to autonomic hyperreactivity, and to attenuation of late components of event-related potentials, especially the P300 wave.

**Individual influences**

*1. Psychiatric co-morbidity.* Studies repeatedly demonstrate high rates of co-morbidity of other psychiatric disorders with alcohol or drug misuse. In hospital studies, 'dual diagnosis' is found in 75% of those with alcoholism, and the epidemiological catchment area (ECA) study showed 'dual diagnosis' rates of nearly 50% in alcoholics in the general population. The most common diagnosis is antisocial personality disorder, followed by affective (major depression or mania) and anxiety disorders. Definite or probable drug dependence is found in 50% of hospitalized alcoholics in some samples who have definite or probable drug dependence (Dinwiddie and Reich, 1991). Premorbidly they are more likely to exhibit conduct disorder, hyperactivity and oppositional disorder as children.

2. *Are there different 'types' of dependence/addicts?* In recent years possible addictive typologies have been suggested. With regard to alcohol addiction, at least two major distinct groups can be delineated by family history and history of dependence (Bohman *et al.*, 1987). Alcohol-related expectancies provide the final common pathway from specific risk factors to later alcohol abuse, but the expectancies are different between the two groups (Wiers *et al.*, 1994).

(a) *Milieu-limited (Type 1)* is the most common group. It is inherited by both sexes from the father or mother, though many cases are 'sporadic'. Onset is later (after the age of 25), and it is dependent for development on long-term exposure to socially sanctioned high levels of alcohol intake. Those in this category are often anxious/dependent personalities, who report alcohol as inducing a sense of calm alertness. Social learning is important in the intrafamilial transmission of this type of alcoholism, with family stress leading to negative affectivity and coping styles emphasizing repression. The expectancies in these drinkers are that 'problems dissolve in alcohol', which is used for its initial psychomotor stimulant effect to counter negative affect. Binge drinking occurs, and is associated with guilt.

(b) *Male-limited (Type 2)* is inherited down the male line. Offspring are at high risk of developing early onset of high alcohol consumption associated with delinquent behaviour. In these people, alcoholism seems to be an expression of a delinquent/antisocial personality, and extremes of temperament, which may relate to an inherited mild dysfunction of the prefrontal cortex. Milieu is relatively unimportant in the genesis of this form of alcoholism, although the expectancies of this type of drinker are that alcohol produces feelings of power and aggression, and is a cognitive and motor stimulant. Female relatives of affected males have a high incidence of somatization disorder.

# Further reading

Bohman M, Sigvardson S, Cloninger CR, von Knorring A-L. Alcoholism: lessons from population, adoption and family studies. *Alcohol and Alcoholism, Supplement*, 1987; **1:** 55–60.

Cloninger CR, Bohman M, Sigvardsson S. Inheritance of alcohol abuse: cross-fostering analysis of adopted men. *Archives of General Psychiatry,* 1981; **38:** 861–8.

Dinwiddie SH, Reich T. Epidemiological perspectives on children of alcoholics. *Recent Developments in Alcoholism,* 1991; **9:** 287–99.

Preble E. Taking care of business – the heroin users life on the street. *International Journal of the Addictions,* 1969; **4:** 1–24.

Reich T, Cloninger CR, Van Eerdewegh P, Rice JP, Mullaney J. Secular trends in the familial transmission of alcoholism. *Alcoholism: Clinical and Experimental Research,* 1988; **12:** 458–64.

Robins LN. Vietnam veterans rapid recovery from heroin addiction: a fluke or normal expectation? *Addiction,* 1993; **88:** 1041–54.

Sher KJ. *Children of Alcoholics: a critical appraisal of theory and research.* London: University of Chicago Press, 1991.

Wagstaff A. Economic aspects of illicit drug markets and drug enforcement policies. *British Journal of Addiction,* 1989; **84:** 513–83.

Wiers RW, Sergeant JA, Gunning WB. Psychological mechanisms of enhanced risk of addiction in children of alcoholics: a dual pathway? *Acta Paediatrica Scaninavica Supplement,* 1994; **404:** 9–13.

# Related topics of interest

# ADDICTION – PHYSICAL AND PSYCHOLOGICAL ASPECTS

The most common drugs to cause problems are alcohol and nicotine. The most frequently used illicit drug is cannabis, on which 80% of all law-enforcement efforts are expended.

**Features of the dependence syndrome**

Central to the conceptualization of addiction is the dependence syndrome. The cardinal features of substance dependence remain similar to those decribed by Edwards and Gross for the alcohol dependence syndrome in 1976. ICD-10 lists the following:

- Compulsion to take the substance.
- Loss of control over onset, termination or levels of use.
- A physiological withdrawal state.
- Evidence of tolerance.
- Progressive neglect of alternative pleasures or interests as a result of substance use.
- Persisting with use despite evidence of associated harm.

Narrowing of the repertoire of substance use is also mentioned as a characteristic feature.

**Physical effects of drugs**

These can be regarded as falling into two categories: direct pharmacological effects (including idiosyncratic reactions), and tolerance/withdrawal phenomena. The latter are caused by neuroadaptation to the effect of the drug, leading to the appearance of a state physiologically opposite to that produced by the substance itself when the drug is withdrawn. Thus sedative drugs generally produce a state of anxiety or agitation on withdrawal, stimulants a state of anergia. The table below lists the major classes of licit and illicit substances of abuse, their modes of action, effects and features of withdrawal.

| Drug | Mode/site of action | Behavioural/ psychological effects | Withdrawal syndromes/adverse effects |
|------|---------------------|-----------------------------------|--------------------------------------|
| Alcohol | GABA receptors. Membrane fluidity altered | *Low doses cause:* overconfidence, lability of mood, initial enhancement of spinal reflexes, raised pain threshold, restlessness *High doses cause*: general CNS depression, leading to coma and death | (a) 'The shakes' (b) ''Rum Fits' (c) Delirium Tremens (d) Alcoholic Hallucinosis |

| Drug | Mode/site of action | Behavioural/ psychological effects | Withdrawal syndromes/adverse effects |
|---|---|---|---|
| Nicotine | Nicotinic receptors. Dopamine release in mesolimbic system via stimulation of ventral tegmental area | Increased sympathetic tone. Increased hedonic tone from nucleus accumbens DA release. Subjective relaxation | Dysphoria, poor concentration |
| Hallu-cinogens LSD Psilocybin Mescaline PCP | PCP acts at NMDA receptor. LSD is serotonin analogue at 5-HT$_2$ receptors | *Most produce:* Dilated pupils, ↑HR and BP, ↑temperature; paranoia in clear sensorium, illusions and hallucinations, depersonalization, anxiety, distortion of time sense, inappropriate affect. *PCP* also causes violent behaviour, extreme hyper-activity, hypervision, mutism, echolalia, coma, ataxia, nystagmus, analgesia, (rarely), intracranial haemorrhage | No physical withdrawal syndromes have been described. 'Flashbacks' (brief re-experiencing of hallu-cinogenic state) may be precipitated by cannabis or antihistamine intake. LSD may cause pro-longed or permanent receptor changes or cell death. Prolonged psychosis, usually schizoaffective, sometimes after single ingestion of LSD (Abraham and Aldridge, 1993). Post-hallucinogen perceptual disorder |
| Caffeine | Increased cellular concentraion of cyclic AMP, due to enzyme inhibition. Increased cerebral blood flow | Alertness, tremor, palpitations | Headache, lassitude, irritability |
| 'Ecstasy' MDMA (Methoxy-desmethyl-ampheta-mine) (Steele *et al.,* 1994) | Stimulates release of 5-HT from corti-cal system originating in raphe nuclei. Some dopamine release. Inhibits monoamine release | Predominantly CNS stimulant. ↑HR and BP, dry mouth, anorexia, ↑alertness, elevated mood, bruxism or jaw clenching, 'alteration of consciousness with sensual and emotional overtones' | *Acute:* flashbacks, anxiety, insomnia, panic attacks, psychosis, hyper-pyrexia (esp. if subject is dehydrated), death. *Subacute (24 hours – 1 month):* drowsiness, depression, anxiety, irritability. *Chronic (> 1 month):* panic disorder, psychosis, flashbacks, major depressive disorder, memory disturbance, |

| Drug | Mode/site of action | Behavioural/ psychological effects | Withdrawal syndromes/adverse effects |
|---|---|---|---|
| | | | permanent irreversible destruction of raphe nuclei 5-HT axons demonstrated in non-human primates – significance in humans uncertain |
| Cocaine | Stimulates dopamine and other central monoamine release | Euphoria, excitement | Psychosis, violence, crawling sensation under skin ('cocaine bugs'). Withdrawal: (a) 'Crash' 24–48 hours extreme lassitude, dysphoria, craving. (b) Depression may follow over the next few weeks |
| Cannabis | Large number of active components. THC probably binds to an endogenous ligand | Euphoria, anxiety, increased appetite, ↑ suggestibility, distortion of time and space, conjunctival injection, normal pupil size | Anxiety, panic, depression, paranoia. Toxic psychosis, precipitation of functional psychosis in vulnerable individuals. Smoke more carcinogenic than cigarettes. Claims of long-term personality deterioration have not been substantiated |
| Opiates | Agonists to endogenous opiate receptors. Cause histamine release | *Mild intoxication:* analgesia, drowsiness and mental clouding, apathy, lethargy, euphoria, nausea/ vomiting, itching, pupillary constriction, constipation, flushed warm skin. *Severe intoxication:* miosis, respiratory depression, often long-lasting, hypotension/shock, pulmonary oedema, depressed reflexes, coma, seizures (propoxyphene/meperidine) | *Withdrawal:* Appear 8–10 hours (up to 48 hours with methadone). Peak 48–72 hours, lasts 7–10 days, (craving lasts much longer). Lacrimation, rhinorrhoea, yawning, sweating, restlessness, irritability, sleepy, gooseflesh, pupillary dilation, insomnia |
| Amphetamine | Stimulates prefrontal dopamine release. Other central monoamines also released | Elevated, anxious or irritable mood, ↑ energy, ↓ appetite, talkativeness, insomnia, tachycardia, hyperthermia. Severe intoxication may produce toxic psychosis, with symptoms indistinguishable from paranoid schizophrenia, though of shorter duration | Agitation, panic, paranoid psychosis. Long-term EEG changes in prefrontal areas, of unknown significance. *Withdrawal:* ↑ sleep, nightmares (REM rebound) fatigue, lassitude, |

| Drug | Mode/site of action | Behavioural/ psychological effects | Withdrawal syndromes/adverse effects |
|------|---------------------|-----------------------------------|--------------------------------------|
| | | | increased appetite, depression (sometimes severe) |
| Benzodiaz-epines | GABA receptor agonist (open chloride channel) | Sedation, disinhibition may lead to violent or impulsive behaviour. Euphoria, especially with IV administration | Insomnia, nightmares (REM rebound) restlessness, anxiety/panic, twitching, convulsions |
| Inhalants (Dinwiddie, 1994) | Fluidization of cell membranes, potentiation of hyperpolarization at GABA-A receptor, ?also act on glutamate receptors | Resembles alcohol intoxication. Stimulation and disinhibition followed by depression and sedation. Distortion of size, colour, passage of time, brief delusions or hallucinations (usually visual or tactile) | Sudden death from cardiac arrhythmias in both first time and long-term users. Central and peripheral nerve damage. Cerebellar damage (esp. toluene). Neuropsychological deficits (also with occupational exposure). Renal, hepatic, pulmonary, bone marrow pathology. Damage to fetus *in utero* |

For more detail, see Robson 1994.

**Psychological features of addiction**

Whilst it is almost certainly possible to produce withdrawal syndromes in any person given sufficient quantities of a drug for sufficient length of time, the fact remains that most people exposed to a drug never become addicted. It might almost be said that the question in addictions is not why so many become addicted, but why so many others do not.

The epidemiological catchment area (ECA) survey in the USA, and other studies of populations and groups of addicts, show that psychiatric disorder is common in those with substance misuse problems. The most common associated conditions are:

- Antisocial personality.
- Depression.
- Anxiety.
- Mania.

and these are often primary (i.e. precede the substance misuse). Evidence from Vietnam, where 40% of GIs experienced drug withdrawals at some point, but the prevalence of persisting drug problems was similar to the normal US population, suggests strongly that high levels of drug use do not predict high levels of subsequent substance misuse problems (Robins, 1994). However, the fact that the overwhelming majority of those with persistent nicotine addiction start smoking before the age of 20 suggests that exposure during adolescence, where neural pathways and coping skills are still developing, may be particularly harmful.

**Classical and operant conditioning**

Drugs of addiction have profound effects on central reward pathways, and can be used to produce conditioning in animals (to the extent that rats will starve whilst self-administering cocaine). Drug-associated paraphernalia, or situations associated with drug use, can precipitate craving and full-blown physical withdrawal syndromes, even in long-abstinent addicts, through classical conditioning (conditioned withdrawal). Some addicts – 'needle freaks' – experience drug-like effects from the act of injecting whatever is in the syringe. It is clear that, once drug use is established, it can reinforce a variety of drug-seeking or using behaviours via operant conditioning. Aversion therapy (a form of classical conditioning), although out of fashion, has been shown in controlled trials to be effective in the treatment of addictions. Clearly, drugs of abuse are powerful operant reinforcers of drug-seeking behaviours, and this may underlie the subjective compulsion to use, the narrowing of repertoire, and the increasing salience of drug-seeking behaviour.

**Expectancies**

It is perhaps not surprising that subjective experience of a drug is shaped by the expectations of its effect. In experimental situations, the expectancy may be more powerful than the nature of the substance being consumed, and this is also known in drug-using circles (a 'bad trip' is often the result of pre-trip anxiety).

# Further reading

Abraham HD, Aldridge AM. Adverse consequences of lysergic acid diethylamine. *Addiction,* 1993; **88:** 1327–34.

Corrigal WA, Coen KM, Adamson KL. Self-administered nicotine activates the mesolimbic dopamine system through the ventral tegmental area. *Brain Research,* 1994; **653:** 278–84.

Dinwiddie SH. Abuse of inhalants: a review. *Addiction,* 1994; **89:** 925–39.

Edwards G, Gross MM. Alcohol dependence: provisional description of a clinical syndrome. *British Medical Journal,* 1976; **1:** 1058–61.

Robins LN. Vietnam veterans rapid recovery from heroin addiction: a fluke or normal expectation. *Addiction,* 1993; **88:** 1041–54.

Robson P. *Forbidden Drugs.* Oxford: Oxford University Press, 1994.

Steele TD, McCann UD, Ricaurte GA. 3,4-methylenedioxymethamphetamine (MDMA 'Ecstasy'): pharmacology and toxicology in animals and humans. *Addiction,* 1994; **89:** 539–51.

## Related topics of interest

Addiction – aetiology (p. 1)
Addiction – strategies of treatment (p. 11)
Learning (p. 171)

# ADDICTION – STRATEGIES OF TREATMENT

Addictive behaviours most commonly refer to problems of alcohol and illicit drug abuse and dependence. However, the general approach can be useful in other conditions, including eating disorders and gambling.

It is important to consider the aim of treatment before considering the strategies which may be employed. The aims can broadly be defined as either abstinence oriented or as harm reduction.

Harm reduction was initially described in relation to injecting drug misuse, when it was recognized that the prevention of harm, predominantly HIV infection, was a higher priority than achieving abstinence. Thus since it was not possible to prevent large numbers of people from using opiates, strategies which reduced injecting, reduced sharing of injecting equipment and promoted improved health in intravenous drug users were developed.

Although the strategies described in this topic may appear to be abstinence oriented, they are applicable in a variety of situations to harm reduction. One may use a motivational approach (see below) to help a patient become abstinent or to change their injecting behaviour.

It is helpful to consider strategies of treatment for this group of patients in terms of the 'Stages of change' model of Prochaska and DiClemente. Different strategies are appropriate at different stages. The following strategies will be considered:

- Changing behaviour.
- Detoxification.
- Relapse prevention.
- Rehabilitation.

**Changing behaviour**

The 'Stages of change' model referred to above is an attempt to describe the behavioural and psychological processes which occur when an individual attempts to change a habit. The following stages can be considered to form a cycle which most people go around several times before exiting:

*1. Precontemplative.* The individual has not started to consider the possibility of change and does not pay any attention to the problems which his/her behaviour causes him/herself or others.

*2. Contemplative.* The individual starts to consider the possibility of change. This stage is likely to be characterized by ambivalence about further action.

*3. Decision.* The individual either alone or with help commits him/herself to a decision.

*4. Action.* The individual takes steps to break the habit.

5. *Maintenance.* The individual tries to sustain the changed situation.

6. *Relapse.* The individual reverts to the previous behaviour or a different but also problematical behaviour. In previously dependent individuals this will be characterized by rapid reinstatement.

Although ambivalence was mentioned at the contemplative stage, it is also likely to be a relevant factor at later stages.

Dealing with ambivalence is at the heart of motivational interviewing. This is a collaborative approach which considers motivation to be the result of a therapeutic interaction rather than a personality trait held by the patient. Reflective listening and Socratic questioning are used to elicit self-motivational statements from the patient and to deal with resistance. The patient is thus enabled to change.

**Detoxification**

Detoxification will be described according to individual drug class. The setting may be in-patient, day-patient, out-patient or at home, depending on local resources and patient needs:

1. *Alcohol.* Chlordiazepoxide is commonly used; alternatives include diazepam and chlormethiazole. In-patient treatment would usually be considered when there is a history of withdrawal seizures, poor physical health, delirium, cognitive impairment, risk of self-harm which would be lessened by admission, severe anxiety and inadequate social support outside hospital. Attention should be paid to the need for thiamine administration.

2. *Benzodiazepines.* If a patient is only on one benzodiazepine the first step may be a gradual reduction in dose. However if this is unsuccessful, impracticable or the patient is on several benzodiazepines, then a long-acting drug such as diazepam should be substituted and gradually withdrawn. Admission may be indicated by a similar range of complications as for alcohol above. Intervention should also be aimed at managing anxiety (see Psychological treatment – cognitive therapy, p. 261), coexistent mood disorder and exacerbating factors, such as caffeine excess.

3. *Opiates.* In-patient treatment has a much higher rate of completion than out-patient treatment. Detoxification is

usually from methadone but may also be from other substances, including heroin, dihydrocodeine and proprietary cough medicines. Several methods are currently used:

(a) Methadone reduction (usually over 10 days followed by a variable period of admission).
(b) Clonidine and naltrexone (5–10 days).
(c) Lofexidine.
(d) Intermittent naloxone infusion.

Methadone is a long-acting oral $\mu$-opiate receptor agonist. Clonidine and lofexidine are $\alpha_2$ agonists which reduce the central noradrenergic activation which is associated with the withdrawal state. Naltrexone and naloxone are opiate antagonists.

All regimens will also make use of supportive adjunctive treatment, which includes:

- Metaclopramide.
- Lomotil.
- Mebeverine.
- Diazepam.

**Prevention of relapse**

1. *Physical methods.*
(a) *Disulfiram.* Inhibits alcohol dehydrogenase, so alcohol ingestion leads to the accumulation of acetaldehyde. Symptoms which result include flushing, nausea, headache and hypotension. Efficacy is greatly improved when a second party, for example spouse, is involved in the daily administration of the drug.
(b) *Naltrexone.* Blocks the action of any opiates ingested.

2. *Psychological.* Relapse prevention strategies as described by Marlatt and Gordon. This is a treatment which shares features of cognitive behaviour therapy. It is a collaborative treatment in which the patient is helped to recognize triggers for relapse and high-risk situations (which may be environmental or emotional states) and to develop protective or avoidant strategies.

3. *Self-help groups.* Twelve-step model of Alcoholics Anonymous (AA) and Narcotics Anonymous (NA). Patients attend regular, and initially frequent, group meetings which aim to provide mutual support. They are required to recognize themselves as addicts and to work towards abstinence.

4. *Social – community reinforcement.* This is a strategy which makes use of community agencies, including the family, to provide rewards for abstinence. These may include contact with key people, work, leisure and housing opportunities.

**Residential rehabilitation**

- Mostly provided by the non-statutory and voluntary sector.
- Concept houses developed from the therapeutic communities of Maxwell Jones which have a structured and hierarchical system in which the patient is expected to remain drug free and to progress by achieving increasing levels of responsibility and privileges.
- Residential programmes based on the 12-step programme.
- Christian-based centres. Some of these consider personal faith to be essential for recovery of the addict.

**Family-based approaches**

- Assessment at any of the above stages may reveal that a vital role in the addictive behaviour is played by a partner or the more general family environment. Intervention with a couple or family whenever possible may therefore be more appropriate than individual treatment.
- A variety of approaches are used, including behavioural, systems and strategic therapies (see Psychological treatment – family therapies, p. 267).

## Further reading

*Addiction,* 1994; **89:** (11), Special Issue.
Marlatt GA, George WH. Relapse prevention: Introduction and overview of the model. *British Journal of Addiction,* 1984; **79:** 261–73.
Miller W. Motivational interviewing with problem drinkers. *Behavioural Psychotherapy,* 1983; **11:** 147–72.
Prochaska JO, DiClemente CC. Stages and processes of self-change of smoking: toward an integrative model of change. *Journal of Consulting and Clinical Psychology,* 1983; **51:** 390–5.

## Related topics of interest

# AFFECTIVE DISORDERS – CLASSIFICATION AND EPIDEMIOLOGY

Few areas in psychiatry have caused more problems in nosology than the classification of affective disorders, particularly depression. Endogenous vs Reactive, Neurotic vs Psychotic, Major vs Minor, are all attempts to divide the syndrome into meaningful categories, with separate aetiological/prognostic/therapeutic implications. Depression is extremely common, and varies from a normal transient mood state to a severe, life-threatening psychotic illness. It is important to exclude organic conditions, as there are many organic causes of low mood. Most functional depressive illnesses have some precipitant, and the differentiation between diagnosis of *acute stress reaction* and *adjustment reaction* depends on the extent to which symptoms are attributable to, and commensurate with, the precipitating stress.

**Definition**
> *In these disorders, the fundamental disturbance is a change in mood or affect, usually to depression (with or without anxiety) or to elation...* (ICD-10)

**Subdivision**

An ideal classification of depression would take into account what is known about the genetics of the disorder, its prognosis, aetiology and response to treatment. It would also attempt to separate mood disturbance of an episodic nature from that due to long-term personality factors. There is insufficient clear knowledge of this to provide an unequivocal subdivision, and ICD-10 and DSM-IV adopt different approaches.

The major (and clearest) subdivision of affective disorder is between manic depressive illness (bipolar disorder) and depression. They are genetically separate to an extent, and are distinct with respect to age of onset (bipolar disorder is earlier). The existence of pure unipolar mania is in doubt, and patients who have suffered a manic episode virtually always suffer from depression at some point. Unipolar depression, by contrast, is very common.

**Epidemiology**

*Bipolar disorder* is rare, with a lifetime incidence of about 0.6%. *Depression* has been called 'the common cold of psychiatry': at any one time, 5% of the population is depressed, and the lifetime incidence is 1 in 5 for women, and 1 in 10 for men. Fifty per cent of depression is recurrent. Worldwide, the incidence of depression may be increasing. *Dysthymic disorder* is stated in DSM-IV to have a lifetime prevalence of 6% and a point prevalence of 3%.

**Mania, hypomania, bipolar disorder, cyclothymia**

ICD-10 and DSM-IV both recognize *hypomania,* which is a degree of mania short of the full-blown syndrome. Symptoms include elevation of mood or irritability, and overactivity, sleep disturbance, and so on but not to the degree of severe disruption of life, or need for hospitalization, and without development of delusions.

Full-blown *mania* is a severe and potentially life-threatening syndrome (judgement of risk is impaired, and exhaustion and dehydration may be severe). The symptoms are of a severe disturbance of biological functioning, involving mood, biological regulation, thought and cognition.

Repeated episodes of affective disturbance, including at least one episode of mania or hypomania, are classified as bipolar affective disorder (in DSM-IV the terms *bipolar 1* and *bipolar 2* are used to distinguish bipolar disorder with (respectively) full-blown mania or only hypomania). Additionally, recurrent episodes can be categorized by the frequency of cycling: 'rapid cycling' bipolar disorder is defined as more than four mood swings per year, ultra-rapid cycling as cycling frequencies of the order of days or weeks and ultra-ultra-rapid cycling bipolar disorder as illness in which swings in mood from mania to depression occur more than once a day. Rapid cycling (Post, 1992) may occur spontaneously or may be precipitated by the use of antidepressants. These groups do seem to have different therapeutic and prognostic implications.

Recurrent mood swings of lesser severity are classified as *cyclothymia*, which characteristically begins in adolescence or early adulthood. The lifetime risk of bipolar disorder in people with cyclothymia is 15–50%. Unlike bipolar disorder, the definition of cyclothymia requires a degree of chronicity of symptoms, reflecting its initial categorization as a form of personality disorder. This lack of clarity may reflect a lack of knowledge, but may also reflect the reality that less severe disturbances of mood regulation shade imperceptibly into normal personality variants.

Bipolar disorder is the most genetically determined psychiatric disorder, with a heritability of 0.8. The offspring of people with bipolar disorder have an increased incidence of both bipolar disorder and unipolar depressive disorder.

**Depression**

The overlap between normal sadness and depressive personality on the one hand, with manic depression and psychosis on the other, has caused problems in psychiatric nosology. Evidence for this has been the variation in the meaning of the term 'manic depressive psychosis' or the status of neurotic depression and depressive personality.

Genetic and family studies show that depression is inherited, and offspring of unipolar depressives tend to suffer from unipolar depression. There may also be some overlap with alcoholism (Winokur's (1979) 'depressive spectrum disorder').

Clinically, the important characteristics are the severity of the depression, the presence or otherwise of psychotic symptoms, and the degree to which biological features are present, as all of these correlate with likely response to electroconvulsive therapy (ECT) or antidepressants; and psychotic depressions respond better if neuroleptics are used in addition to antidepressants. The old distinction between 'endogenous' and 'reactive' depressions is less useful, as most depressions have some precipitant, and are thus to an extent reactive. There is some evidence that 'atypical' depressions, with a reversal of the usual biological symptoms (i.e. hypersomnia, hyperphagia, hypersexuality), panic attacks, and premorbid rejection-sensitive personality may have a preferential response to monoamine-oxidase inhibitors (Liebowitz *et al.,* 1988).

ICD-10 broadly conforms to the above, specifying single or recurrent episodes of mild, moderate or severe nature, and coding for the presence or absence of somatic (biological) symptoms. The category of dysthymia is used to describe a persistent depressed state lasting at least 2 years, never or rarely of sufficient severity to fulfil criteria for depressive disorder. Recurrent brief depression is included as a separate category, as is postpsychotic depression.

DSM-IV is altogether less satisfactory, and divides unipolar depression into major depressive disorder (with or without psychotic symptoms) and dysthymia. This latter category is a most unsatisfactory mixture of minor, neurotic depression and depressive personality disorder, being defined in terms of 'depressed (or irritable) mood for most of the day, more days than not, ... for at least 2 years'. DSM-IV recognizes that major depression commonly occurs in those suffering dysthymia – so called 'double depression'. It also includes minor depression, as a less severe variant of major depression. This failure to separate clearly minor degrees of depression from lifelong constitutional factors is a serious deficiency, as the prognostic and therapeutic implications of the two are different.

Another area of controversy surrounds the debate about the existence of seasonal affective disorder (SAD). Clinically this is characterized by a tendency to become depressed in the winter (particularly with atypical features) and often hypomanic in the spring, but the episodes are generally not severe enough to come to medical attention. This should be distinguished from episodes for example precipitated by anniversaries. SAD is included in DSM-IIIR but not ICD-10.

## Further reading

Liebowitz MD, Qutikin FM, Stewart JW, McGrath PJ, Harrison WM, Markowitz JS, Rabkin JG, Tricamo E, Goetz DM, Klein DF. Antidepressant specificity in atypical depression. *Archives of General Psychiatry,* 1988; **45:** 129–37.

Post RM. Rapid cycling and depression. In: Montgomery S, Rouillon (eds) *Long term Treatment of Depression.* Chichester: John Wiley, 1992.

Winokur G. Unipolar depression: is it divisible into autonomous subtypes? *Archives of General Psychiatry,* 1979; **36:** 47–52.

## Related topics of interest

# AFFECTIVE DISORDERS – IN THE ELDERLY

**Epidemiology**

- Results from several studies give a prevalence amongst those aged over 65 in the community of 1–3% for major depression and at least 10% for depression which is significant though does not satisfy criteria for major depression.
- Higher levels are found in those in residential care, nursing homes and general hospitals, especially those with Parkinson's disease or cerebrovascular accidents.
- Rate of first admission with affective disorder increases with age.

**Aetiology**

- Genetic contribution becomes less marked in old age.
- Age-related changes in brain metabolism and ventricular enlargement have been demonstrated and may play a role in the development of depression.
- Life events may have particular meaning for the elderly, who may have less hope of reversing misfortune in the future. Specific events to be negotiated at this stage of life include: bereavement, conflicts with children, marital problems, loss, dependency, social isolation, housing problems and financial hardship. A capacity for intimacy is protective.

A recent study by Green *et al.* (1992) identified three factors which were significantly associated with development of depression 3 years later: lack of satisfaction with life, feelings of loneliness, and smoking. (Also female gender and bereavement in mulitivariate analyses.) Another study showed that persistence or remission of depression could be predicted by changes in health, sleep disturbance and addition of formal support services.

**Presentation**

- Symptom presentation is diverse and may be less readily recognized than in younger age groups. Examples include: pain, persecutory symptoms, acute loneliness and anxiety, recent alcohol abuse, shop-lifting and accentuation of previous personality trait. Although somatic symptoms are important, they can be difficult to evaluate in the presence of physical disease. A recent change in global functioning can be an important clue. Attention should be paid to the development of agitation, retardation, loss of interest or pleasure, feelings of worthlessness, self-reproach or guilt, delusions may characteristically be nihilistic or with poverty, guilt or punishment as a theme.

- An apparent dementia may be caused by depression ('pseudodementia'). Features which suggest depression include: short rapid course, clear onset, complaints of poor memory and lack of effort on memory testing. The coexistence of both conditions (co-morbidity) is common, especially in multi-infarct dementia. Reversible dementia occurring in the course of late-life depression is a predictor for a four-fold increase in the rate of later development of irreversible dementia.
- Hypochondriacal features can be difficult to evaluate because of high levels of physical illness, and co-morbidity is common. Depression can be a response to physical illness or a side-effect of treatment.
- Rates of attempted suicide are significant: 8.7% of 126 patients following hospital admission for major depression. Completed suicide is higher in the elderly than in younger people.

Recognition has traditionally been less than optimum because of the tendency to attribute symptoms to a normal sadness consequent on reduced circumstances or loss. Rather these factors should be regarded as particular precipitating or maintaining factors. As with all cases involving the elderly, assessment should be at home and include relevant family members and the multidisciplinary team.

**Treatment**

- *Antidepressants.* There are increasing problems with drug interactions and risk of side-effects with age, particularly postural hypotension and delerium with tricyclics. Large numbers in placebo-controlled trials with selective serotonin reuptake inhibitors are yet to be performed. The advantages of SSRIs are the lack of anticholinergic symptoms but there may be some increase in other unwanted side-effects, for example, extrapyramidal symptoms. Full doses of drugs should be used following gradual and careful introduction. There is controversy about the optimum length of treatment. Some authors maintain that treatment should be indefinite to reduce an otherwise high rate of relapse. Over a 2-year follow-up of major depressive disorder, relapse is 2.5 times more likely with placebo than with dothiepin 75 mg daily. Another author puts forward evidence that long-term treatment reduces risk of suicide in those with mood disorders.
- *Electroconvulsive therapy* may be safer than prolonged or high-dose tricyclic antidepressants. It is effective in old age. Some studies indicate it may be more effective than

in younger age groups, although on the other hand a longer course of up to 20 treatments may be necessary and the elderly are more vulnerable to confusion as a side-effect.

- *Psychological approaches* include family therapy and education, life review therapy and cognitive behavioural therapy. These and less specific support may be provided by attendance at a day hospital.
- *Social approaches* are important and social and health services should work together to provide optimum care. Provision includes support to carers, day centres and practical support in the home.

**Outcome**

A 12-month follow-up study by Murphy in 1983 showed a high mortality and poor prognosis, roughly quoted as '.. a third get better, a third stay the same and a third get worse'. Some recent studies have shown a better prognosis but generally rates of relapse increase with follow-up period. Most studies show an increased mortality in late-life depression compared with age-matched controls which is not accounted for by suicide deaths. A 12-month follow-up in 1991 used some helpful categories and gave the following results: complete recovery without further relapse, 47%; complete recovery with further relapses, 18%; varying degrees of 'depressive invalidism' with or without further relapses, 13%; continual depression, 11%; development of dementia, 0; death, 11%.

# Further reading

Burvill PW. Prognosis of depression in the elderly. *International Review of Psychiatry,* 1993; **5:** 437–43.

Green BH, Copeland JRM, Dewey ME, Sharma V, Saunders PA, Davidson IA, Sullivan C, McWilliams C. Risk factors for depression in elderly people: a prospective study. *Acta Psychiatrica Scandinavica,* 1992; **86:** 213–17.

Murphy E. The prognosis of depression in old age. *British Journal of Psychiatry,* 1983; **142:** 111–19.

Old Age Depression Interest Group. How long should the elderly take antidepressants? A double blind placebo control study of continuation/prophylaxis with dothiepin. *British Journal of Psychiatry,* 1993; **162:** 175–82.

Wilkinson AM, Anderson DN, Peters S. Age and the effects of ECT. *International Journal of Geriatric Psychiatry,* 1993; **8:** 401–6.

# Related topics of interest

# AFFECTIVE DISORDERS – LONG-TERM TREATMENT

Bipolar disorder is almost always a recurrent illness. Over the past few years there has been increasing recognition of the degree of long-term morbidity associated with depressive disorders. This is of two types:

(a) 'Chronic depression' caused by or occurring as a consequence of a failure to recognize or adequately treat depressive illness.

(b) Recurrent depressive episodes. After one episode, there is a 50% chance of recurrence; after two or more, the risk is over 90%.

The lifetime mortality from suicide in affective disorder is of the order of 10–15%, and there is also considerable psychological and social morbidity associated with depression.

The reduction of hidden morbidity from depression is a major public health and educational task. Campaigns such as the 'Defeat Depression' in the UK aim to:

(a) Raise the awareness of depression in both health professionals and the general public.

(b) Change attitudes towards depression and its treatment. These may sometimes be a serious barrier to effective treatment (e.g. in a recent survey, 80% of respondents believed that antidepressants were addictive).

In addition, education of GPs in the correct treatment of depression has been demonstrated to be effective, and may also reduce the incidence of suicide (see Suicide – prevention, p. 343).

## Maintenance treatment for affective disorders

**Bipolar disorder**

The prophylactic efficacy of lithium in bipolar disorder has been known for some time. Its long-term use should probably be considered in any patient with more than one episode of mania, and after single episodes if these are severe and difficult to treat. Lithium should never be used as a short-term treatment, as at least 50% of patients suffer an illness similar to the original one on withdrawal of medication. The incidence is much higher than expected due to relapse, and is more in the nature of a withdrawal syndrome (Goodwin, 1994). For this reason, use of lithium for less than 2 years increases the overall episode frequency, and should be discouraged.

**Unipolar disorder**

Chiefly because of the high risk of suicide in recurrent depressions, the World Health Organization (WHO) now recommends that maintenance antidepressant medication be considered for those with more than one episode of severe depression, particularly within a period of 5 years. A period of at least 2 years' prophylaxis is recommended, before a trial of discontinuation, with the patient being followed up at least every 2 months during and after treatment (WHO, 1992).

# Which maintenance treatment for prevention of relapse?

**Lithium or other mood stabilizers**

Lithium is the treatment of choice for recurrent bipolar disorder. Blood levels for lithium maintenance can in general be lower than those required for treatment of the acute episode, though there is no absolute rule, and both 'subtherapeutic' (i.e. <0.4 mmol⁻¹) and higher levels are needed in some patients. There is some work to suggest that alternate day dosage, using one and a half times the daily dose, is as effective, and causes fewer side-effects than daily dosage (though the effect on compliance has not been studied). As an alternative, carbamazepine or sodium valproate are as effective in prophylaxis as lithium, and may be better tolerated, so that some authorities now recommend carbamazepine as first-line treatment. Both these anticonvulsants are also effective in rapid-cycling bipolar disorder, unlike lithium. In those patients who cannot be controlled by a single agent, the combination of lithium and carbamazepine, or lithium and a neuroleptic is more effective than either alone (Peselow *et al.*, 1994). Thyroid supplementation may be helpful in rapid-cycling patients (Hopkins and Gelenberg, 1994).

In recurrent unipolar depression, lithium may be a better long-term prophylactic than antidepressants, as the latter may cause receptor down-regulation (though the clinical significance of this is uncertain). Studies of patients in long-term lithium clinics have shown that suicide mortality may be reduced below that of the general population (Coppen, 1994). This may be a consequence of the high levels of supervision in these clinics, but it may also be that lithium itself protects against suicide, possibly by modulation of 5-hydroxytryptamine (5-HT) systems, which are implicated in suicide.

**Antidepressants**

If a patient with recurrent depression has been successfully treated using antidepressants, then it is possible to maintain them on these in the long term. The full therapeutic dose should be used, as reduction in dose causes increased relapse. If long-term treatment is a possible outcome, then consideration of the therapeutic agent, and particularly its range of side-effects, should be made at the onset of treatment. The older tricyclics, with their prominent anticholinergic side-effects, are probably less acceptable. Sexual dysfunction is common with most classes of antidepressant, and should be specifically enquired about before embarking on long-term treatment.

**Psychological therapy**

Few trials exist of long-term outcomes. Early claims that psychological therapy reduced relapse in the first 5 years when compared to drug treatment (although having face validity) have not been confirmed. Both cognitive behaviour therapy (CBT) and interpersonal therapy (IPT) have been shown to be as effective as maintenance antidepressants in recurrent depressive disorder (Frank *et al.,* 1992)

**Neuroleptics**

These might be considered in patients who have had a psychotic episode, or bipolar patients who do not wish to take, or are intolerant of, mood-stabilizing drugs. Low doses of oral or depot medication may be helpful, but the long-term side-effects (particularly tardive dyskinesia) make these drugs a second choice. There is some indication that clozapine may be effective in refractory affective disorder, particularly mania (Banov *et al.,* 1994).

# Further reading

Banov MD, Zarate CA, Tohen M, Scialabba D, Wines JD. Clozapine in refractory affective disorders: polarity predicts response in long-term follow-up. *Journal of Clinical Psychiatry,* 1994; **55:** 295–300.

Coppen A. Depression as a lethal disease: prevention strategies. *Journal of Clinical Psychiatry,* 1994; **55:**(4, suppl), 37–45.

Frank E, Johnson S, Burger DJ. Psychological treatments in the prevention of relapse. In: Montgomery S, Rouillon F. (eds) *Prevention of Relapse in Long Term Treatment of Depression.* Chichester: John Wiley, 1992; 197–228.

Goodwin W. Recurrence of mania after lithium withdrawal: Implications for the use of lithium in the treatment of bipolar affective disorder. *British Journal of Psychiatry,* 1994; **164:** 149–52.

Hopkins HS, Gelenberg AJ. Treatment of bipolar disorder: how far have we come? *Psychopharmacology Bulletin,* 1994; **30:** 27–38.

Peselow ED, Fieve RR, Difiglia C, Sanfilipo MP. Lithium prophylaxis in bipolar illness. The value of combination treatment. *British Journal of Psychiatry,* 1994; **164:** 208–14.

WHO. Pharmacotherapy of depressive disorders. A consensus statement. *Journal of Psychopharmacology,* 1992; **6:** (suppl), 343–4.

# Related topics of interest

# AFFECTIVE DISORDERS – NEUROTRANSMITTER CHANGES

**Neurotransmitters**

The monoamine theory of depression states that depressive disorder (and possibly mania) are due to an abnormality in monoamine neurotransmitters. Initially it was suggested that this abnormality was in the absolute level of neurotransmitter available. More recent versions of the theory have postulated a change in receptor numbers or sensitivity. The neurotransmitters serotonin (5-hydroxy-tryptamine, or 5-HT), noradrenaline and dopamine have been studied and the evidence supporting a role for each of these in affective disorder will be considered in turn.

*1. Serotonin/5-HT.* Studies have been performed in both healthy controls and depressed subjects. The evidence supports a reduction in 5-HT neurotransmission in depressive disorder, although it is not clear whether this is a causal factor or a marker of the disorder.

(a) *Studies in healthy controls.* Studies using the technique of tryptophan depletion imply a role for 5-HT in the regulation of mood. A drink is administered which contains all the essential amino acids, but lacks tryptophan (TRP). This results in a reduction in plasma tryptophan, probably through induction of protein synthesis. TRP enters the brain via a transport system where it competes with other large neutral amino acids (LNAAs). Therefore if the plasma concentration of TRP falls relative to other LNAAs, brain TRP will also fall. As TRP hydroxylase is not saturated, lowering brain TRP will lower brain 5-HT. These effects have been confirmed in animals. In normal volunteers, TRP depletion appears to lower mood, but only in those with a vulnerability to depression (e.g. those with a strong family history) or in those who have some depressive symptoms prior to the procedure.

(b) *Studies in depressed subjects.* It is important to remember that most of the methods used to measure 5-HT function are indirect, but the following have been found in studies of depressed patients:
- A small reduction in plasma TRP (more likely if melancholic features are present).
- Decreased platelet 5-HT uptake compared to controls.
- Platelet imipramine binding may be decreased.

- Decreased 5-hydroxyindoleacetic acid (5-HIAA) levels in the CSF but only in a subgroup of depressed patients (approximately 35%) who have a history of suicide attempts (particularly violent attempts). This abnormality of 5-HIAA is not confined to depressive disorder but seems to be a feature of impulsive behaviour and is seen in schizophrenia and personality disorder.
- Post-mortem studies show conflicting results and have methodological difficulties (death by suicide is over represented and there is a delay before examination).
- Neuroendocrine tests. These provide a functional assessment of brain 5-HT neurotransmission. Activation of 5-HT pathways produces an increase in prolactin, growth hormone, and adrenocorticotrophic hormone. Depressed patients show blunted prolactin responses to TRP, clomipramine and fenfluramine.
- TRP depletion causes temporary relapse in patients who have recently recovered from a depressive disorder and are maintained on antidepressants. This is particularly marked in those on antidepressants which affect 5-HT.
- Most antidepressants increase brain 5-HT function. This does not necessarily mean that altered brain 5-HT function is the cause of depression. Although 5-HT is increased within a few hours of starting antidepressants, significant clinical effects take several weeks to develop. This may be because the clinical effect requires neuroadaptive changes to occur or because the effect is mediated by other neurotransmitter systems which are affected by 5-HT.

2. *Noradrenaline.* Again the evidence supports a reduction in noradrenergic function in depressive disorder, for example:

- Reduced growth hormone response to clonidine (which suggests a downregulation in post synaptic noradrenergic receptors).
- Reduced MHPG (3-methoxy-4-hydroxyphenylethylene glycol, a metabolite of noradrenaline) in the CSF of depressed patients.
- Post-mortem findings are inconsistent.
- Antidepressants and electroconvulsive therapy (ECT)

cause a reduction in the number of beta-noradrenergic binding sites in the cortex, which might be a primary finding or secondary to increased noradrenaline turnover.

- Some antidepressants such as desipramine have purely noradrenergic effects and are clinically effective.

*3. Dopamine.* There is little evidence for an abnormality of dopaminergic function in depressive disorder.

- HVA (homovanillic acid) levels are not altered in depression.
- Neuroendocrine testing does not reveal consistent changes suggestive of abnormalities of dopaminergic function.
- L-dopa does not have a consistent antidepressant effect.

**Endocrine abnormalities**    A variety of neuroendocrine changes have been reported in patients with mood disorders. The most consistent have been seen in the production of cortisol. The following findings have been noted:

- About half of patients with depressive disorder have increased cortisol levels. This increase in cortisol is not specific and is also seen in mania and schizophrenia. It is not just a simple stress reaction to being ill, because the diurnal pattern is altered as well (remaining high in the afternoon and early evening when it would normally decrease).
- Dexamethasone suppression test. Dexamethasone is a synthetic analogue of cortisol. A significant proportion of patients with depression do not show the normal cortisol suppression in response to dexamethasone. Again this effect is not specific to depression, but is found in a wide variety of other psychiatric disorders namely mania, schizophrenia and dementia.
- Mood disorders are associated with diseases involving an abnormality of cortisol levels. Using the Present State Examination (PSE) there is a 50% rate of depressive disorder in Cushing's disease. A higher than expected rate is also seen in Addison's disease. Administration of exogenous steroids can precipitate elated mood.

These abnormalities of cortisol may represent a marker of other changes rather than a cause of the disorder. The hypothalamus is central to the regulation of the neuroendocrine axis and it receives many neuronal inputs that use monoaminergic transmitters.

There are also abnormalities seen in thyroid hormones in depressive disorder:

- Approximately one-third of patients with depressive disorder have reduced thyroid stimulating hormone (TSH) response to an infusion of thyroid releasing hormone (TRH). However again this is not specific and has been reported in other psychiatric disorders.
- Hyper and hypothyroidism are associated with affective changes.

**Water and electrolytes**

'Residual' sodium (similar to intracellular sodium) has been reported as increased in both depression and mania. There have also been reports of changes in red blood cell sodium-potassium ATPase (adenosine triphosphatase) in both disorders.

**Sleep abnormalities**

Early morning wakening is the classic sleep abnormality associated with depression but initial insomnia and interrupted sleep are also common. The sleep electroencephalogram (EEG) shows:

- Delayed sleep onset.
- Shortened REM latency (time from onset of sleep to the start of rapid eye movement sleep).
- Decreased slow wave sleep.
- Increased first period of REM.

It is also of interest that sleep deprivation can temporarily improve depression.

**Brain imaging**

Structural brain imaging with computer tomography (CT) and magnetic resonance imaging (MRI) has yielded inconsistent results. Functional brain imaging: SPECT (single photon emission tomography) and PET (positron emission tomography) studies have shown reduced blood flow particularly in frontal areas.

# Further reading

Delgado PL, Price LH, Heninger GR, Charney DS. Neurochemistry. In: Paykel ES (ed.) *Handbook of Affective Disorders*. Churchill Livingstone, 1992.

# Related topics of interest

# ALZHEIMER'S DISEASE – NEUROBIOLOGY

**Neuropathology**

The brain at post-mortem shows gross atrophy. Gyri are shrunken and sulci widened. These changes may also be seen on computerized tomography (CT) and magnetic resonance imaging (MRI). There is increasing evidence that these investigations can show temporal lobe abnormalities in life which correlate with the presence of the disease.

*1. Neurofibrillary tangles.* In the brain it is necessary to see those tangles for a histological diagnosis: they only occur rarely in non-demented patients.

Neurofibrillary tangles are intracellular paired helical filaments. They are composed of paired helical filaments tau of (PHF-tau). Tau protein is normally associated with microtubules. The transformation of tau to PHF-tau, which occurs by phosphorylation, is central to the cytoskeletal pathology of AD. It is believed to be caused by mutated amyloid precursor proteins (APP).

*2. Amyloid plaques.* These occur more commonly in the cortex of non-demented patients than do tangles; in Alzheimer's disease (AD), however, their density correlates with severity of disease.

Amyloid plaques are extracellular and consist of a dense core of amyloid fibrils. They consist of beta amyloid protein for which the DNA/mRNA coding has been identified. Precursors of beta amyloid protein have characteristics of transmembrane proteins and occur mostly in layers III and V of the cortex and throughout all layers in the hippocampus. It is thought that deposition of beta amyloid results from neuronal dysfunction, since the distribution of the precursors is neuronal. Plaques contain markers for acetylcholine (ACh), gamma-aminobutyric acid (GABA), neuro-peptide Y (NPY), somatostatin and substance P (SP).

Both tangles and plaques are found in the cerebral cortex, hippocampus, amygdala, nucleus basalis of Meynert and locus coeruleus in AD.

*3. Pyramidal cell loss.* This occurs consistently in AD, in cortical layers III and V. Tangles occur most commonly in these neurons and they receive ascending projections from the basal forebrain (ACh), raphe nuclei (serotonergic) and from the brainstem (noradrenergic). Interneurons containing GABA and several neuropeptides interconnect pyramidal cells.

**Cortical neurotransmitter systems**

*1. Cholinergic function.*

(a) There are significant reductions in nicotinic receptors in cortex and hippocampus.

(b) Evidence about change in the level of muscarinic receptors is equivocal; since the relevant neurotransmitter levels are reduced, it may be that the unchanged level of receptors represents a compensatory response to presynaptic cholinergic hypofunction.

(c) Reduced levels of choline acetyltransferase (ChAT) are found in the cerebral cortex of AD patients.

(d) In addition, neuron loss occurs in the nucleus basalis of Meynert, diagonal band of Broca and medial septal nuclei. These basal forebrain structures provide cholinergic innervation to the cortex and hippocampus.

(e) It is thought the cell loss in these nuclei is secondary to cortical events rather than vice versa.

(f) Cholinergic dysfunction, though common in AD, is not a prerequisite for dementia since Pick's patients have cell loss in the nucleus basalis without cortical ChAT dysfunction.

(g) In olivopontocerebellar atrophy (which is not a dementing condition) levels of cortical ChAT dysfunction are similar to those in patients with AD. Both demented and non-demented Parkinson's patients have reduced levels of ChAT.

*2. Serotonergic function.*

5-hydroxytryptamine$_2$ (5-HT$_2$) receptors are found to be consistently reduced in frontal, temporal, parietal cortex and hippocampus in AD. This loss is thought to reflect cortical pyramidal cell loss. The level of 5-HT2 receptors has been found to correlate inversely with the number of tangles. No consistent picture has been found for the other serotonergic receptors.

*3. Adrenoreceptors.*

(a) $\alpha$-adrenoreceptors are unchanged in the temporal and frontal cortex; in the hippocampus $\alpha_2$ receptors are reduced and $\alpha_1$ receptors unchanged.

(b) $\beta_2$ receptors are increased and $\beta_1$ receptors reduced in the prefrontal cortex in AD, with an associated reduction in noradrenaline (NA). In the hippocampus one study has shown increased numbers of $\beta_2$ and decreased numbers of $\beta_1$, while another showed increases in both subtypes.

4. *Cortical interneuron transmitter receptors.*
(a) GABA levels in interneurons are reduced in AD.
  - Cortical plaques contain glutamic acid decarboxylase immunoreactivity.
  - The cortex in AD shows a loss of GABA reuptake markers.

(b) Cortical glutaminergic innervation comes from pyramidal interneurons and from the thalamus. Binding of radioactive ligands for glutamate uptake systems is reduced by 30–60% in the cerebral cortex and hippocampus in AD. It is thought that glutamate has a role in the progression of AD rather than in primary aetiology. Although some studies indicate specific *N*-methyl D-aspartate (NMDA) receptor deficits, homogenized preparations which measure the NMDA glutamate receptor specifically have found no significant difference between brains of those with AD and controls. Disparities may be explained by differences in local neuropathology. Autoradiography of kainate glutamate receptors has also shown anatomically discrete changes in receptor binding.

(c) Somatostatin co-localizes with GABA in non-pyramidal neurons and reduced cortical concentrations of this chemical have also been reported.

(d) NPY containing neurons are reduced in the hippocampus and temporal cortex.

(e) Vasoactive intestinal peptide (VIP) levels are unchanged or modestly reduced in the cerebral cortex.

(f) Corticotrophin releasing factor (CRF) is reduced in the cortex, though immunoreactivity is preserved in the hippocampus.

(g) Cholecystokinin (CCK) shows no consistent change.

(h) Substance P shows no consistent change.

5. *Second messenger systems.* Radioligand results are not reliable indicators of the functional situation since disruption of cells, for example by plaques, may affect functional integrity. Study of the second messenger systems associated with receptors gives an insight into functional capabilities in the AD brain. Second messenger systems include:

(a)  *Adenylate cyclase.* Stimulated by β-adrenergic, $D_1$, adenosine $A_2$, $5HT_1$ and VIP containing neurons. Autoradiographic studies of the stimulatory G-protein linked to adenylate cyclase using ($^3$H)forskolin show decreased binding in the frontal cortex, but not in the hippocampus and show inconsistent results in the temporal cortex.

(b)  *Phosphoinositide* mediates action of muscarinic receptors, $5HT_2$, $\alpha_1$ and a number of peptide receptors and excitatory amino acid receptors. The activity of this system appears to be reduced in the frontal cortex in AD.

Studies have revealed an increasingly complex picture over the last decade. It is not unusual for studies of the same brain area to reveal contradictory results. Discrepancies could be explained by methodological differences or by morphological differences between brains studied. Tangles and plaques can interfere with transmitter synthesis or release, and thus receptor measurement can be influenced by morphological status.

In summary, there are many neurotransmitter and receptor abnormalities in AD. There needs to be an improved understanding of the interactions between neurochemical changes and the diverse structural changes. Even though AD is a degenerative condition, the brain may remain plastic and therefore capable of compensatory responses.

# Further reading

Dewar D. Neurotransmitter system abnormalities associated with the neuropathology of Alzheimer's disease. In: Kerwin R (ed.) *Neurobiology and Psychiatry*, Vol 1. Cambridge: Cambridge University Press, 1993; 61–94.

Gallo JM. The biochemistry of tau proteins in Alzheimer's disease. In: Kerwin R (ed.) *Neurobiology and Psychiatry*, Vol 2. Cambridge: Cambridge University Press, 1993; 27–42.

Hardy J. Alzheimer's disease and the beta amyloid precursor protein. In: Kerwin R (ed.) *Neurobiology and Psychiatry*, Vol 2. Cambridge: Cambridge University Press, 1993; 19–26.

# Related topics of interest

# ANTIPSYCHOTIC MEDICATION

## Mode of action

**The dopamine hypothesis**

The dopamine hypothesis of schizophrenia states that the positive symptoms of psychosis are due to a functional overactivity of dopamine in the brain, and some extremely attractive theories have been proposed as to how this relates to positive symptoms (McKenna, 1987). For conventional neuroleptics, it has long been known that efficacy in alleviating the symptoms of psychosis is proportional to the strength with which the drug binds to central dopamine receptors, particularly in the mesolimbic system.

**Atypical antipsychotics**

Atypical antipsychotics, of which clozapine and risperidone are the currently available examples, have a different mechanism of action. Whilst they do blockade $DA_2$ receptors, and also adrenergic and histaminergic receptors (as do classical neuroleptics), the major difference is their powerful blockade of 5-hydroxytryptamine (5-HT) receptors. They are the only drugs which have been shown in clinical trials to be superior to conventional neuroleptics such as chlorpromazine or haloperidol (Marder and Meibach, 1994); they seem to be effective against the negative symptoms of schizophrenia, in which conventional neuroleptics are largely ineffective. They are also relatively free of extrapyramidal side-effects (EPSE), certainly at lower doses. Both are expensive, and clozapine causes a potentially fatal agranulocytosis in 1–2% of patients, and so frequent blood monitoring is necessary.

## Indications for use of antipsychotic medication

**Control of severely disturbed behaviour**

Severely disturbed behaviour has many possible causes, and may result in injury to the individual concerned, or to others. Neuroleptics are a useful adjunct to behavioural control, which involves containment in a safe environment with low levels of stimulation. Sedation is the effect desired, and is an effect somewhat separate from the antipsychotic one. Haloperidol or droperidol orally, IM or IV (with caution, cardiac arrhythmias may occur, particularly with haloperidol) are used. Chlorpromazine can be given orally, but its IM use is complicated by the need to give large volumes, and the fact that the injection is irritant and painful. It should be avoided by this route.

**Treatment of psychotic conditions**

This is the most common indication. Neuroleptics are the mainstay of the short- and long-term treatment of schizophrenia and the paranoid psychoses, and are also used in the treatment of acute mania, in which haloperidol is said to be especially efficacious. The use of high doses, or 'megadose' therapy is probably justified in fewer cases than it is used (Thompson, 1994). Those who fail to respond to 6–8 weeks' treatment with adequate doses should be tried on another neuroleptic, or an atypical antipsychotic (e.g. risperidone or clozapine), or adjunctive lithium or benzodiazepines. Electroconvulsive therapy (ECT) may be effective in resistant delusional states. In long-term treatment, continuous antipsychotic treatment has been shown to be more effective than intermittent use of medication in the prophylaxis of psychotic recurrence (Jolley *et al.*, 1990).

**Treatment of personality disorders**

Long-term treatment with low doses of antipsychotics may be helpful, particularly in 'Cluster B' patients, with labile affectivity, and a tendency to repeated self-harm (see Self mutilation, p.306).

**Other uses**

Recurrent brief depression and Tourette's syndrome are both indications for neuroleptics (see appropriate topics, pp. 283 and 347).

**Atypical antipsychotics**

Current indications for their use (Edwards, 1994) are:

- Patients with severe negative symptoms who have not responded to conventional neuroleptics.
- Those with severe unwanted extrapyramidal side-effects, including dyskinesia.
- Treatment-resistant schizophrenia and affective disorders (Kimmel *et al.*, 1994).

However, as experience with their use becomes more widespread, the significant advantages in terms of side-effect profile (particularly the rarity of tardive dyskinesia in long-term usage) and therapeutic efficacy may lead to drugs like risperidone becoming first-line treatments.

**Drawbacks of antipsychotic medication**

*1. Short-term problems.* Acute side-effects, which may be problematic, particularly with high doses, can be related to the receptor group primarily involved:

(a) *Dopamine.* Receptors are found in the mesolimbic and nigrostriatal areas of cortex, the chemoreceptor trigger zone of the medulla (metoclopramide, domperidone, prochlorperazine all blockade dopamine here), and the pituitary.

- *Pseudoparkinsonism.* Dose related, and worse with drugs with less anticholinergic action.
- *Acute dystonic reaction.* Classically with young men on haloperidol.
- *Akathisia.* The 'largactil shuffle'. A feeling of psychic and/or motor restlessness, which may be intolerable, and lead to determined non-compliance or suicide. In acutely disturbed patients, it may cause a paradoxical worsening of behaviour. Treatment (usually unsatisfactory) is with propranolol or benzodiazepines, or, better still, by dose reduction as soon as possible.
- *Neuroleptic malignant syndrome (NMS).* Caused by excessive dopamine blockade of the extrapyramidal system. A triad of:
  (a) Hyperthermia.
  (b) Muscular rigidity.
  (c) Clouding of consciousness.
  Muscle creatine phosphokinase (CPK) is usually greatly elevated. In its full-blown form, NMS can be fatal. Treatment should be in the intensive care unit, using bromocriptine and dantrolene sodium. The chances of recurrence on re-challenging with neuroleptics after recovery are only about one in three, even if the same antipsychotic is used, and the risks of NMS are probably increased in physically compromised (exhausted, infected or dehydrated) patients.
- *Hyperprolactinaemia and galactorrhoea.* These result from dopamine blockade in the pituitary, where it acts as a prolactin release inhibitory factor. It is particularly common with sulpiride.

(b) *Anticholinergic:*
- *Dry mouth, blurred vision, constipation, problems with micturition.*
- *Hyperthermia and heatstroke* are more likely in patients on neuroleptics, especially those with pronounced anticholinergic action, due to inhibition of sweating (sympathetic, cholinergic). This is a particular danger in highly disturbed, active patients, who may also be dehydrated.

(c) *Antiadrenergic:*
- *Hypotension.*
- *Ejaculatory problems.*

(d)  *Antihistaminergic:*
  - *Sedation* (may be useful therapeutically).
  - *Antinauseant* (prochlorperazine is marketed for this).

Lowered seizure threshold, cardiac conduction problems and idiopathic blood dyscrasias or liver problems may occur. Photosensitivity is a problem with many of the older agents.

*2. Long-term problems.* The unwanted acute side-effects of drug treament will all be less tolerable in the long term. In addition, those causing most problems are:

- *Weight gain.* Thirty per cent of people on long-term neuroleptic treatment are morbidly obese, compared with 5% of the normal population. Obesity results from an increase in appetite caused by neuroleptic action on the hypothalamus.
- *Loss of hedonic tone.* Chronic dopamine blockade in the nucleus accumbens lowers mood and reduces pleasurable feelings in response to reward. The chronic smoking of people on neuroleptics may be an attempt to overcome this affective deadening (nicotine causes dopamine release in the nucleus accumbens).
- *Apathy.* By blockading dopamine receptors in the prefrontal cortex, neuroleptics may reduce motivation and drive.
- *Tardive dyskinesia (TD).* A serious long-term complication of dopamine blockade. Tardive dyskinesia consists of choreiform or athetoid movements, or tics, which have an onset years or more after the onset of treatment, and are more common in elderly women. They are thought to result from postsynaptic receptor upregulation resulting in supersensitivity. Although TD has been described in drug-naive schizophrenics, and may therefore be part of the syndrome, it is much more common in those treated with neuroleptics. Higher doses, and probably also concomitant treatment with anticholinergics, worsen TD. For this reason, anticholinergics should not be prescribed routinely. TD may be irreversible, but at least two-thirds recover if antipsychotics are stopped. Clozapine may reverse established TD.

# Further reading

Edwards JG. Risperidone for schizophrenia. *British Medical Journal,* 1994; **308:** 1311–12.

Jolley AG, Hirsch SR, Morrison E, McRink A, Wilson L. Trial of brief intermittent neuroleptic prophylaxis for selected schizophrenic outpatients: clinical and social outcome at two years. *British Medical Journal,* 1990; **301:** 837–42.

Kimmel SE, Calambrese MD, Wayshville MD, Meltzer HY. Clozapine in treatment-refractory mood disorders. *Journal of Clinical Psychiatry,* 1994; **55:**(9, suppl B) 91–3.

Marder SR, Meibach RC. Risperidone in the treatment of schizophrenia. *American Journal of Psychiatry,* 1994; **151:** 825–35.

McKenna PJ. Pathology, phenomenology and the dopamine hypothesis of schizophrenia. *British Journal of Psychiatry,* 1987; **151:** 288–301.

Thompson C. Consensus statement. The use of high-dose antipsychotic medication. *British Journal of Psychiatry,* 1994; **164:** 448–58.

# Related topics of interest

# ANXIETY AND PANIC

**Definitions**

A *panic attack* is defined as a discrete period of intense fear or discomfort (classically a 'feeling of impending doom'), accompanied by somatic symptoms of anxiety, such as sweating, shaking, palpitations, shortness of breath. There is often an intense urge to flee or escape. Onset is sudden, and the peak is usually within 10 minutes, after which the feelings subside. Between attacks the subject may be normal, or experience anticipatory anxiety.

*Anxiety* may be a normal healthy response to a situation in which there is a perception of threat, either physical or psychological. It can be an important motivational drive, and attention and speed of response follow an inverted 'U'-shaped curve with increasing anxiety and arousal (the Yerkes–Dodson law). 'Optimal arousal' is the level at which performance is maximized, and is at lower levels of arousal, the more complex the task.

Anxiety disorders are characteristically divided into *panic disorder* (episodic paroxysmal anxiety), with recurrent attacks of severe anxiety (panic) which are not restricted to any particular situation or set of circumstances, and *generalized anxiety disorder* (GAD), characterized by anxiety, which is generalized and persistent but not restricted to any particular environmental circumstance (i.e. it is 'free-floating'). In GAD 'the intensity, duration or frequency of the anxiety and worry is out of proportion to the likelihood or impact of the feared event' (DSM-IV). There are associated physical symptoms such as fatiguability, poor concentration, irritability, disturbed sleep or muscle tension, and the subject finds it difficult to control the worry.

**Epidemiology**

- Anxiety and panic are some of the most common symptoms in the general population. Generalized anxiety disorder has a 1-year prevalence of 3% and a lifetime prevalence of 5%, and panic disorder a 1-year prevalence of 1–2% and a lifetime prevalence of 1.5–3.5%.
- Co-morbidity is common: two-thirds of patients with panic disorder have associated depression, which begins before the panic disorder in one-third of cases, and coincident with or subsequent to it in the other two-thirds. Agoraphobia and social phobia are also commonly associated, and DSM-IV separates panic into two categories, depending upon whether there is associated agoraphobia.

- Generalized anxiety disorder is frequently accompanied by other anxiety disorders and by depression, which is so common in both clinical and epidemiological samples that it can be regarded as the rule rather than the exception (Wittchen *et al.*, 1991). Co-morbidity of depression and anxiety worsens prognosis.
- Longitudinal studies suggest that persons with mixed anxiety–depression symptoms may represent a population who are at increased risk for more severe mood and anxiety disorders (Katon and Roy-Byrne, 1991). Substance misuse or dependence is also extremely common.

**Aetiology**

Genetic causes are thought to be important in anxiety disorders of all kinds because the concordance for anxiety disorders is greater among monozygotic than dizygotic twins. However, the relevant studies do not distinguish clearly between the different kinds of anxiety disorder.

*1. Hypotheses about the origin of panic disorder.*
(a) The biochemical hypothesis is based on three sets of research observations:
- Certain chemical agents can induce panic attacks more readily in patients with panic disorder than in healthy people, for example, yohimbine, sodium lactate.
- Panic attacks are reduced by drugs such as imipramine and other antidepressants which could be acting on a biochemical abnormality.
- Panic disorder is more frequent among relatives of panic disorder patients than among the general population.

To explain the effects of these chemical agents, it has been proposed that regulation of the adrenergic system is abnormal in panic disorder.
(b) The hyperventilation theory is that panic attacks are caused by overbreathing. Although some patients with panic attacks hyperventilate, measurement of $pCO_2$ during these attacks shows that hyperventilation does not occur in every such patient (see related topic on 'Hyperventilation', p. 159).
(c) The cognitive model is based on the theory that patients with panic disorder misinterpret physical sensations such as palpitations as a medical catastrophe (heart attack) and panic as a consequence. This will lead to further physical symptoms such as hyperventilation,

which, in turn, leads to more anxiety. There is some experimental evidence to support this hypothesis.

It seems likely that the first and third set of causes combine, so that panic disorder develops in a person with poorly regulated autonomic responses to stressors when he becomes afraid of the consequences of symptoms of autonomic arousal.

In GAD, the cognitive distortions make a person prone to interpret a wide range of situations as threatening. Most relate to issues of acceptance, competence, responsibility, control and the anxiety symptoms themselves. In panic, by contrast, there is a specific tendency to misinterpret a variety of bodily sensations in a catastrophic manner, as signifying immediate impending physical or mental catastrophe. The subject may not be aware of these antecedent sensations, and so may experience the panic attacks as spontaneous.

*2. Treatments.*

(a) *Biological.*

- Tricyclic antidepressants such as imipramine have been shown to be effective in both anxiety and panic disorder. They are also useful in GAD when (i) there is an associated depressive disorder, and (ii) long-term anxiety has to be controlled.
- There is evidence that depression with prominent anxiety and panic responds to monoamine oxidase inhibitors (MAOI), but these drugs should be reserved for the occasional patients for whom other drugs and psychological treatments have been tried without success.
- The use of short (a few weeks at most) courses of high-dose benzodiazepines to break the cycle of anxiety and panic has been found to be effective, but risks include withdrawal symptoms and potential dependency when the drug is stopped.
- Beta blockers can be used to treat somatic symptoms of anxiety, for example, palpitations, trembling.

(b) *Psychological.*

- The most effective psychological treatment for panic disorder is a form of cognitive therapy. There is evidence that cognitive therapy is at least as effective as imipramine in panic disorder (Clark *et al.*, 1994), and it has also been shown to be effective in GAD (Butler *et al.*, 1987).

# Further reading

Butler G, Cullington A, Hibbert G, Klimes I, Gelder M. Anxiety management for persistent anxiety disorder. *British Journal of Psychiatry*, 1987; **151:** 535–42.

Clark DM. Anxiety states: panic and generalised anxiety. In: Hawton K, Salkovskis PM, Kirk J, Clark DM (eds) *Cognitive Behaviour Therapy for Psychiatric Problems*. Oxford: Oxford University Press, 1989; 52–96.

Clark DM, Salkovskis PM, Hackmann A, Middleton H, Anastasiades P, Gelder M. A comparison of cognitive therapy, applied relaxation and imipramine in the treatment of panic disorder. *British Journal of Psychiatry,* 1994; **164:** 759–69.

Katon W, Roy-Byrne P. Mixed anxiety and depression. *Journal of Abnormal Psychology,* 1991; **100:** 337–45.

Wittchen H-U, Essau CA, Kreig J-C. Anxiety disorders: similarities and differences of comorbidity in treated and untreated groups. *British Journal of Psychiatry,* 1991; **159**(suppl. 12): 23–33.

# Related topics of interest

# BEHAVIOURAL DISTURBANCE IN CHILDHOOD

**Classification**

ICD-10:AXIS I = behavioural and emotional disorders with onset usually in childhood or adolescence:

- Hyperkinetic disorders.
- Conduct disorders (see Delinquency and antisocial personality, p. 81).
- Mixed disorders of conduct and emotions.
- Emotional disorders with onset specific to childhood, for example, separation anxiety, phobias, school refusal, depression.
- Disorders of social functioning.
- Tic disorders.
- Other emotional and behavioural disorders, for example, enuresis, encopresis.

In DSM-III-R, Axis I is organized in a similar manner, but also includes eating disorders and gender identity disorders. Many other psychiatric disorders can occur in childhood or adolescence but are not classified by age, for example, other major adult disorders.

**Individual disorders**

Preschool children tend to exhibit delays or deviations from normal development rather than psychiatric syndromes as such.

*1. Temper tantrums.* These are normal in toddlers and are reinforced if the behaviour achieves something. If the behaviour is persistent or troublesome, limit-setting and a clear plan of management can be helpful.

*2. Sleep disorders.* Most children have an established sleep pattern by the age of one year. Problems can be related to temperament, family stress factors and parental problems, for example, depression. The underlying problems should be dealt with and the parents should avoid rewarding waking. Night terrors, sleep-walking and nightmares are common in young children. Night terrors are characterized by absence of waking and lack of memory for the dream. These tend to resolve with age.

*3. Eating disorders.* Eating difficulties are common in children. Disorders include food refusal and faddiness, non-organic failure to thrive, pica and obesity.

**Attention deficit disorder (hyperkinetic syndrome)**

Hyperkinesis is characterized by overactivity, restlessness and poor attentiveness and it is often associated with delays in language development, motor clumsiness and lower IQ. Rates range from 0.1–10% in different populations, and with different diagnostic criteria. The sex ratio is 3M:1F. Aetiological factors include social and family (including genetic) aspects. The prognosis is related to the severity of hyperactivity, to low IQ and aggressive behaviour. Hyperkinesis may predict later antisocial behaviour and can affect development.

**Disorders of social functioning**

*1. Reactive attachment disorder.* This describes social, emotional and behavioural difficulties related to parental neglect, abuse or mishandling. Mental retardation and autism should be considered in the differential diagnosis.

*2. Social disinhibition syndrome or primary attachment disorder.* This is characterized by superficial relationships with any adult and is often related to disrupted early experiences, particularly an institutional upbringing. The disorder can be improved by a change in environment but difficulties often persist which may jeopardize future placements (i.e. fostering or adoption).

**Emotional disorders**

These may be an exaggeration of normal range of behaviour in terms of duration and effects on social functioning and development.

*1. Separation anxiety disorder.* Separation anxiety is common in preschool children and those just starting school.

*2. Phobic disorder of childhood.* Phobias are common in early childhood, decline in middle childhood, although school and social fears are commonest at this age.

*3. School refusal* (cf. truancy which is a conduct disorder). The child is unable to go to school or stay there but the parents know where the child is. It is commonest at times of changing school (especially around 11 years of age), or is associated with change in family or school circumstances. It can often be seen in terms of separation anxiety or 'school phobia'. It represents less than 3% of children with psychiatric disorders (i.e. 1 in 1000) and has an equal sex incidence. It may be related to family problems, for example marital discord, maternal depression (20%), overprotection and parental neurosis (whereas truants tend to come from a lower social class where there is inconsistent discipline, antisocial behaviour and paternal absence). It is important to assess the effect on schoolwork and on family. The most crucial aspect of management is to get the child back to school as soon as possible, and to be most effective this should involve the parents, school and educational social worker (ESW). Any other contributory problems should be dealt with, for example maternal depression. If this fails, there may be a need for teaching in an interim unit, or, more rarely, home tuition; in-patient treatment should be reserved for the most refractory cases. The prognosis is better in younger children, where the problem is identified and dealt with early on.

*4. Social sensitivity disorder and sibling rivalry disorder.* These are generally self-limiting but can be helped by reducing stresses and improving coping skills.

*5. Obsessive-compulsive disorders (OCD).* These obsessional symptoms are common in childhood and adolescence but OCD is rare.

*6. Depression.* This is difficult to assess and diagnose in early childhood but can occur in prepubertal children. It may be related to concurrent stresses and parental depression. Physical illness, bereavement and sadness should be considered in the differential diagnosis. The efficacy of treatments is unclear as yet but family therapy (and cognitive behavioural therapy (CBT) or individual psychotherapy) may be most appropriate in this age group. Depression is generally self-limiting.

*7. Recurrent abdominal pain and somatization.* These are common presentations of emotional difficulties, and represent 8–10% of attenders in primary care.

**Elimination disorders/other emotional and behavioural disorders**

*1. Enuresis.* This is defined as involuntary emptying of the bladder over the age of 5 years without physical cause and may be primary or secondary. At 5 years 3% are wet during the day and 10% at night. At 14 years 1% are wet at night. Boys are affected slightly more often, as are those in the lower social classes. It may be related to delays in the development of the autonomic nervous system. It may also present or be precipitated by acute stresses.

Management: physical causes should be excluded. Star-charts can be effective in recent onset cases. The pad and bell method is effective for children over six years old. Imipramine can be useful but the symptoms usually recur once it is stopped. The majority of cases resolve by adolescence.

*2. Encopresis.* Faeces are passed inappropriately. This may be primary or secondary (i.e. following a period of continence), and may be caused by constipation. Boys are more commonly affected and it occurs in 3% of four year olds and 1.5% of seven year olds. It may be related to abnormalities of toilet training, or to emotional disturbance, especially sexual abuse. Management may be best carried out in conjunction with the paediatricians, and physical causes should be dealt with. Underlying psychological problems should be addressed and behavioural techniques may be effective. Encopresis generally resolves by adolescence but psychological problems may persist.

*3. Tics.* Tics occur in about 10% of children and generally disappear without treatment.

# Further reading

Black D, Cottrell D (eds). *Seminars in Child and Adolescent Psychiatry.* London: Gaskell (Royal College of Psychiatrists), 1993.

Graham P. *Child Psychiatry: a Developmental Approach*, 2nd Edn. Oxford: Oxford Medical Publications, 1991; 166–90, 210–21.

Rutter M. Relationships between mental disorders in childhood and adulthood. *Acta Psychiatrica Scandinavica*, 1995; **91:** 73–85.

# Related topics of interest

# BEREAVEMENT AND GRIEF COUNSELLING

**Stages in the grieving process**

*1. Numbness* occurs before the onset of acute grief. It may last from only a few hours to 2 weeks.

*2. Disbelief* is also common within the first few days. Once a person feels and knows the death has occurred, the process of grieving begins. It may take months to completely accept the finality of the death.

*3. Acute grief* – the events which occur during this stage are understandable in terms of loss of attachment:

- Urge to cry out.
- Searching.
- Anxiety.
- Agitation.
- Pining.
- Somatic responses.
- Anger can be borne and appropriately dissipated or it may be displaced onto self (guilt), family (family rows), professionals (litigation), God (loss of faith) or suppressed (depression, psychosomatic illness).
- Awareness of the presence of the deceased. Illusions of seeing or hearing the deceased can occur and hallucinations of the deceased are also normal at this stage.
- Taking on attitudes and mannerisms of the deceased as a way of identification with them.

*4. Acute grief* gradually subsides and is replaced by depression and despair.

*5. Resolution.* In this phase the bereaved person may always remain lonely but also discover new or old abilities or interests. Psychological readjustment is termed 'grief work'.

**Abnormal grief**

*1. Delayed grief.* More than 2 weeks passes before the onset of the grieving process.

*2. Inhibited grief.* The bereaved person may develop avoidance strategies. For example they may become hyperactive, irritable or develop depression. They may retain an idealized version of the deceased. When this occurs in young children it may predict later psychiatric illness. Inhibited grief may be a more normal response to loss in older people, perhaps as a consequence of the natural preparation for further loss and death in old age.

*3. Chronic grief.* The grieving process endures for longer than expected (although it is not possible to set a rigid definition of the precise duration of normal grief). It occurs when the person becomes 'stuck' with features of recent bereavement although years have elapsed. It can serve as a defence against recognizing another problem or as a mechanism for keeping other family members close by.

*4. Complicated grief.* This is more likely in the following situations:

- Death of a fully grown child.
- Sudden death.
- Suicide.
- An ambivalent relationship before death.

**Psychiatric associations**

1. In the recently bereaved there is an increased morbidity from stress-related conditions and mortality. Widowers aged over 54 years have a 40% rise in mortality, most of the excess being due to cardiovascular disease.

2. The bereaved are also at increased risk of developing:

- Hypochondriasis.
- Phobias.
- Alcoholism.
- Depression.
- Mania.

**Treatment**

*1. Grief counselling.* This aims to facilitate the tasks of mourning in the recently bereaved.

*2. Grief therapy.* This aims to identify and resolve the conflicts of separation which underlie aspects of the grieving process which are abnormal because they are absent, delayed, excessive or prolonged. It is usually time limited, for example to 10 sessions, focused and follows these procedures:
(a) Rule out physical disease.
(b) Set up a contract of treatment and establish an alliance.
(c) Revive memories of the deceased. If the deceased is remembered in an idealized way, the groundwork of remembered positive memories should be set and then more mixed and gradually negative memories are

revived. If the patient has negative memories the task is to revive some positive ones.

(d) Deal with affect or lack of affect stimulated by memories.

(e) Assess which of the following four grief tasks are not completed:

- Accepting the reality of the death.
- Development of affect in response to the death.
- Ceasing to feel helpless without the deceased.
- Developing freedom from the attachment in order to cultivate new relationships.

(f) Explore and defuse linking objects. These are objects which have special meaning about the deceased and are similar to transitional objects in an earlier developmental stage.

(g) Deal with fantasies which the patient may have about ending grieving.

(h) Help the patient to say a final goodbye.

(i) Change following grief therapy may occur in subjective experience, behaviour or symptom relief.

## Further reading

Melges FT, De Maso DR. Grief resolution and therapy: reliving, revising and revisiting. *American Journal of Psychiatry,* 1980; **34:** 498–512.

Parkes CM. *Bereavement: studies of grief in adult life.* Harmondsworth: Pelican Books, 1975.

Stedeford A. Bereavement. *Medicine in Practice,* 1983; **25:** 702–7.

## Related topic of interest

# BRAIN AREA DYSFUNCTION

**Frontal lobes**

The primary observed effect of frontal lobe dysfunction from any cause is on personality. The central pathophysiological dysfunction is *disinhibition,* which leads to a loss of normal control over emotion, behaviour and cognition. In cases following an acute event the changes will be obvious, but causes such as benign tumours can have an insidious onset with changes at first being subtle and only noticed by those who know the patient well. Although features may occur after damage to one lobe, most severe forms involve damage to both.

Symptoms include:

- Disinhibition.
- Euphoria.
- Blunting of emotional responsiveness.
- Egocentricity.
- Interference with others.
- Irresponsibility.
- Lack of tact and concern.
- Childishness.
- Purposeless drive.
- Loss of initiative.
- Loss of judgement.
- Apathy.
- Inertia.
- Aggressiveness.
- Learning disabilities due to frontal lobe dysfunction are due to increased distractibility, perseveration and lack of attention to environmental cues.

Examination may reveal:

- Re-emergence of primitive reflexes such as the palmar reflex and oral rooting reflex.
- Decreased ability in trail-making tests.
- Decreased verbal fluency (naming of as many objects as possible in a certain category in 1 minute).
- Perseveration is detected by the Wisconsin Card Sorting Test in which the subject is required to modify behaviour on the instruction of the examiner.

Causes include:

- Cerebrovascular – infarction or haemorrhage.
- Tumour, for example, meningioma.

- Myxoedema.
- Pick's disease.
- Syphilis (general paralysis of the insane).

In cases where insight has been preserved, some improvement in symptoms may be achieved by behavioural techniques.

**Temporal lobes**

*1. Bilateral lesions.* In the medial temporal lobe these cause a pure amnesic syndrome (see Memory, p. 185):

(a)  A dense loss of memory for recent events.

(b)  The inability to retain new information.

(c)  Preserved intelligence and personality distinguish this condition from a dementing process.

Causes of bilateral lesions include:

- Thiamine deficiency in alcoholics, leading to Korsakov's psychosis.
- Head injury, the effects may be temporary or permanent.
- Epileptic seizure, which has a temporary effect that may nevertheless persist for some time after the seizure.
- Parapituitary tumours.
- Encephalitis, herpes simplex.

*2. Unilateral lesions.* Lesion of the dominant lobe leads to:

(a)  Disorders of communication which may involve speech, reading and/or writing.

(b)  Contralateral homonymous upper quadrantic vision defect (due to involvement of lower fibres of the optic radiation).

Lesion of the non-dominant lobe also leads to this visual field defect, but may not cause any other detectable symptoms.

Causes of unilateral lesions include:

- Cerebrovascular infarction and haemorrhage.
- Tumours.
- Head injury.

**Parietal lobes**

Damage in these areas leads to the following phenomena:

*1. Cortical sensory loss.*

- Astereognosis. The ability to identify objects by palpation alone is lost.
- Agraphaesthesia. The ability to recognize numbers or

letters written on the palm of the hand and the ability to discriminate separation of two points on the finger pad is lost.
- Sensory and visual inattention.

2. *Disturbances of body image (agnosia).*

- A non-dominant lesion causing a left hemiparesis may also result in neglect of the left side of the body and lack of awareness of the disability.
- Non-dominant lesions also result in prosopagnosia, which is the failure to recognize the faces of others.

3. *Disturbances of visuospatial functions (apraxias).*

- *Ideomotor* – loss of the ability to imitate gestures despite retention of the ability to carry out the same action automatically.
- *Dressing apraxia* – may result from an ideomotor apraxia or an agnosia, causing neglect of the left side of the body.
- *Constructional apraxia* – the inability to copy two-dimensional designs or to construct a three-dimensional model. There may also be loss of topographical orientation and memory. It results in difficulty with everyday tasks and the liability to get lost.

These problems more commonly occur in right-sided lesions.

- Gerstmann's syndrome – consists of right/left disorientation, agraphia, acalculia and finger agnosia.
- Parietal defects – cause loss of temporal awareness, such that patients have difficulty in judging the time of day.
- Inferior homonymous quadrantic field visual defect – occurs when the optic radiation is involved.

Causes of parietal lobe defects include:
(a) Cerebrovascular infarction and haemorrhage.
(b) Tumours.
(c) Head injury.

**Occipital lobe**

Damage will primarily cause visual problems, but these may result in disturbed behaviour in the case of cortical blindness. This results from bilateral occlusion of the posterior cerebral arteries, which leads to the patient being unable to see but denying this blindness.

**Speech defects**

Speech defects involve the frontal, temporal and parietal lobes:

- The posterior two-thirds of the inferior frontal gyrus.
- The posterior one-third of the middle and central temporal gyri.
- The adjacent parietal lobe.

*1. Nominal dysphasia.*
(a) Leads to difficulty in finding words while the ability to describe the function of objects and to recognize when the correct word is preserved.
(b) Resultant speech is telegraphic but with correct grammar.
(c) Difficulty in comprehension occurs only in severe cases and disability may be less marked in free-flowing speech than in the test situation.
(d) The lesion is usually in the temporal lobe.

*2. Broca's dysphasia – motor/expressive dysphasia.*
(a) Motor control of the muscles of articulation is disrupted by the cerebral lesion.
(b) Words are mispronounced but the patient retains awareness of what he/she wants to say, leading to frustration.
(c) There is usually a partial rather than a complete loss of speech.
(d) The ability to read and write may also be affected, depending on the size of the lesion.
(e) The lesion is in the middle and inferior frontal gyri.

*3. Receptive aphasia.*
(a) Speech is fluent, rambling and incoherent.
(b) Patients are unable to repeat words or phrases.
(c) Grammar is abnormal.
(d) Speech contains neologisms.
(e) Reading and writing are also impaired.
(f) It is less common than motor aphasia.
(g) The lesion is in the white matter of the posterior temporal parietal areas.

Despite the distinctions described above, about 60% of patients with aphasia have a mixture of problems.

# Further reading

Bond MR. Organic disorders. In: Kendell RE, Zealley AK (eds) *Companion to Psychiatric Studies*. Edinburgh: Churchill Livingstone, 1988; Chap. 14.

Marsden CD, Fowler TJ (eds). Examination of the nervous system. In: *Clinical Neurology*. London: Hodder and Stoughton, 1989; Chap. 3.

# Related topics of interest

# CHILD SEXUAL ABUSE – ASSESSMENT AND CONSEQUENCES

**Prevalence**

- Estimates of the incidence of child sexual abuse (CSA) in females vary from less than 10% to over 30%, depending on the definition of abuse (see below), but when only incidents involving genital contact are involved the rates are approximately 10% (Mullen *et al.*, 1988).
- The underlying prevalence of CSA appears to have remained steady over the past four decades at approximately 12% for females.
- In the USA the lifetime prevalence of any sexual assault for one site (Los Angeles) of the Epidemiological Catchment Area (ECA) Study was 13.2%.

**Definition and assessment of sexual abuse**

(a) The definitions used for sexual abuse have varied among studies. Some have included experiences that did not involve physical contact with the subject.
(b) Most definitions include any sexual experience that involves physical contact that is against the subject's will, which includes the subject being touched or being made to touch the abuser in any sexual way, including oral sex or rape.
(c) The age at which abuse occurred also varies; some studies explore abuse before the age of 12, others up to the age of 16 or 18.

**Assessment and management (child)**

Sexual abuse can become apparent in various ways:

- Direct report by the child or someone else (e.g. family member).
- Physical symptoms in the genital and anal area which may indicate that abuse has taken place.
- Sexually precocious or inappropriate behaviour.
- Otherwise unexplained pregnancy.
- Behavioural or emotional problems, and scholastic difficulties. In particular, acting out, deliberate self-harm, anorexia nervosa and substance abuse in teenagers is a common presentation.

The definitions and estimated prevalence of sexual abuse are outlined above. Sexual abuse can occur in all socio-economic classes, but especially in socially deprived families in cramped housing with marital difficulties. Incest is generally father–daughter. In incest, approximately 25% of the mothers were victims of incest themselves. The abuser may suffer from a psychiatric disorder, personality disorder or substance abuse.

The details of the assessment of what has or may have happened, and of the child and family depends on how the problem has presented itself. It is a multidisciplinary procedure involving social services, the GP, child psychiatrists, paediatricians and police, and concentrates on the level of ongoing risk, need for care, and longer term issues.

Social services must be informed, and they have a statutory duty to investigate reports of abuse. Social services then consult with other agencies – police, the child's family or carers, the child, and paediatricians/psychiatrists as appropriate. They would then consider whether an emergency protection order (Children Act 1989) is required to remove the child from immediate danger. Subsequent management involves child protection conferences to coordinate all those involved in the child's care in making further decisions. Psychiatrists have a particular input in assessing the occurrence of sexual abuse (facilitated for example by the use of anatomically correct dolls), assessing the child's behaviour and the likely consequences of the abuse, and making decisions about their placement and other specific management issues.

In the longer term psychiatrists have a key role in reducing the emotional consequences of sexual abuse. This varies but generally includes supporting the child within the family if possible, with techniques appropriate to the child's age. For older children, groups can be helpful for support and sharing of experiences.

**Assessment and management (adult)**

- Many abuse researchers tend to overlook other forms of maltreatment that a child might experience in a given family, despite the fact that physical, psychological, and sexual child abuse frequently occur together.
- There are many different methods used to elicit information about sexual abuse, including interviews, symptom-rating scales, case note studies and questionnaires.
- Many researchers prefer to use an interview rather than self-report questionnaires. The following procedure is recommended:
  —— Questions about sexual abuse within a wider context in which other topics are also addressed, so that rapport can be established before the topic of CSA is broached.

- — Using interviewers of the same gender as the subject.
- — Adopting an interview style in which a series of clear, unambiguous questions are asked about different types of adverse sexual experience, rather than broad closed questions such as 'Have you ever been sexually abused?'.
- — Requesting the subject's permission to ask questions about her experiences with confidentiality being stressed.
- A validated, structured sexual trauma interview has been used in many general population studies (Russell, 1983).
- Many studies distinguish between childhood (younger than 14 years of age) and adult occasions of trauma as well as degrees of severity. The operational definition of 'severe' sexual trauma often includes any form of penetration.

**Adult consequences of child sexual abuse**

- Childhood molestation is associated with multiple short- and long-term psychological difficulties.
- These occur in both clinical and non-clinical samples and are present in both men and women.
- Among the problems that have been associated repeatedly with CSA history are:
  - — Symptoms of post-traumatic stress.
  - — Low self esteem and guilt.
  - — Anxiety.
  - — Depression.
  - — Somatization.
  - — Dissociation.
  - — Interpersonal dysfunction.
  - — Eating disorders.
  - — Sexual problems.
  - — Substance abuse.
  - — Suicidality.
- Women with a history of being abused are significantly more likely to have raised scores or measures of psychopathology on tests such as the General Health Questionnaire (GHQ) and Present State Examination (PSE), and to be identified as psychiatric cases (Mullen *et al.*, 1988).
- Depressive, anxiety and phobic symptoms characterize the clinical syndromes found in abused women.
- The experience of CSA may explain why women are overrepresented among those with depressive and anxiety disorders.

**Methodological problems in the study of the psychological effects of CSA**

- Varying definitions of use (see above).
- Most research has been retrospective, cross-sectional and correlational rather than longitudinal.
- Report biases. Some abused subjects may truthfully report no knowledge of having been abused. If these subjects are included in 'no abuse' comparison groups, between group differences will be obscured.
- There is no satisfactory way to ensure the validity of the subject's recollection of childhood sexual abuse.
- Because sexual abuse is often correlated with other variables, special attention must be paid to the comparison group's status on these factors.
- Other forms of abuse, for example, physical abuse, neglect, often co-vary with CSA but are not always enquired after (see above).
- Conclusions regarding causality. Reliance on retrospective, non-longitudinal design generally precludes definite inferences regarding abuse effects. It is important to determine which 'effects' are likely to be epiphenomena of sexual abuse (i.e. arising from third variables, including other forms of maltreatment).
- Generalization of findings. The type and extent of CSA reported by subjects often differs significantly from group to group. For example, clinical subjects typically report more frequent molestations by more perpetrators, a longer abuse duration, a greater likelihood of intercourse, and more symptomatology than do non-clinical samples. As a result, findings derived from clinical groups may not generalize well to general population samples or to other individuals with less severe abuse histories.

## Further reading

Briere J. Methodological issues in the study of sexual abuse effects. *Journal of Consulting and Clinical Psychology*, 1992; **60**: 196–203.

Mullen P, Romans-Clarkson SE, Walton VA, Herbison GP. Impact of sexual and physical abuse on women's mental health. *Lancet*, 1988; **i**: 841–5.

Phillips C. Child abuse and disorders of parenting. In: Black D, Cottrell D (eds) *Seminars in Child and Adolescent Psychiatry*. Royal College of Psychiatrists, London: Gaskell, 1993.

Russell DEH. The incidence and prevalence of intrafamilial and extrafamilial sexual abuse of female children. *Child Abuse and Neglect*, 1983; **7**: 133–46.

Wyatt GE, Peters SD. Methodological considerations in research on the prevalence of child sexual abuse. *Child Abuse and Neglect*, 1986; **10**: 241–51.

## Related topic of interest

Psychiatric disorders – life events (p. 246)

# CHRONIC FATIGUE SYNDROME

**Terminology**

This term has been used to describe patients who have disabling mental or physical fatigue (usually both) which has lasted for at least 6 months. Medical investigation will have produced no adequate explanation.

'Chronic fatigue syndrome' is not an ICD-10 category but it is closely related to the syndrome of neurasthenia (F48.0) which is classified under the 'neurotic, stress-related and somatoform disorders'. Other terms which are used to describe this presentation are 'myalgic encephalomyelitis' and 'postviral fatigue syndrome'.

**Symptoms**

These include the following:

- Mental fatigue.
- Physical fatigue with no impairment of muscle function.
- Poor sleep.
- Sore throat.
- Headache.
- Muscle pain.
- Subjective fever.
- Swollen joints.
- Swollen lymph glands.

**Prevalence**

Chronic fatigue is common in primary care, and in the UK approximately 10% of GP attenders will admit to chronic fatigue. It is a smaller number of patients (perhaps 1% of GP attenders) who suffer from chronic disabling fatigue and no diagnosis other than that of an idiopathic chronic fatigue syndrome who are likely to be referred to hospital.

**Aetiology**

The cause is not known but there is usually a combination of physical, psychological and social contributory factors. Prolonged inactivity often aggravates the condition. Research in the topic comes from several medical disciplines, including neurology, psychiatry and virology, and controversy persists about the underlying mechanisms. Much of the relevant research suffers from serious methodological flaws, such as poor case definition or biased selection. An example of the latter would be the study of a population sampled from a highly specialized hospital unit.

Important treatable differential diagnoses include anaemia, asthma, anxiety disorders, cancer, depression, myasthenia gravis and polymyalgia rheumatica.

**Outcome**

There is some evidence that, of patients referred to a general hospital with unexplained fatigue and followed up (median period 1 year) a number of factors are associated with ongoing functional impairment; belief in a viral cause of the illness; limiting exercise; avoiding alcohol; changing or leaving employment; belonging to a self-help organization, and current emotional disorder (Sharpe *et al.,* 1992).

**Treatments**

1. Those based on the assumption of an underlying physical cause have not been successful.

2. There is some limited evidence of the efficacy of antidepressants (both tricyclics and monoamine-oxidase inhibitors) but the evidence is not extensive.

3. Cognitive behavioural therapy has been shown to be useful in a randomized controlled trial (Sharpe *et al.,* 1995). Underlying physical or psychological causes are not pursued but an explanatory model of the aetiology and maintenance of the condition is presented to the patient. This hypothesis states that the patient probably had an acute illness but that the chronic symptoms are due to a behavioural vicious cycle: inactivity during the initial illness leads to lack of fitness and the symptoms of unfitness (tachycardia, tachypnoea, fatigue, etc.) are attributed to ongoing illness. Patients then fail to pursue exercise long enough to become fit again. Further symptoms of demoralization and depression may then occur and exacerbate the whole picture. The therapist works collaboratively with the patient to explore and test this hypothesis. Engagement in treatment is vital, since many patients may naturally resent being sent to a psychiatrist or psychologist with what they believe to be a physical condition. This approach specifically avoids concepts which split psyche and soma, and initial joint consultation with a physician can often be useful in breaking down this division in the patient's mind. Patients are helped gradually to extend their physical and mental activity and are also given supportive psychotherapy and in some cases antidepressant medication.

Education and involvement of the family is often vital to the success of this approach. While the patient may be successful in breaking free from the strictly physical interpretation of the symptoms and disability, family members, friends or peers in self-help groups may have very strongly held views and advise her/him to rest at all costs.

Involvement of family and friends in the treatment plan is usually helpful and in some cases will be vital to its success.

Initial experience shows that the above approach is useful but this is an area where more research will continue to update our knowledge in terms of case definition, natural course and outcome of specific treatment approaches.

## Further reading

Sharpe M. Chronic fatigue syndrome: can the psychiatrist help? In: Hawton K, Cowen P (eds) *Dilemmas and Difficulties in the Management of Psychiatric Patients.* Oxford: Oxford University Press, 1990; 231–40.

Sharpe M, Hawton K, Seagroatt V, Pasvol G. Follow up of patients presenting with fatigue to an infectious diseases clinic. *British Medical Journal*, 1992; **305:** 147–52.

Sharpe M, Hawton K, Simkins S *et al.* Cognitive behaviour therapy for chronic fatigue syndrome: a randomized controlled study. *British Medical Journal*, 1995; in press.

Wessely S, Powell R. Fatigue syndromes: a comparison of chronic 'post-viral' fatigue with neuromuscular and affective disorders. *Journal of Neurology, Neurosurgery and Psychiatry,* 1989; **52:** 940–8.

Wessely S, Sharpe M. Chronic fatigue, chronic fatigue syndrome, and fibromyalgia. In: Mayou R, Bass C, Sharpe M (eds) *Treatment of Functional Somatic Symptoms.* Oxford: Oxford University Press, 1995; 285–312.

## Related topics of interest

Medically unexplained symptoms (p. 180)
Neurosis divisible? (p. 206)
Psychological treatment – cognitive therapy (p. 261)

# CHRONIC PAIN

**Definition**

Pain is defined as:

*An unpleasant sensory and emotional experience associated with actual or potential tissue damage, or described in terms of such damage...*

*... activity induced in the nociceptor and nociceptive pathways by a noxious stimulus is not pain, which is always a psychological state...'*
(International Association for the Study of Pain)

Chronic pain which is not due to an underlying physical diagnosis may relate to a number of psychiatric conditions:

*Persistent somatoform pain disorder (F45.4; ICD-10).* Persistent severe and distressing pain which is not fully explained by a physiological process or physical disorder. Occurs in association with emotional conflict or psychosocial problems which are sufficient to allow the conclusion that they are causally linked. Results in increased support and attention, either personal or medical.

*Behavioural Syndrome (BS; ICD-10).* Psychological and behavioural factors associated with disorders or diseases classified elsewhere. This category should be used to record the presence of psychological or behavioural influences thought to have played a major part in the aetiology of physical disorders such as asthma and ulcerative colitis.

*Depression.* Pain can be a symptom *de novo,* or a pre-existing pain can be perceived as worse during a depressive episode.

*Delusional disorders.*

In the latter two situations the psychiatric condition should be recognized and treated on its own merits. This topic is concerned in the main with pain which falls within the domain covered by PSPD and BS.

**Aetiology**

(a) Findings show increased levels of both present and previous anxiety and depression in patients with chronic pain. The effect of pain on reporting bias makes unequivocal interpretation of these results inappropriate.

(b) There are increasing reports of a history of sexual abuse in patients presenting with chronic pelvic pain and irritable bowel syndrome, although the methodology in these studies does not lead to problem-free interpretation.

(c) The onset of chronic pain may often follow a stressful event.

(d) When a patient presents with chronic pain it is very rarely an 'either or' argument between a physical and a psychogenic cause. Chronic pain is usually multifactorial, and results from a combination of organic, psychiatric, personality and sociocultural factors.

(e) Pain characteristics which increase the likelihood of a contribution from psychological factors include:
- Multiple body sites.
- Increase in area over time.
- Described in emotional terms, for example 'frightful', 'dreadful', 'punishing', 'awful'.
- Not affected by specific movements.
- Does not wake patient from sleep.
- Barely affected by analgesia or transcutaneous electrical nerve stimulation (TENS).
- Over-reaction on examination.
- Weakness of all muscle groups in a body region.
- Superficial tenderness.

(f) Personal and psychiatric history characteristics which increase the likelihood of a contribution from psychological factors include:
- Adoption of adult role early in life.
- History of chronic illness in close relative.
- Past history of conversion symptoms.
- Difficulty in expressing emotions.
- Excessive use of analgesics.
- Repeated requests for surgery.
- Assumption of invalid role.
- 'Doctor shopping'.

**Assessment**

*1. Assessment of pathology.* Initially requires accurate investigation of degree and extent of organic pathology – current and past tissue damage.

*2. Pain history.*

(a) Using a developmental perspective explore past pain, investigations and disability. There may be considerable anxiety or other distress as a result of misinterpretation of previously given information, or as a result of how it was delivered.

(b) Patient's belief about cause of pains. The patient's cognitive interpretation of what the pain means is important, as is the doctor's reaction to the patient's beliefs.

(c) Circumstances at onset of pain.

(d) Description of pain. Adjectives to describe pain fall into categories of sensory (burning, crushing, sore...), emotional (agonizing, dreadful, sickening....) and intensity (weak, intense, severe....).

(e) Intensity, using verbal or visual 10-point scale.

(f) Location of pain.

(g) Temporal pattern.

(h) Precipitating and relieving factors.

(i) Behavioural outcome of pain.

(j) Effect of mood on pain.

(k) Effect of drugs on pain.

*3. Assessment instruments* (see Benjamin and Main, 1995).

(a) McGill Pain Questionnaire. Checklist of 78 words which can be used to describe pain. Intensity of pain corresponds to number of words ticked.

(b) Mood scales; for example, Hospital Anxiety and Depression Scale.

(c) Illness beliefs rating; for example, Whitely Index.

(d) Pain coping questionnaire.

(e) Locus of control.

**Treatment**

- Engaging the patient in treatment is vital as in other somatoform disorders, because the patient will often present with a disagreement with her/his doctors about the cause of the pain. The patient may have a long history of fruitless investigation or unconvincing reassurance. A critical factor in building confidence and rapport can be the physical examination by the pain specialist. A patient is far more likely to accept a reassuring explanation from a doctor who has examined her/him than to accept a secondhand explanation.
- There is evidence for the efficacy of cognitive behavioural treatment of chronic pain and also for biofeedback techniques (Mendelson, 1991).
- It is important to work collaboratively to allow the patient to stop searching for 'the cause'. Rather, the aim is to develop effective strategies in everyday living to minimize the pain or the behavioural consequences of it.
- Antidepressants are often useful, both for an intrinsic analgesic effect (tricyclic at low doses) and in treating underlying or superimposed depression.

- There is an argument for preventative work, and as shown in a recent study where early intervention using behavioural techniques in acute musculoskeletal pain led to a better outcome (Benjamin and Main, 1995).

## Further reading

Benjamin S, Main CJ. Psychiatric and psychological approaches to the treatment of chronic pain: concepts and individual treatments. In: Mayon R, Bass C, Sharpe M. (eds) *Treatment of Funcational Somatic Symptoms*. Oxford: Oxford University Press, 1995.

Mendelson G. Psychological and social factors predicting responses to pain treatment. In: Bond MR, Charlton JE, Woolf CJ. (eds) *Proceedings of the VIth World Congress on Pain*. Amsterdam: Elsevier, 1991.

Romano JM, Good AB. Recent advances in chronic pain. *Current Opinion in Psychiatry,* 1994; **7:** 494–7.

Tyrer S. Psychiatric assessment of chronic pain. *British Journal of Psychiatry,* 1990; **160:** 733–41.

## Related topics of interest

Illness behaviour and associated concepts (p. 162)
Medically unexplained symptoms (p. 180)

# COGNITIVE FUNCTION – ASSESSMENT

This may be appropriate in a variety of clinical situations:

- As part of the assessment of a person with a dementing illness, both in diagnosis and in follow-up as the disease develops.
- In a patient with brain injury which may be traumatic, secondary to cerebrovascular disease or following surgery.
- In a patient with learning disability.
- For child development assessment.

**Clinical interview**

Cognitive function assessment should be a routine part of all mental state examinations, but is of particular importance in the above situations.

Subjective memory problems should be enquired after and then permission gained for testing of the patient's memory:

- Orientation:
  Time, date and place.
- Information registration and short-term memory:
  Name and address registration and recall at 5 minutes.
- Immediate memory:
  Increasing strings of numbers forwards and backwards.
- Recent memory:
  Recent events, for example, admission to hospital.
- Attention and concentration:
  Serial sevens, months of the year forwards and backwards, also judged on general behaviour during the interview.
- General knowledge:
  Prime minister, what is in the news.

Detailed contemporaneous recording of these tests in the patient's notes provides important information for later comparison. This type of test is formalized in the Mini Mental State Examination of Folstein *et al.* (1975), which also includes assessment of parietal function.

Effective clinical examination of an elderly person depends in large part on technique. A cognitively impaired person can have a catastrophic reaction to persistent and insensitive questioning, and a gentle even 'meandering' approach can yield better results. Performance may vary greatly from day to day and with time of day, so repeated assessment is often informative. Environment is also crucial and, whenever possible, the assessment is best carried out in the patient's own home. Information from family, care workers and other members of the multidisciplinary team should be elicited. These will allow the results of formal testing to be set in context and thus improve the meaningfulness of the overall assessment.

**Specialized tests**

*1. Intelligence tests.* These are usually designed to indicate the ability of the subject in relation to the rest of the population from which he/she is drawn. They can be powerfully affected by situation and culture, and care should always be taken in administration and interpretation of the test. Misuse of IQ tests has been said to underlie apparent racial differences in IQ in the USA. Results can also be affected by motivation, anxiety or hostility towards testing. They are by necessity limited and may miss an aspect of a patient's overall functioning which adds to or detracts from their everyday ability. Risks and dangers of testing in children include using purpose- or age-inappropriate tests, unsatisfactory conditions, over-generalization of conclusions and labelling as a result of the tests. The tests most commonly used in the UK are detailed below, for children and adults.

*2. Children.*
(a) Wechsler Pre-school and Primary School Intelligence Scale. Applicable between ages 4 and $6^1/_2$ years. Verbal, non-verbal and combined scores.
(b) Wechsler Intelligence Scale for Children. Ages 6–14 years. Verbal and non-verbal scales. Overall score computed so that mean is 100 with standard deviation of 15. Often used in definitions of mental retardation.
(c) Stanford–Binet Intelligence Scale. Aged 2 years to adulthood. Assesses verbal reasoning, abstract/visual reasoning, quantitive reasoning and short-term memory. Intelligence quotient by comparison with normative data.
(d) Others include the British Ability Scale and Goodenough–Harris 'draw a man' test, in which one child's picture of a man in compared against standardized criteria for age.
(e) There are also tests of educational attainment including the Word reading Subtest of the British Ability Scale, Neale Analysis of Reading Ability, Schonell Graded Word Spelling Test and the Wide Range Achievement Test.

3. *Adult.*
(a)   Wechsler Adult Intelligence Scale (WAIS). Has 11 subtests, six dealing with words or numbers to give verbal IQ and five with spatial patterns to give performance IQ.
(b)   Mill Hill Vocabulary Test and Raven's Progressive Matrices (MHV–RPM). These are respectively a vocabulary test involving recall and recognition and a diagram-completion test.
(c)   National Adult Reading Test (NART). Subjects are required to read a list of words which have variations from the usual rules of pronunciation and are therefore difficult to read correctly when unfamiliar (e.g. ache, aisle, campanile, drachm, syncope). This is taken to represent 'premorbid' IQ and often used in the assessment of patients with dementia.
Further details of assessment in dementia are given in Dementia – assessment (p. 89).

Tasks involving mental speed begin to be performed less well after the age of 25, but many other cognitive functions show no real decline until 60 and the changes in non-dementing persons are not great. There is no evidence that affective mental illness has any permanent effect on IQ, although chronic schizophrenia may do so.

# Further reading

Folstein ME, Folstein SE, McHugh PR. 'Mini-Mental State': a practical method for grading the cognitive state of patients for the clinician. *Journal of Psychiatric Research*, 1975; **12:** 189–98.

Graham P. Assessment. In: *Child Psychiatry – a developmental approach*, 2nd Edn. Oxford: Oxford University Press, 1991; 2–9.

# Related topics of interest

# CULTURE AND PSYCHIATRY

Culture represents aspects of a society characterized by its customs, beliefs and norms of behaviour. Culture-bound disorders are those which are only found in particular cultures.

Certain psychiatric disorders are found in all cultures at a similar frequency, although the context can affect the presentation and outcome. However, some disorders only occur in certain settings, and even these may not be seen as illness in those cultures. The transition from one culture to another can increase the incidence of certain disorders, and complicate treatment.

**Presentation**

Aspects of culture which affect presentation include:

- Beliefs: for example, religious beliefs, beliefs in witchcraft, political context, family structure. An understanding of the cultural context can help explain the content of delusional ideas, and even clarify whether the beliefs are delusional. In China, food represents family attention but thinness does not carry the same social desirability. This may be related to the observation that those with anorexia nervosa tend to lose weight without having distorted body image.
- Language: this especially applies to emotion, for example in Eastern cultures, there are few words for, low mood and so this tends to be expressed in terms of somatic symptoms.

**Frequency and outcome**

Several major studies have found that:

- The incidence of major psychiatric disorders (schizophrenia, affective psychoses) are similar in a wide range of countries.
- The instruments used can affect the measurements, which raises the issue of the appropriateness of instruments developed in one culture or language.
- There are differences in outcome, which may be true effects or artefacts of the method of measurement.
- The US–UK study found that the definition of schizophrenia was broader in the US than the UK, and that it included mania, depressive illness, neurotic and personality disorders.
- The International Pilot Study of Schizophrenia (IPSS) was carried out in nine countries. The study compared the clinical diagnosis of schizophrenia with the diagnosis from the Present State Examination (PSE) and Catego programme. The investigators concluded that these were in broad agreement except in the US and Russia. It also

looked at outcome and found that this was better in developing countries, an observation that has also been seen in other studies (for example 59% had a good outcome (i.e. full recovery) after 12 years in Mauritius).

**Culture-bound syndromes**

*1. Koro.* This is an anxiety state found in S.E. Asia. The principal symptom is the belief that the penis is disappearing into the abdomen and that this will be fatal (cultural belief). There are associated anxiety symptoms and it often occurs in epidemics. In non-Chinese people it is often associated with other psychiatric disorders rather than occurring in isolation.

*2. Windigo (Wihtigo).* This is a depressive reaction found in North American Indians. Cultural antecedents include: cold winters lead to possibility of starvation; cultural taboos against cannibalism; belief in the wihtigo, a cannibalistic ice spirit. The syndrome starts with an aversion to normal foods, nausea and vomiting. These are followed by anxiety symptoms and the belief that the individual has been possessed by the wihtigo. If they cannot be healed by the community, then they ask to be killed (and used to be).

*3. Amok.* This is a dissociative state seen in the Philippines and Malaysia. A male villager receives a real or imagined slight. He leaves the village then returns to kill every living thing he encounters, and stops only when killed or captured. He is not held responsible or punished. If admitted to hospital, individuals often have other major psychiatric disorders. (Berserker is a similar entity.)

*4. Latah.* This is a form of hysteria, usually seen in females in Malaysia (but part of a group of startle reactions found in a variety of cultures). Latah antu (spirit) enters the body leading to a hyperstartle response to unexpected gestures or contact, especially tickling. This response includes imitative behaviour, coprolalia and automatic obedience to commands. It is often culturally accepted as non-psychiatric behaviour.

*5. Anorexia nervosa/bulimia.* These are commonest in developed countries. The presentation varies, for example, absence of distorted body image in cultures where thinness is less desired.

*6. Frigophobia.* An obsessive-compulsive neurosis characterized by a fear of cold, and loss of vitality, with compulsive wearing of multiple layers of clothing.

7. *Possession states.* These are not generally seen as illness in indigenous culture, and are transient. Sufferers believe they are possessed by a spirit leading to overactivity and voice changes. A ritual can be used to induce them. It can be important to consider possession states in the differential diagnosis of psychoses (e.g. with delusions of control).

8. *Dhat.* An anxiety state in Hindus characterized by fear of loss of semen with associated somatic and psychological symptoms.

9. *Voodoo.* This is a phobic neurosis, particularly in Haiti. Violation of the taboo may be fatal.

10. *Evil eye.* Another phobic neurosis, seen in Mexico and North Africa. Strong glances are harmful, so individuals take precautions to avoid or counteract evil eye.

11. *Acute transient psychosis.* This is more common in Africans and Afro-Caribbeans, and its nature is under debate.

**Effects of migration**

The key issues are whether there are different rates of psychiatric morbidity in immigrants, and, if so, whether these are due to constitutional differences, to selective migration, to the stress of migration or initial adaptation, or to the stresses of living in a foreign culture and associated social factors.

Particular groups that have been studied include Norwegians in USA and Afro-Caribbeans and Asians in the UK. General conclusions are that the incidence of psychiatric disorders as a group are not increased (general practice and general population studies), but that the incidence of schizophrenia and the affective psychoses are (although this varies in different cultural groups). Likely mechanisms include selective migration and longer-term effects of living in a different culture interacting with specific disorders, but complicating factors are differences in presentation and social factors associated with migration such as poverty and unemployment.

**Treatment issues**

- Specific cultural treatments may be appropriate, for example, faith healers, medicine man, which are based on cultural beliefs.
- Drugs: Asians appear to have increased sensitivity to drugs, and conversely, Afro-Caribbeans are often given larger doses.

- Psychotherapy: there are cultural issues of access to and the appropriateness of psychotherapy which is offered in one culture to those from another.
- Mental Health Act: this is used more often, for example, in Afro-Caribbeans, but this is not entirely accounted for by the increase in cases of schizophrenia.
- Services: consider access, acceptability, liaison with community and language.

## Further reading

Leff J. *Psychiatry Around the Globe*. London: Gaskell, 1981.

Lipsedge M. Cultural influences on psychiatry. *Current Opinion in Psychiatry*, 1993; **6:** 274–9.

Moodley P. Transcultural psychiatry. In: Appleby L and Forshaw D (eds). *Postgraduate Psychiatry*, 1st Edn, Oxford: Heinemann, 1990; 414–22.

## Related topics of interest

# DANGEROUSNESS ASSESSMENT

As with the assessment of suicidal risk, it is useful to know the demographic and psychiatric variables which contribute to dangerous behaviour, and careful history taking is vital. As a fundamental principle, all patients should be assumed to have the potential to be dangerous, particularly if they are not known to the psychiatrist. It is important to see patients in a room which is within earshot of other staff, and which preferably has a panic button. Ideally, a room should be arranged so that the doctor is sitting nearer to the door than the patient, in case a quick exit is needed (see Violent patients, p. 353).

**Categories of mental disorder associated with dangerousness**

*1. Organic brain impairment.* Organic mental disorder may lead to violent behaviour, either through general disinhibition and loss of control, or through the production of psychotic states (e.g. delusional misidentifications). Epilepsy, particularly of the temporal lobes, brain infections such as meningitis or encephalitis, focal brain damage (especially to the prefrontal and frontal cortex) and more general medical illness indirectly affecting brain function (e.g. hypoxia, hepatic encephalopathy), may all lead to violent behaviour (often of an unpredictable nature).

*2. Intoxication and withdrawal states.* Alcohol has a dose-related effect on human aggression, and any person intoxicated with alcohol should be regarded as at increased risk of impulsive violence. Short-acting barbiturates may have a similar effect. Certain other drugs, such as PCP (phencyclidine), amphetamine and cocaine (particularly in the form of 'crack'), have been associated with serious and unpredictable violence (Sudbury and Ghodse, 1991). Users of anabolic steroids may experience 'steroid rage' in which otherwise stable characters may become extremely violent with minimal provocation (Pope and Katz, 1990). Amphetamines and anabolic steroids may also cause a psychosis-like picture which can result in violent behaviour.

Withdrawal states from many substances (e.g. alcohol, benzodiazepines) may cause irritability or severe craving (e.g. cocaine) which can lead to impulsive or desperate behaviour.

*3. Psychosis.* Psychotic illness may be associated with violence, which may be bizarre. In people with schizophrenia, two groups can be identified. The first is those with hallucinations (sometimes command hallucinations) or paranoid delusions. The violent or dangerous acts committed by these psychotic patients are because paranoid and confused patients believe that they are about to be attacked, and act in what they see as self-defence. The second group is the longer-term patients in whom violence results from psychotic disorganization or general excitability. Akathisia as a result of neuroleptic treatment may also cause restlessness and lead to violence.

Manic patients may become extremely violent with little warning. This is particularly so early in treatment, when limit-setting is first attempted.

*4. Morbid jealousy.* Morbid jealousy has a number of different causes, and is associated with violence against the person to whom the jealousy is directed, or others associated with that person (Shepherd, 1961). It is an important cause of domestic homicide.

*5. Personality disorder.* Individuals with sociopathic personality disorder commit acts of violence which are repeated, often serious, and for which they characteristically feel no remorse, and which are part of a spectrum of antisocial behaviours. Those with borderline personality disorder show repeated acts of aggression against self and others as part of a range of poorly controlled unstable behaviours. Explosive personality disorder is characterized by uncontrollable outbursts of rage, often with subsequent remorse. Individuals with anankastic personality disorder can occasionally become severely violent when their rituals or habits are challenged. Psychotic patients with concurrent personality disorder are at increased risk of disturbed behaviour of all types.

Personality problems, particularly low self-esteem, sexual problems, and often financial and other social conflicts, are characteristic of individuals showing repeated non-psychotic violence, usually towards family members, particularly the spouse, but sometimes a child.

**General demographic variables**

The majority of violent acts are committed by young men between the ages of 14 and 24, but violent or dangerous acts can be committed by people of any age or sex. In long-term hospital patients, violence is equally common in men and women. There are no racial differences in the level of violence among psychiatric patients (Tardiff, 1992).

**History and mental state**

In the history, it should be remembered that the best predictor of future behaviour is past behaviour, and that past acts of dangerousness or aggression are the surest sign of further dangerousness. The patient may be asked directly whether they have ever considered harming someone, and what stopped them from doing so. A childhood history of severe emotional neglect, physical abuse, and conduct disorder during childhood and adolescence may support a diagnosis of sociopathic or dissocial personality disorder. The triad of bedwetting, firesetting and cruelty to animals is said to have predictive value with regard to later repeated violence against humans (Felthous and Kellet, 1987). Specific enquiry should be made about use of illicit drugs (including anabolic steroids) or alcohol, and subsequent behaviours. Other impulsive behaviours, such as self-harm, gambling, etc., should be enquired after.

In the mental state, suspicion or paranoia should be noted, and hallucinations or delusions relating to threats to the self from others should be asked about.

**Management of dangerous patients**

The acute management of violent patients is dealt with elsewhere (see Violent patients p. 353). The management of dangerousness involves the use of appropriate containment coupled with treatment of the underlying conditions contributing to it. Where risk to others is felt to be a serious concern, a forensic opinion should always be sought with regard to the appropriateness of referral to special hospital or medium secure unit. Short-term containment on a locked ward, or continuous/regular observation, should be considered. If a patient considered to be a danger to others absconds, or their whereabouts is unknown, the police should be informed, as should anyone thought to be particularly at risk.

## Further reading

Felthous AR, Kellet JR. Childhood cruelty to animals and later aggression against people. A review. *American Journal of Psychiatry,* 1987; **144:** 710–17.

Pope HG, Katz DL. Homicide and near homicide by anabolic steroid users. *Journal of American Psychiatry,* 1990; **51:** 28–31.

Shepherd M. Morbid jealousy: some clinical and social aspects of a psychiatric symptom. *Journal of Mental Science,* 1961; **107:** 687–705.

Sudbury PR, Ghodse AH. Substance misuse and antisocial behaviour. *Current Opinion in Psychiatry,* 1991; **4:** 440–7.

Tardiff K. The current state of psychiatry in the treatment of violent patients. *Archives of General Psychiatry,* 1992; **49:** 493-9.

## Related topics of interest

# DEFENCE MECHANISMS

*The conceptualisation of the ego mechanisms of defense*(sic) *remains one of the most valuable contributions that psychoanalysis has made to medicine* (George Vaillant, 1971)

Defence mechanisms and coping styles are habitual, unconscious and, sometimes, pathological mental processes employed to avoid the psychic pain or conflicts between instinctual needs, internalized prohibitions and external reality.

**Purposes of defence mechanisms**

(a) To keep affects within bearable limits during sudden alterations in emotional life (e.g. object loss).

(b) To restore psychological equilibrium by postponing or deflecting sudden increases in biological drives (e.g. sexual awareness) ('instinctual anxiety').

(c) To gain 'breathing space' to integrate changes in self-image (e.g. puberty, disfigurement, illness).

(d) To handle unresolvable internal conflicts with important people (dead or alive), or their representations as objects in the internal psychic world from which one cannot part ('object anxiety'). Whilst defence mech-anisms may be useful, they may, by preventing the experience of psychic pain, actually obstruct the resolution of conflicts.

(e) To defend against the internal psychic conflict resulting from instinctual (Id) feelings towards others.

**Mechanisms of action**

The use of defence mechanisms serves to alter perception, cognition, etc., in a way which may be more or less adaptive or maladaptive. They may achieve this in a variety of ways:

• Action, often towards others, which serves to release feelings or impulses (*action* defences).

• Distortion of self and object images to conform with subjective emotional state or desired meaning (*borderline* defences).

• Disavowal of undesired aspects of self (*disavowal* defences).

• Regulation of self-esteem or mood by focusing on under- or overvalued aspects of experience (*narcissistic* defences).

• Neutralization of affects without distortion of reality (*obsessional* defences).

• Open acknowledgement of affect, and constructive adaptation thereto (*mature* defences).

All defences can be used in adaptive 'coping' ways, which aid accommodation with reality, or maladaptive 'defensive' ways, which seem to obstruct rather than facilitate this change.

**Natural history of defence styles**

Long-term studies in adults show that defence styles are remarkably stable over time (Vaillant *et al.*, 1986), but this is not to say that they are fixed. There is a natural process of maturation of defences with age and psychological development. Defences such as denial, which are normal responses to stress in small children, are replaced by more sophisticated defences such as repression or dissociation in older children, and by sublimation in adults. Similar shifts in defence style may occur during recovery from psychological disorder. Although the most rapid changes occur during childhood and adolescence, defences continue to mature in later years.

**Individual defences**

Following Vaillant's (1971) classification, these can be grouped into four categories: narcissistic (image-distorting), immature, neurotic and mature. Brief descriptions of some of the commoner ones follow.

*1. Narcissistic/borderline (or image-distorting).* Common in healthy individuals before 5 years of age, and in dreams and fantasy of adults.
(a) *Delusional projection.* Perception of one's own feelings in another person, and acting on the perception.
(b) *Projective identification.* The projection of unconscious material on to another person, who then unconsciously identifies with and acts as that material.
(c) *Psychotic denial.* Denial of external reality, including use of fantasy as substitute for other people.
(d) *Distortion.* Gross reshaping of external reality to suit inner needs.
(e) *Splitting (of self or others).* Perception of complex or contradictory elements of self or others as separate, avoiding ambivalence or conflict.

*2. Immature defences.* Common in healthy individuals of 3–16 years, and also personality disorders, affective disorders and adults in psychotherapy.
(a) *Projection.* Attributing one's own unconscious feelings to others.
(b) *Schizoid fantasy.* Use of fantasy and autistic retreat to resolve conflict or gratify unmet needs for intimacy.

(c) *Hypochondriasis.* Transformation of anger or reproach towards others into self-reproach and then complaints of pain, illness or neurasthenia. Introjection of aspects of others, often of their illness symptoms, is part of this defence mechanism.

(d) *Passive aggression.* Aggression towards others expressed via actions which often seem to harm the individual more, such as passivity, masochism and self-reproach.

(e) *Acting out.* Direct expression of wishes via impulsive actions in order to avoid being conscious of accompanying affect, and to avoid or release tension.

*3. Neurotic defences.* Common in healthy individuals from childhood onward in mastering acute stress and neurotic disorders.

(a) *Intellectualization* (includes isolation, rationalization, undoing, magical thinking). Thinking about (not acting on) desires in formal, affectless ways.

(b) *Repression.* Unconscious inhibition of wishes or desires, resulting in their temporary or permanent loss.

(c) *Displacement.* Redirection of feelings from significant to less emotionally significant people or circumstances, for example, practical jokes, 'kicking the cat', 'hostile' wit, caricature, most phobias.

(d) *Reaction formation* (includes identification with the aggressor, altruistic surrender). Replacement of unacceptable desires or actions with their opposites; for example, extreme prudishness as a response to sexual desires.

(e) *Dissociation* (neurotic denial). Temporary change of character or sense of personal identity to avoid emotional distress; for example, 'dissociation hysteria', short-term use of intoxicants.

*4. Mature defences.* Common in healthy individuals from adolescence onwards. Integrated uses of other defences in a reality-seeking way may reflect the increasingly complex cognitive integration of adolescence. Includes some behaviours which are consciously deployed, but this deployment is reflex, as with other defences.

(a) *Altruism* (includes constructive reaction formation, philanthropy). Partial gratification through genuine service to others.

(b) *Humour.* Overt expression of feeling, directly acknowledging painful or difficult emotions, including other people, without causing them or oneself discomfort.

(c) *Suppression.* Conscious or semiconscious postponement of attending to a conscious impulse or conflict. 'Looking on the bright side', the 'stiff upper lip' and postponement without avoiding the issue are all examples.

(d) *Anticipation.* Anticipation or planning for future inner discomfort, before it becomes necessary to face it.

(e) *Sublimation.* A rechannelling of instincts into productive endeavour, allowing the instincts to be to an extent satisfied.

**Significance of defence styles**

The major significance of defence styles is their association with both physical and psychological health and illness. It is a general finding that the persistent use in adulthood of immature, narcissistic or borderline types of defence is associated with poorer long-term psychological health, interpersonal functioning and social success. Use of neurotic defences is uncorrelated with psychosocial functioning, with the exception of the obsessional defences, isolation, intellectualization and undoing, which seem to be positively correlated with higher psychosocial functioning in psychiatric patients, but whose importance is overshadowed by mature defences in normal samples. Whilst the direction of causality is impossible to determine, Vaillant's (1971) study indicated that the association of mature defence styles with positive psychosocial outcomes was strongest for those with the worst family backgrounds, suggesting that they might be protective.

Even more interesting is the growing body of literature reporting associations of coping style with long-term physical health, and adaptation to illness. It is interesting to note that denial has been shown to be an adaptive mechanism, at least in cancer patients, where it is correlated with length of survival, better self image and less mood and sleep disturbance (Fricchione *et al.*, 1992) and in patients with end-stage renal disease, but not in rheumatoid arthritis, where denial of emotional significance correlates with worse outcome (McFarlane *et al.*, 1987).

# Further reading

Fricchione GL, Howanitz E, Jandorf L, Kroessler D, Iannis Z, Wojnicki RM. Psychological adjustment to end-stage renal disease and the implications of denial. *Psychosomatics,* 1992; **33:** 85–91.

McFarlane AC, Kalucy RS, Brooks PM. Psychological predictors of disease course in rheumaoid arthritis. *Journal of Psychosomatic Research,* 1987; **31:** 757–64.

Vaillant GE. Theoretical hierarchy of adaptive ego mechanisms: a 30-year follow-up of 30 men selected for psychological health. *Archives of General Psychiatry,* 1971; **33:** 766–70.

Vaillant GE, Bond M, Vaillant CO. An empirically validated hierarchy of defense (*sic*) mechanisms. *Archives of General Psychiatry,* 1986; **43:** 786–94.

# Related topic of interest

Psychological treatment – general principles (p. 270)

# DELINQUENCY AND ANTISOCIAL PERSONALITY

Delinquency is a legal term used when a young person commits a criminal offence. It is the behavioural expression of multiple factors, both within the individual and society. A degree of 'delinquent' behaviour for example experimental drug taking, vandalism, arson, and fire-setting, as well as minor breaches of the peace, is so common as to be regarded as a normal part of adolescence, and 80% of adolescents self-report having committed an indictable offence. Persistent delinquent behaviour is indicative of an abnormal process of development, and it should be examined in terms of both antecedent and subsequent life course.

**What are the childhood antecedents of delinquency?**

*1. Difficult children.* The New York study of Chess and Thomas identified a group of children, about 5% of the total, whom they classified as 'difficult'. Their characteristics were:

- Withdrawal from novelty.
- Irregular rhythmicity.
- Slow to warm up.
- Emotional intensity.
- Predominantly negative affect.

The biological basis of this behaviour pattern probably relates to a low threshold for limbic stimulation and a decrease in inhibitory centres of the CNS (Sperry, 1995).

There is a two-way interaction between parents and children, therefore difficult children, by taxing their parents more, create an environment for themselves which may further reinforce their difficult behaviour.

'Externalizing' behaviour at age 3 predicts behavioural problems at 5, which in turn predicts 'uncontrolled' behaviour at 11 and antisocial personality traits by age 13 (Robins, 1991).

*2. Conduct disorder.* Defined as persistent antisocial, aggressive and defiant conduct, or socially disapproved of behaviour, often involving damage to property, and lack of response to normal sanctions. Two thirds of children with conduct disorder have problems which persist into adulthood. There is a marked male predominance (3:1), and prevalence in the Isle of Wight study (Rutter *et al.*, 1976) was 4%.

*Socialized* conduct disorder occurs in individuals who are generally well integrated into their peer group, but whose moves are against those of society.

*Unsocialized* conduct disorder is a solitary activity, often occurring against a background of parental neglect and poor social relations with peers. Emotional problems are common.

There are four contributory factors to conduct disorder, of which the first is the most important:

- *Family*. Often large, characterized by lack of affection, rejection, marital disharmony (including divorce and separation), ineffective or inconsistent discipline, and parental violence and aggression. Children are at high risk of conduct disorder if either parent, but particularly the mother, has a history of criminality or alcoholism.
- *Peer group*. Oppositional attitudes (especially in older children and adolescents).
- *Neighbourhood.* Urban deprivation, poor schooling.
- *Constitutional.* Low intelligence, learning difficulties, overactivity, impulsiveness.

These factors clearly interact within and across generations; for example, inherited temperamental traits of overactivity and impulsiveness in parents, which impair their parenting ability, are also inherited by their children, who are thus constitutionally more difficult to care for. The family environment outlined above is conducive to the formation of anxious avoidant attachments, which are associated with persistent delinquency in later life (Bowlby, 1988). Attachment patterns that are formed in the first year of life are usually stable over time, and become increasingly a core feature of the individual rather than environmentally determined by his or her interactions with others during the first few years of life.

**Does delinquency in adolescence predict adult criminality?**

The available evidence strongly suggests that delinquency in childhood and adolescence predisposes to adult antisocial behaviour. The stability of aggression through development rivals that of IQ (i.e. it is very stable). Follow-up studies have shown that children with extremes of temperament at the age of 11 are at increased risk of adult criminality, and that temperamental traits predict a variety of areas of social adjustment (Sigvardsson *et al.*, 1987), with 15% of the variance in adult outcome being explained by childhood temperament. Studies of aggressive adolescents show that they exhibit abnormalities in a number of domains of personality function, considered from the viewpoint of various different theoretical approaches (Davis and Boster, 1992).

*1. Social-environmental and behavioural.*

- *Family background* as described above: Parents are neglectful, erratic and harsh in punishment; child uses aggression as an escape from or avoidance of unwanted family intrusions.
- *Family stressors* such as substance abuse, poverty, divorce and domestic violence.
- *Family modelling* of aggression as a means to control others.
- *Rejection by peer group* because of aggression, leads to isolation or deviant group membership.

*2. Cognitive.* IQ tends to be lower than average, particularly in cases of earlier onset.

- Abnormalities in appraisal of the environment, in which neutral situations are viewed as hostile, and the self-image is as a person to be feared.
- Abnormal expectations of outcomes of specific behaviour, with positive expectancies of aggression as a problem-solving behaviour.
- Restricted patterns of fantasy and imagination. There is a focus on violent outcomes in fantasy life. Unable to anticipate negative consequences of aggression.
- Deficit in positive empathy towards others.
- Concrete operational style of information processing, with little generation of alternative courses of action and constricted range of problem-solving, no use of abstract reasoning.
- Little ability to learn from aversive situations.

*3. Affective.*

- High level of cognitive arousal.
- Restricted range of emotional expression.
- Concrete and dichotomous (black-or-white) perceptions of own emotions.
- Difficulty modulating affective expression.
- Often dysphoric.
- Either undercontrolled or overcontrolled in expression of anger.

- Possibly, a mixture of aggression and shyness or rejection by peers has predictive value (Robins, 1991).

**Antisocial personality and other adult outcomes**

The adult form of delinquency is antisocial personality disorder (ASP), and many of the criteria used in its diagnosis are the same as those for conduct disorder. Data from the Epidemiological Catchment Area (ECA) study strongly suggest that conduct disorder is predictive of later antisocial personality. The more severe the conduct disorder, and the earlier it presents, the more likely is an eventual diagnosis of ASP (Robins, 1991). Nevertheless, the majority with conduct disorder do not progress to ASP, but the time course or mechanism of recovery is not known.

History of conduct disorder before 15 years gives a poor prognosis for both psychological and social well-being. There is a strong association with later substance abuse, and with high rates of psychiatric morbidity, as measured by the General Health Questionnaire (GHQ) and Present State Examination (PSE). There are also increased rates of mania, schizophrenia, obsessive-compulsive disorder and hypochondriasis. Socially, marital breakup, poor work history, and even death by violence are associated with a childhood history of aggression (Robins, 1991).

**Interventions and treatment**

Little is certain regarding the treatment of delinquency or conduct disorder. Attachment behaviour in children can be altered in early life by a change in parenting style, and interventions aimed at teaching better parenting skills may reduce the anxious avoidant attachments which are predictive of later delinquency (Bowlby, 1988). Attendance at nursery school, where attention can be given to encouraging patterns of behaviour based on concern for others, and exposure to conforming peer groups achieved, can be effective. Delinquent adolescents may respond to interventions aimed at the cognitive and affective deficits discussed above (Davis and Boster, 1992). There is increasing optimism that multiple interventions in pharmacological, behavioural, cognitive, interpersonal and dynamic modalities may help some people with ASP, particularly those with a concurrent Axis 1 syndrome (Sperry, 1995).

# Further reading

Bowlby J. Developmental psychiatry comes of age. *American Journal of Psychiatry*, 1988; **145:** 1–10.

Davis DL, Boster LH. Cognitive-behavioural-expressive interventions with aggressive and resistant youths. *Child Welfare*; 1992; **6:** 557–73.

Robins LN. Conduct disorder. *Journal of Child Psychological Psychiatry,* 1991; **32**(1) 193–212.

Rutter M, Tizard J, Yule W, Graham P, Whitmore K. Isle of Wight Studies 1964–1974. *Psychological Medicine*, 1976, **6:** 313–32.

Sigvardsson S, Bohman M, Cloninger CR. Structure and stability of childhood personality: prediction of later social adjustment. *Journal of Child Psychological Psychiatry,* 1987; **28**(6): 929–46.

Sperry L. In: *Handbook of diagnosis and treatment of the DSM–IV personality disorders.* New York: Brunner-Mazel, 1995; Chapter 2, 15–34.

# Related topics of interest

# DELUSIONAL DISORDERS

A *delusion* is defined as an abnormal belief held with utter conviction against contrary evidence, and not consistent with the person's social or cultural background. The term *paranoia* has two slightly different meanings. Colloquially, and in the way it is normally used by psychiatrists, it means persecutory. However, as a technical term, it may be broadened to include all self-referential ideas or thoughts.

Delusional disorders are those in which the presenting symptom is one or more fixed delusions, with other symptoms characteristic of schizophrenia being either absent or of very minor significance. DSM-IV has five criteria:

- Non-bizarre delusions (i.e. those relating to things which can happen in real life) lasting for at least 1 month.
- The characteristic symptoms for schizophrenia have never been present.
- No marked impairment of functioning or behaviour, except in areas of life directly impacted by the delusions.
- Any disturbance of mood must be brief compared to the duration of the delusions.
- No organic cause.

**Aetiology and incidence**

Delusional disorder is uncommon, accounting for 1–2% of in-patient admissions. The population prevalence is probably around 0.03% and lifetime morbidity up to 0.1%. Predisposing factors are:

*1. Age.* These disorders are much more common in middle-aged or older patients.

*2. Immigrant status.*

*3. Being a member of a minority group.*

*4. Deafness.* Characteristically long-standing severe bilateral deafness; this is probably because it produces social isolation.

*5. Paranoid or sensitive premorbid personality traits.*

*6. Marital status.* Single, divorced or widowed – the first two factors are probably secondary to the personality type described above, which is not conducive to stable long-term relationships.

**Diagnostic subtypes**

DSM-IV has seven categories:

*1. Erotomanic type.* This is a delusional belief that another person is in love with the individual. The person is characteristically of higher status and may or may not be personally known to, or acquainted with, the patient. Patients in this category are probably more often female. They may be very persistent in their pursuit of the object of their desires, and can on occasions resort to violence in response to a perceived threat to the other, or against those they believe to be preventing the other from declaring their love (e.g. spouses).

2. *Grandiose type.* This is characterized by delusions of inflated worth, power, knowledge, identity, or relationships with special or exalted people.

3. *Jealous type.* Morbid jealousy may have many causes, including mood disorder, substance misuse (particularly alcohol) or as part of a more general psychotic illness. It is probably more common in men. Whatever the aetiology, it is characterized by obsessive searching for evidence of a partner's infidelity. Personal possessions and clothing may be searched for notes or letters, underwear examined for signs of sexual activity, and sometimes private detectives hired to follow the partner. Morbid jealousy is a serious condition, particularly because it may be associated with violence towards the partner or even murder.

4. *Persecutory type.* Here the delusions are paranoid in the colloquial sense, in that the person believes they are being malevolently treated. These delusions may be 'encapsulated', and the person, being suspicious of others, may not mention them unless they are directly touched upon in an interview.

5. *Somatic type.* Delusions relating to physical defectiveness or the presence of organic disease. Clearly these types of delusional disorder border on hypochondriasis, on the one hand, and also conditions such as anorexia nervosa, which may both contain beliefs of an almost delusional intensity. This category would include the monosymptomatic hypochondriacal psychosis described by Munroe (1980). The belief that one's viscera have rotted away (Cotard's syndrome) would not be included in this category, because the delusion is bizarre (see below).

6. *Mixed type.* These are delusions from more than one of the above categories.

7. *Unspecified type.*

**Other paranoid psychosis**

*1. Cotard's syndrome.* This is characterized by florid nihilistic delusions involving the patient having lost everything, including the insides of their body. The patient may repeatedly express the view that his/her bowels are rotting or missing.

*2. Capgras syndrome (illusion of doubles, or illusion de soises).* This is more common in women than men. The patient believes that someone, usually a close friend or relative, has been replaced by a double who is an exact replica. This syndrome is of interest only because it is eponymous, and in fact it is only found as a symptom of another illness, usually schizophrenia.

*3. Induced delusional disorder* (folie à deux). This describes the situation in which a second person comes to believe in, and cooperate with, the delusional system of someone with a paranoid illness. The second sufferer (who is not psychotic) is usually living in close proximity with the proband, and is often relatively isolated. Treatment is said to be geographical: separation works very well.

**Treatment and prognosis**

These illnesses are often persistent and difficult to treat. Antipsychotic medication is the treatment of choice, and will usually have the effect of reducing the intensity of the delusions, although these often remain within the patient's mind but at an intensity which is tolerable and does not interfere with their lives or the lives of others around them.

# Further reading

Enoch MD, Trethowan WH. *Uncommon Psychiatric Syndromes.* 3rd Edn, Oxford: Butterworth Heinemann, 1991.
Munroe A. Monosymptomatic hypochondriacal psychosis. *British Journal of Hospital Medicine*, 1980; **24:** 34–8.

# Related topics of interest

# DEMENTIA – ASSESSMENT

**Definition**

*Global deterioration of intellectual function in a clear consciousness*

The function of assessment in a patient presenting with this condition is fourfold:

- To establish the diagnosis. Dementia must be distinguished from aphasia, amnesia, delirium and mental retardation.
- To identify treatable causes or exacerbating factors.
- To make predictions about the course of the illness.
- To plan care and services which will be necessary for the patient and his/her family.

**Causes of dementia**

*1. Dementia due to primary neuronal damage*

(a) Senile dementia of the Alzheimer Type (SDAT).
(b) Alzheimer's disease.
(c) Lewy body dementia.
(d) Parkinson's disease.
(e) Pick's disease.
(f) Huntington's chorea.
(g) Steele–Richardson syndrome.
(h) Striatonigral degeneration.
(i) Subacute sclerosing panencephalitis.
(j) Progressive multifocal leucoencephalopathy.
(k) Creutzfeld–Jacob disease.

*2. Dementia secondary to disease process elsewhere*

(a) Vascular – multi-infarct dementia, vasculitides, cerebral anoxia.
(b) Trauma – non-penetrating head injury, subdural haematoma.
(c) Structural – tumours, primary and secondary, cerebral lymphoma.
(d) Inflammatory – multiple sclerosis, encephalitides, syphilis, AIDS, sarcoid, Whipple's disease.
(e) Metabolic/toxic – chronic renal failure, portosystemic encephalopathy, alcohol, Wilson's disease, heavy metal poisoning.
(f) Endocrine – hypothyroidism, Cushing's disease, Addison's disease, panhypopituitarism.
(g) Vitamin deficiency – $B_{12}$, pellagra, thiamine.
(h) Hydrocephalus – communicating, non-communicating.

**Investigation**

Results from several studies suggest that the yield rate of assessment in patients presenting with dementia is as follows – in 1025 patients, a clinical diagnosis of dementia was confirmed in 100%; 105 patients (12%) were found to have a treatable cause, in descending order of frequency:

- Depression, 22 (pseudodementia).
- Normal pressure hydrocephalus, 20.
- Other psychiatric disorder, 15.
- Drug toxicity, 13.
- Space-occupying lesion, 13.
- Hypothyroidism, 6.
- Alcohol abuse, 2.
- Other disorders, 14 (= vitamin $B_{12}$ deficiency, 3; hyperparathyroidism, 2; hypoparathyroidism, 1; hyponatraemia, 2; hypoglycaemia, 1; severe anaemia, 1; uraemic encephalopathy, 1; sarcoidosis, 1; neurosyphilis, 1).

Pseudodementia has a clearly defined onset and shorter course than organic dementia. Patients complain of cognitive impairment, emphasize their disability and failures, and show affective change and distress. Nocturnal confusion is rare. Patients answer 'I don't know' when undergoing cognitive testing, show variability in carrying out tasks of comparable difficulty and have a smaller verbal/performance IQ discrepancy on the Wechsler Adult Intelligence Scale. A proportion of elderly depressed patients go on to develop dementia.

Investigation can also reveal a coexisting physical illness. One study identified abnormal findings in 20% of patients undergoing routine screening in a psychogeriatric service; not all the findings affected the subsequent treatment of the patient.

The clinical interview will contain the following components:

*1. Medical history.* This is taken from both the patient and an informant. Attention should be paid to change in functioning, abilities at home, alteration in mood and behaviour, getting lost, failure to recognize familiar individuals and failure at work.

*2. Drug history.* Phenothiazines, lithium, tricyclic antidepressants, haloperidol, benzodiazepines, anticholinergics, anticonvulsants and antihypertensive agents can not only cause reversible cognitive impairment, but also worsen cognitive function in those already suffering from dementia. However, almost any prescribed drug can affect cognitive functioning in the elderly.

*3. Mental state.* This should include cognitive function (see Cognitive function – assessment, p. 66) and enquiry to reveal functional psychiatric conditions. The mini-mental state examination (MMSE) of Folstein *et al.* (1975) is often used to assess cognitive function.

*4. Physical examination.* This should be comprehensive, but pay particular attention to:
(a)  Gait, coordination, reflexes, proprioception.
(b)  Cranial nerves, hearing, sight.
(c)  Cardiovascular system.

*5. Routine laboratory tests.*
(a)  Full blood count, erythrocyte sedimentation rate.
(b)  Urinalysis, urine culture.
(c)  Urea, calcium, potassium, sodium, phosphate.
(d)  Liver function tests.
(e)  Serum $B_{12}$, serum folate.
(f)  Serum proteins.
(g)  Serum glucose.
(h)  Thyroid stimulating hormone.
(i)  Chest X-ray.
(j)  Electrocardiogram.
(k)  Wasserman reaction or other appropriate test for syphilis.

*6. Other investigations.* The following may also be helpful, and in some centres are carried out routinely.
(a)  Skull X-ray.
(b)  Computerized tomography (CT) may be an aid in differential diagnosis and to detect change over time.
(c)  Electroencephalogram.

*7. Specialized investigations.*
(a)  Evoked potentials (EP) from auditory, somatosensory or visual events provoke waves (e.g. P300) which are thought to reflect speed of cognition. The latency of these increases with age and in AD, although there is no useful specificity for the condition.
(b)  Regional cerebral blood flow (RCBF). Reduction of hemispheric blood flow has been demonstrated to be

commensurate with the degree of cognitive impairment, and in multi-infarct dementia (MID) there are changes in autoregulation and oxygen consumption.

(c) Positron electron tomography (PET) measures glucose utilization in the living brain and can be used to make quantitive measurements during psychological manipulation as well as in the resting state. In a comparative study it has been shown to reflect neuronal pathology better than CT or nuclear magnetic resonance imaging (NMR).

(d) NMR has great potential in the differential diagnosis of dementia.

8. *Diagnostic interviews.*

(a) *Geriatric mental state (GMS).* This is derived from the present state examination (PSE) and is used with the computerized diagnosis AGECAT. This brings 157 items into eight diagnostic clusters, gives the principal diagnosis, an alternative diagnosis and the degree of diagnostic confidence which can be held.

(b) *CAMDEX,* which comprises:
   - A structured psychiatric interview.
   - The ischaemic score of Hachinski.
   - The Dementia score of Blessed.
   - A cognitive examination, which includes the MMSE with extra items to detect abnormalities of abstract thinking, perception, orientation, language, memory, praxis, attention and calculation.
   - A standardized schedule to record interviewer observations on mental state.
   - A structured interview with a relative or other informant.
   - Physical examination.
   - Record of laboratory tests.

(c) *Psychometric testing* can be helpful both in making the diagnosis and in detecting deterioration, but it is not routinely necessary (see Cognitive function – assessment, p. 66). Automated cognitive assessment can be more acceptable to the elderly than one might think. Simple initial tests can allow a feeling of mastery of a new phenomenon to those who are not familiar with computers.

(d) *The behaviour rating scale* of the Clifton Assessment Procedures for the Elderly, if carried out, also results in assessment which has immediate relevance to daily life and practical implications for treatment packages.

# Further reading

Boyd WD, Christie JE. Psychiatry of old age. In: Kendell RE, Zealley AK (eds) *Companion to Psychiatric Studies*. Edinburgh: Churchill Livingstone, 1988; Chap. 27.

Folstein ME, Folstein SE, McHugh PR. 'Mini-Mental State': a practical method for grading the cognitive state of patients for the clinician. *Journal of Psychiatric Research*, 1975; **12:** 189–98.

Marsden CD, Fowler TJ. Dementia. In: *Clinical Neurology*. London: Edward Arnold/Hodder and Stoughton, 1989; Chap. 10.

# Related topics of interest

Alzheimer's disease – neurobiology (p. 30)
Cognitive function – assessment (p. 66)

# DEMENTIA – BEHAVIOURAL ABNORMALITIES

Behaviour can be defined as observable acts which can be measured. It can be further helpful to consider behaviour as described simply in terms of observed actions (topographic), or described with some reference to the reasons for and effects of the action (functional). It is helpful to consider behaviours as occurring somewhere on a spectrum between the two extremes.

The development of a limited number of new behaviours in a person with dementia may easily be conceived as behaviour rather than 'personality change'. However, more pervasive behavioural abnormality may lead to consideration of a personality change. It is argued that assessment of the situation even in these latter cases should occur within the framework of behaviour change, in order to avoid judgemental reactions which could prejudice the quality of an individual's care.

**Types of behavioural change in dementia**

*1. Aggressive behaviour.* This is common and a distinction may exist between verbal and physical aggression. Common forms are resisting help, being uncooperative, irritability, other verbal aggression, biting, scratching, kicking, hitting. Destroying property and sexual aggression are uncommon. It may be useful to describe aggression in terms of the setting rather than actual activity.

*2. Activity disturbance.* Activity may be reduced or increased in dementia, the former less often giving rise to clinical concern. Increased activity should be described in terms of description and severity. Examples include pottering, checking, inappropriate walking. Severity may be described in terms of frequency, length of time spent on the activity or degree of disturbance caused.

*3. Eating behaviour.* Reduction in food intake is most common and may occur more frequently in Alzheimer's disease than multi-infarct dementia. Increased food intake may also occur, as may development of sweet preference, chewing and swallowing abnormalities.

*4. Diurnal rhythm.* Normal age-related changes of reduced sleep time and decrease in slow wave sleep (SWS) are exaggerated in dementia. Electroencephalogram (EEG) and sleep changes occur early in dementia. Later in dementia the sleep–wake cycle of the EEG becomes disorganized or even completely broken down and this may relate to increased activity in the latter part of the day and inappropriate night time activity.

5. *Sexual behaviour.* Includes inappropriate sexual talk, hugging, kissing, self-exposure, fondling. More extreme forms such as public masturbation and sexual aggression are rare. There is some tentative evidence of reduced sexual drive and impotence in dementia.

6. *Other.* Includes screaming, picking at clothes or furniture and repositioning small domestic objects.

**Assessment**

- Physical health.
- Family relationships.
- Information collected from patient. Likely to be a difficult and unreliable source but a semi-structured interview may be helpful, for example, Sandoz Clinical Assessment-Geriatric (Shader *et al.*, 1974).
- Information collected from carers. Biases again likely to intervene, such as level of stoicism of the carer (e.g. present behavioural examination; Hope and Fairburn, 1992).
- Direct observation. Potentially the most accurate method. Attention must be paid to setting, preparation of patient and observer, definition of observed events and so on. Events can be recorded according to frequency, duration, occurrence at predetermined time points, occurrence within predetermined time periods, frequency and time duration.
- Indirect objective measures: for example, pedometers for walking, EEG recording for sleep disturbance, weight change for eating disturbances.

Good definition and measurement of behavioural changes opens the way to pharmacological manipulations and neuroimaging to increase our understanding of brain abnormalities in dementia.

# Further reading

Hope RA, Fairburn CG. The present behavioural examination (PBE): The development of an interview to measure current behavioural abnormalities. *Psychological Medicine*, 1992; **22:** 223–30.

Hope T, Patel V. Assessment of behavioural phenomena in dementia. In: Burns A (ed.) *Ageing and Dementia, a Methodological Approach.* London: Edward Arnold, 1993; 221–36.

Shader RI, Salzman C, Harmatz JS. A new scale for clinical assessment in geriatric patients (SCA-G). *Journal of the American Geriatrics Society*, 1974; **22:** 223–30.

# Related topics of interest

# DEMENTIA – DEFINITIONS AND CATEGORIES

Epidemiological studies of dementia have been difficult owing to the problems of case definition. However the situation has been clarified recently by the adoption of several specific systems of definition. The major ones which are in current use are detailed below.

**ICD-10**

'Dementia is a syndrome due to disease of the brain, usually of a chronic or progressive nature, in which there is disturbance of multiple higher cortical functions, including memory, thinking, orientation, comprehension, calculation, learning capacity, language and judgement. Consciousness is not clouded. Impairments of cognitive function are commonly accompanied, and occasionally preceded, by deterioration in emotional control, social behaviour, or motivation. This syndrome occurs in Alzheimer's disease, in cerebrovascular disease, and in other conditions primarily or secondarily affecting the brain.'

**DSM-III-R**

'Loss of intellectual abilities sufficient to interfere with social functions, memory impairment, one of the following: impairment of abstract thinking/deterioration in judgement/aphasia/apraxia/personality change, consciousness not clouded, other disorders excluded.'

**NINCDS-ADRDA**

The National Institute of Neurological and Communication Disorders and Stroke, and the Alzheimer's Disease and Related Disorders Association define dementia as a 'Decline in memory and other cognitive function (history and examination), delirium excluded.' (These criteria were developed at a workshop of international experts in the field.)

**CAMDEX**

'Global deterioration of intellectual, emotional and motivational behaviour in clear consciousness for 6 months. Progressive failure in everyday life, memory impairment, deterioration in one of the following; intellectual ability, judgement, higher cortical function, deterioration of personality or general behaviour', is the definition given by the Cambridge Mental Disorders of the Elderly Examination.

**Epidemiology**

A recent study of a representative sample of 1042 people over 65 in the UK has given these results:

- 4 year cumulative incidence 3.7% (95% CI 2.4%–5.0%).

- Age specific rates:

| 65–69 | 70–74 | 75–79 | 80–84 | 85–89 | years |
|-------|-------|-------|-------|-------|-------|
| 0.9% | 2.8% | 5.2% | 9.0% | 8.7% | |

**Underlying pathological diagnoses**

This section considers the final pathological diagnosis which may underlie a case of dementia. It is not an exhaustive list of causes (see Dementia – assessment, p. 89) but gives further details on some.

*1. Alzheimer's disease (AD)* (see Alzheimer's disease – neurobiology, p. 30).

(a) Initial presentation of slowly developing memory impairment, personality or mood change.

(b) Dyspraxias and agnosias may develop with a consequent decline in everyday living skills.

(c) Up to 10% develop epilepsy.

(d) Dysarthria and dysphasia are late manifestations.

(e) Muscle rigidity may develop.

(f) Eventually intellectual function is severely impaired and neurological disability great.

*2. Multi-infarct dementia (MID).* Effects of infarction depend on size, location and number of infarcts. Usually the intellectual function deficit is accompanied by multiple small infarcts, indeed individual infarcts may be too small (lacunae) to show on computer tomography (CT) scan. A lesion occurring on the dominant angular gyrus in hippocampus may simulate AD.

(a) A major cause is atheroma and hypertension.

(b) Lacunar infarcts are particularly associated with hypertension and have a predilection for the basal ganglia and upper pons, resulting in slowing, dysarthria, clumsiness, gait disturbance and extra-pyramidal features.

(c) Presentation tends to be stepwise rather than gradual.

(d) Epilepsy occurs in 20%.

(e) Personality and insight may be more preserved than in AD, perhaps leading to more emotional disturbance.

*3. Subcortical dementia.* A term originally coined by Albert to describe the cognitive deficits in progressive supranuclear palsy. Use of this term has extended to include Parkinson's disease associated dementia and Huntington's chorea, diffuse Lewy body dementia and senile dementia of Lewy body type (SDLT).

Clinical features of subcortical dementias include: bradyphrenia, visuospatial disorder, mood disturbance, abnormal motor function and relatively mild impairment of memory and cognition (which may improve with training), less language disturbance but more speech disturbance (dysarthria/hypophonia), as opposed to: aphasia, agnosia, amnesia and more severe impairment of memory and cognition which are described for cortical dementias. Depression is common, as is psychosis, delusions tending to be more complex than in AD.

However this division can be challenged by considering neurochemical abnormalities (see Alzheimer's disease – neurobiology, p. 30). While different pathological causes of dementia have different neuropathological and neuro-transmitter abnormalities, the neurotransmitter abnormalities do not fit a subcortical/cortical demarcation. In addition the two cannot be distinguished on electroencephalogram (EEG) abnormalities, cerebral blood flow and metabolism studies or neuro-psychological tests.

*4. Lewy body dementia.* A recently described condition in which Lewy bodies, which were previously recognized as a pathological finding in the basal ganglia in Parkinson's disease, are found in the cortex of patients with dementia. Patients are thought to have higher incidence of extra-pyramidal symptoms and in particular to be more susceptible to the side-effects of neuroleptic medication.

*5. Pick's disease.* The brain shows mild generalized atrophy with marked atrophy of frontal and temporal lobes. Atrophy affects white and grey matter, leading to a characteristic 'knifeblade appearance'. There is no excess of plaques and tangles compared with normal age matched brains. Thirty per cent show Pick's bodies which are dense structures found in neuronal cytoplasm.

- Onset usually 50–60 years.
- Early changes in character and social activity followed by intellect, memory, language (circumlocution and vocab-ulary restriction), apathy, euphoria and extra-pyramidal phenomena.
- Predominance of frontal lobe features such as euphoria, emotional blunting, disinhibition, apathy or restlessness. There is relative preservation of memory, mathematical ability and parietal function.

- Behavioural change often precedes memory impairment and may be sufficiently severe to resemble the Kluver–Bucy syndrome (loss of emotional response, altered sexual activity, bulimia and apparent visual and sensory agnosia).

6. *Creutzfeld–Jacob disease (CJD)*. One of the spongiform encephalopathies. Cause is thought to be a transmissible protein (prion) but there is also genetic inheritance of vulnerability to replication of prions.

- Triphasic EEG changes and myoclonic jerks are specific to the condition.
- Onset typically aged 50+ but may be any adult age.
- Disease progression is rapid.
- Extensive neurological signs include myoclonic jerks, spastic paralysis in limbs and extra-pyrimadal signs, including tremor, rigidity and choreoathetosis.

7. *Huntington's disease (HD)*. This is autosomal dominant though sporadic cases can occur. The gene is now identified and so members of affected families can be offered counselling and genetic testing before making a decision about child-rearing.

- Onset usually 30–40+ but may be at any stage.
- Disease progression is usually slow, leading to many years of disability.
- Early psychiatric manifestation may be depression, anxiety, paranoid illness or personality change.
- Later there are memory defects with predominant frontal lobe symptoms.
- Choreioform movement disorder usually precedes the cognitive impairment.

8. *Parkinson's disease (PD)*. Dementia may develop in course of established PD. It can be an integral feature of PD itself but because all three conditions are relatively common, it may be co-morbid AD or MID.

9. *Human Immunodeficiency Virus (HIV)* (see HIV, p. 155).

10. *Head injury* (see Head injury, p. 151). Frontal and temporal lobes are particularly at risk in non-penetrating head injury.

- Dementia may result from single episode but recurrent trauma as in boxing can also be the cause.
- 'Dementia pugilistica' is characterized by: ataxia, dementia, extra-pyramidal features, dysarthria and personality change.

*11. Clinicopathological studies.* These attempt to develop methods of predicting the final pathological diagnosis of a case of dementia during life. This is a task fraught with methodological difficulty. Clearer understanding of neuropathology during life would allow better case definition for studies of proposed treatments. In addition there would be benefits for clinical management and planning of service provision. The current definitions of dementia make the following clinical distinctions between AD and MID.

- *AD:*
  - *NINCDS-ADRDA criteria.* Dementia as assessed on the Mini-Mental State Examination of Folstein *et al.* and on the Blessed dementia criteria. Deficits in at least two areas of cognition, progressive decline, onset at 40–90 years; absence of other aetiological factors.
  - *CAMDEX criteria.* Dementia of gradual onset. Absence of other aetiological factor. Early dysphasia, agnosia, apraxia.
  - *DSM-III-R criteria.* Dementia of insidious onset with uniformly progressive deteriorating course. Exclusion of all other specific causes.
- *MID:*
  - *NINCDS-ADRDA criteria.* Generally a diagnosis of exclusion, Alzheimer's being considered unlikely if there is sudden onset, focal signs or gait disturbance.
  - *CAMDEX criteria.* Dementia of sudden onset with stepwise deterioration. One or more strokes or transient ischaemic attacks. Focal neurological signs. Two of the following; patchy psychological deficits, emotional lability, insight loss, depression/anxiety, fits, hyper-tension, headache or dizziness and gait abnormality.
  - *DSM-III-R criteria.* Dementia with a stepwise deteriorating course, focal neurological signs, evidence of aetiologically significant cerebrovascular disease.

# Further reading

Brayne C. Clinicopathological studies of the dementias from an epidemiological viewpoint. *British Journal of Psychiatry,* 1993; **162:** 439–46.

Fleminger S. Subcortical dementia-defining a clinical syndrome. In: Kerwin R (ed.) *Neurobiology and psychiatry.* Cambridge, Cambridge University Press, 1991; 137–54.

Morgan K, Lilley J, Arie T, Byrne J, Jones R, Waite J. Incidence of dementia in a representative British sample. *British Journal of Psychiatry,* 1993; **163:** 467–70.

# Related topics of interest

Alzheimer's disease – neurobiology (p. 30)
Dementia – assessment and causes (p. 89)
Head injury (p. 151)
HIV (p. 155)

# DEPRESSION IN THE MEDICALLY ILL

Major depression is a common disorder, with an estimated prevalence of 6.7% in the general population (NIMH – ECA Study, Regier *et al.,* 1984). However, depression in the medically ill (co-morbid depression) is even more common. Up to one-third of all medical patients, both in hospital and in the community, have some degree of co-morbid depression.

There are four possible explanations for the high rates of depression in medically ill patients:

- Coincidental primary depressive disorder.
- Symptoms of a medical disorder; for example, hypothyroidism.
- Iatrogenic effect of treatment; for example, methyldopa.
- Reaction to the stress of physical illness; for example, rheumatoid arthritis.

Depression is most strongly associated with certain types of medical condition (see table below), and the elderly are also at particular risk; physical illness is the most frequent precipitant for depression in geriatric patients and, in this group, the rate of depression is substantially higher in the more severely ill.

| Type of condition | Examples |
|---|---|
| Cardiovascular disease | Congestive heart failure, myocardial infarction, hypertension |
| Endocrine disorders | Diabetes mellitus, hyperthyroidism |
| Infections | Hepatitis, pneumonia |
| Neoplasms | Cancer of central nervous system, lung cancer |
| Neurological disorders | Dementia, multiple sclerosis, Parkinson's disease, stroke |
| Others | Alcoholism, arthritis |

| | |
|---|---|
| **Harmful effects** | • Depressed, medically ill patients perceive themselves as more ill than non-depressed patients. |
| | • As a consequence, they tend to use health services more (patients with depression visit their doctors almost four times as often as non-depressed individuals; depressed patients stay in hospital over 25% longer than non-depressed patients with equally severe medical illness, and undergo more procedures and incur significantly greater medical costs). |
| | • Increased levels of functional disability. |
| | • Poor compliance with treatment regimes. |
| | • Depression can lead to an 'amplification' of the physical symptoms of medical illness, and failure to recognize the concomitant psychopathology may lead the physician to suspect worsening of the physical illness, which could |

lead to unnecessary investigations and inappropriate treatment.

- There is a clear link between depression and increased morbidity and mortality in patients with physical illness.

**Detection**

- Suicide is raised in those with physical illness, particularly chronic neurological illness or cancer. Depression is probably important in its causation.
- Among medical in-patients, at least one-third of those with psychiatric symptoms remain undiagnosed throughout their hospitalization.
- One reason for this is that measurement of depression in the medically ill is very difficult; somatic symptoms of depression such as change in appetite and weight, disturbed sleep, fatigue and energy loss may all be caused by physical illness.
- Diagnosis, therefore, depends on symptoms without a physical bias (see below):
  — *Fearful or depressed appearance.
  — *Social withdrawal or decreased talkativeness.
  — Psychomotor retardation or agitation.
  — Depressed mood, subjective or observed.
  — Marked diminished interest or pleasure in most activities, most of the day.
  — *Brooding, self-pity or pessimism.
  — Feelings of worthlessness or excessive or inappropriate guilt.
  — Recurrent thoughts of death or suicide.
  — *Mood is non-reactive to environmental events.

  At least five of these nine symptoms for at least 2 weeks suggests co-morbid depression.

  *These four symptoms replace those somatic symptoms of depression listed above.

**Risk factors for co-morbid depression**

A number of factors can trigger or increase the risk of co-morbid depression:

- Previous history of depressive illness.
- Sudden recrudescence of chronic condition.
- Diagnosis or recurrence of cancer.
- Stress of surgery.
- Certain treatments and therapies (e.g. chemotherapy, radiotherapy, corticosteroids, antihypertensives).
- Physical and psychological losses.
- Poor social support.
- Chronic pain.
- Progressive disability.

**Treatment**      Both pharmocotherapy and psychotherapy have a role and
they may act synergistically.

*1. Tricyclic antidepressants.* These cause side-effects
which can affect compliance, which is often a problem in the
medically ill. Sedation, postural hypotension and adverse
effects on cardiac conduction may limit the use of these
drugs.

*2. Drug interactions.* These can occur, and are summarized
in the table below.

| Class | Effect of interaction |
|---|---|
| Anticholinergic drugs | Increased anticholinergic effects |
| | Increased risk of delirium |
| Antihypertensive agents | Potentiate antihypertensive effects, |
|   Calcium antagonists | causing orthostatic hypotension |
|   Methyldopa | |
|   α-adrenergic blockers | |
| Diuretics | Reduce antihypertensive efficacy |

*3. Selective serotonin reuptake inhibitors (SSRI).* The newer
SSRI drugs offer hope of effective treatment for co-morbid
depression because they have fewer side-effects. The effects
and cost of these drugs are shown in the table below.

| Drug | Anticholinergic effect | Sedative effect | Orthostatic effect | Fatal toxicity | Cost (£)[a] |
|---|---|---|---|---|---|
| Amitriptyline | +++ | +++ | +++ | 46 | 4.3 |
| Imipramine | +++ | ++ | +++ | 28 | 5.7 |
| Dothiepin | ++ | ++ | ++ | 50 | 8.2 |
| Lofepramine | + | + | + | 0 | 10.27 |
| Fluoxetine | 0 | 0 | 0 | Low | 20.77 |
| Fluvoxamine | 0 | 0 | 0 | Low | 19.00 |
| Paroxetine | 0 | 0 | 0 | Low | 18.69 |
| Sertraline | 0 | 0 | 0 | Low | 28.40 |

[a]Cost of 30 days treatment (adapted from Series 1992).
+At lowest recommended dose, most are used in higher doses.

# Further reading

Katon W, Sullivan MD. Depression and chronic medical illness. *Journal of Clinical Psychiatry,* 1990; **51**(Suppl. 1): 3–11.

Levenson JL, Hamer RM, Rossiter LF. Relations of psychopathology in general medical inpatients to use and cost of services. *American Journal of Psychiatry,* 1990; **147:** 1498–503.

Series HG. Drug treatment of depression in medically ill patients. *Journal of Psychosomatic Research,* 1992; **36:** 1–16.

# Related topics of interest

# DEVELOPMENTAL DISORDERS

Development is a lifelong process with the expectation of orderly change. It is influenced by the interaction between heredity and environment. Motor development is generally a matter of maturation (of the nervous system), whereas language, intelligence and personality can be significantly and irreversibly altered by early experience.

**Classification and stages of normal development**

1. *Motor milestones.*

2. *Piaget (cognitive development).* Development requires maturation of the nervous system, interactions with inanimate objects, opportunities for social interactions, and construction of an internal representation of the world. The stages are:

- Sensorimotor (0–2 years).
- Pre-operational (2–7 years).
- Concrete operations (7–12 years).
- Formal operations (12 years and upwards).

3. *Freud (psychoanalytic theory).*

- Oral (0–1 years).
- Anal (1–2 years).
- Phallic (2–5 years).
- Latency (5–12 years).
- Genital (12 years onwards).

4. *Kohlberg (moral development).*

- Pre-conventional morality.
- Conventional morality.
- Post-conventional morality.

5. *Bowlby (social and emotional development).* Development of attachments.

6. *Erikson (social development).*

- Trust v. mistrust (0–1 years).
- Autonomy v. shame and doubt (1–3 years).
- Initiative v. guilt (3–5 years).
- Industry v. inferiority (6–12 years).
- Identity v. identity confusion (12–15 years).
- Intimacy v. isolation (early adulthood).
- Generativity v. stagnation (middle adulthood).
- Integrity v. despair (late adulthood).

**Classification of developmental disorders**

*1. Axis II (both ICD-10 and DSM-III-R)*

- Motor function.
- Speech and language.
- Scholastic skills.
- Mixed.
- Pervasive (see Mental handicap – autism, p. 189).

**Developmental disorders**

As a group the developmental disorders have a mixed aetiology, including genetic factors (from family and twin studies), family factors such as family size, and other environmental factors such as lower social class, urban living and deprivation. These factors often also contribute to the prognosis of the developmental disorder. They are often associated with emotional and behavioural problems, which may be the main mode of presentation.

*1. Motor.* Severe motor coordination problems can occur in the presence of normal intelligence, and perceptual abnormalities are common. There are often secondary educational, emotional and behavioural problems. Assessment includes drawing, hopping and catching a ball and testing with the WISC which shows a discrepancy between performance and verbal IQ. Management is by explanation and reassurance, and professional input if necessary (physiotherapists, speech therapists and occupational therapists).

*2. Speech and language.* In normal language development, children can join words at the age of 21–24 months and speak in sentences by the age of three years. Stuttering and stammering are common at 3–4 years but persist in 3% (often related to parental over-concern). Expressive or receptive language, or both, can be affected in developmental language disorders, but social development and intelligence are not. Expressive disorders are by far the most common (5–6 per 1000; 2M:1F). This disorder may be secondary to:

- Hearing problems.
- Delayed maturation (of the nervous system).
- Familial factors (i.e. history of delayed speech development).
- Effects of the social environment (e.g. deprivation and lower socio-economic class, institutions, child sexual abuse, being a twin).

The differential diagnosis includes autism, mental retardation, deprivation, deafness, elective mutism (refusal to speak, often at school, which has a good prognosis in 50% with behavioural and family therapy).

*3. Scholastic skills.* These are complex acquired skills. Scholastic skills require normal language (short words by 6–7 years; newspapers by 10–12 years) and cognitive development.

(a) *Reading and writing.*
- General reading backwardness: often due to mild mental handicap.
- Specific reading retardation (SRR): (includes dyslexia). SRR was found in 4% of 9–10 year olds on the Isle of Wight compared to 10% in London. The sex ratio is 3M:1F. The prevalence is greater in lower social classes. It is frequently associated with psychiatric problems and often presents as anxiety symptoms or conduct disorders. SRR is associated with:
  - Delay in acquisition of speech.
  - Family history.
  - Conduct disorder (30%).
  - Brain injury.
  - Left/right confusion.
  - Large family size.
  - Poor concentration, impulsiveness.
  - Visual and hearing problems.
  - Low birth weight.
  - Epilepsy (but not with neurological abnormalities).

  Management involves remedial teaching and addressing secondary (psychiatric) problems. Most continue to have scholastic and psychiatric problems into adulthood but the prognosis is better for those with high IQ, higher social class and absence of conduct disorder.

(b) *Arithmetic.*
- Specific arithmetic retardation describes impaired arithmetic skills in the presence of normal intelligence. It is generally less handicapping than problems in reading or writing, although it is becoming increasingly important.

# Further reading

Black D, Cottrell D. (eds) *Seminars in Child and Adolescent Psychiatry.* London: Gaskell (Royal College of Psychiatrists), 1993.
Graham P. *Child Psychiatry: a Developmental Approach,* 2nd Edn. Oxford: Oxford Medical Publications, 1991; 103–26.

# Related topics of interest

Mental handicap – autism (p. 189)
Personality – development (p. 223)
Personality – psychological models (p. 234)

# DIFFICULT TO HELP PATIENTS

*Admitted or not, the fact remains that a few patients kindle aversion, fear, despair or even downright malice in their doctors*
 (Groves 1978)

*The sufferer who frustrates a keen therapist by failing to improve is always in danger of meeting primitive human behaviour disguised as treatment*
(Main 1957)

'Heartsink' patients are those whom their carers find in some way unpleasant to treat, and should be distinguished from the occasional patients with whom an individual health professional will have a personality clash.

**Negative attitudes towards patients**

The subject of hatred of patients was first addressed by Winnicott in 1949, who examined the phenomenon of counter-transference (i.e. the feelings consciously or unconsciously stirred up in the therapist by the patient).

Tom Main (1957), approached heartsink patients through a group exploration of patients who had caused near-breakdown in their therapists. These patients (all female, many with medical or nursing backgrounds), were 'decompensated creative masochists', and showed many of the features now described as those of borderline personality disorder. He noted the unconscious needs of therapists which are satisfied when their patients recover, and that failure of the patient to recover could result in increasingly passionate, immature, and sadistically motivated treatment attempts by the carer (e.g. 'Heroic surgical attack'). He noted the pathological behavioural spiral of:

- Induction by the patient of sympathetic concern and feelings of massive responsibility.
- Increasing guilt, which becomes intolerable for the therapist, and is projected onto others.
- Compulsive reparative attempts, and omnipotent attempts to be ideal.
- Further increasing guilt at the failure of the patient to improve, tinged by hatred of the patient.
- Increased use of sedation and other treatment to quieten the patient's 'reproachful distress', followed ultimately by transfer of the patient, abandonment of treatment, and often breakdown of the staff member.

**Groves' classification**

Writing from the viewpoint of a North American Consultant liaison psychiatrist, Groves (1978) divides patients into 4 categories, with characteristic clinical features, needing specific management.

*1. Dependent clingers.* These are very similar to the patients described by Tom Main above.

- Patients progress from normal to pathological degrees of dependency on their doctors.
- Their self-perception is of a bottomless need, and of the physician as an inexhaustible caregiver.
- The physician may initially feel powerful and 'special', before later becoming resentful and despairing.

*Management*

- At the earliest opportunity, firm limits should be set regarding the human limits to the physician's knowledge and skill, time and stamina.
- Follow-up appointments should be given in writing, with no calls allowed outside office hours.

*2. Entitled demanders.*

- They are similar to clingers in their depth of need.
- They use bullying to force the therapist into the role of 'inexhaustible supply depot'. Both patient and therapist are unaware of the deep dependency and terror of abandonment underlying the behaviour.

*Management*

- The therapist should repeatedly emphasize that the patient is indeed entitled to what is realistically good care, and that this will continue for as long as necessary.

*3. Manipulative help-rejecters.* Also have similarities with patients described by Tom Main.

- Have a quenchless need for emotional supplies.
- Feel that no regimen can help them.
- Their 'manipulativeness' is an expression of a desire to be at once close to but at the same time at a safe distance from emotional support.
- The therapist feels initially anxiety, then irritation and depression as therapeutic efforts fail.

*Management*

- Firm limits are set on expectations, and the degree of hostility to be tolerated.

- It is important to share with the patient the pessimism that symptoms will not improve, at the same time promising continuing help and support in dealing with them; this may well result in dramatic improvement of symptoms or frequency of complaints.
- A consistent firm manner is required to balance the 'need/fear dilemma'.

*4. Self-destructive deniers.* These are not simply those (Major deniers) who deny illness, often because of fears of its consequences, and continue to behave as though it did not exist.

- These patients are grossly self-destructive.
- Their behaviour is described as 'unconsciously self-murderous': a form of suicidal behaviour.
- They are highly dependent, but have given up hope of having their needs met

*Management*

- Depressive illness should be assessed and treated if present.
- Otherwise, management is essentially palliative: 'work with diligence and compassion to preserve the denier as long as possible, just as one does with any other patient with a terminal illness'.
- Caregivers need to recognize and tolerate their own wish that the patient would die.

**Frequent hospital attenders**

Many 'heartsink' patients habitually present to hospital doctors and GPs with physical symptoms that cannot be explained by organic disease. These patients often provoke negative feelings in their care givers.

In a recent study of patients attending specialist secondary care clinics, Sharpe *et al.* (1994) found a 20% of repeat attenders were rated by doctors as severely or extremely 'difficult to help'.

Many of these patients have *chronic somatization*, and present to doctors with predominantly physical symptoms. The most well-known diagnostic category in this group is somatization disorder, characterized by persistent and enduring somatic complaints that date from early life and lead to frequent unsatisfactory interactions with doctors. Its prevalence in the community is estimated to be between 0.4 and 0.5%.

This group of patients has a high priority for psychiatric assessment because it is a potential economic burden on hospital resources. It is important therefore for these patients to be appropriately assessed by a psychiatrist and for the psychiatrist to co-ordinate hospital and primary care in the management of these patients.

Explicit recognition and review of 'difficult to help' patients is likely to be more constructive than labelling them as 'heartsinks'. It is important for both the GP and psychiatrist to be consistent in their approach to management. A simple management strategy has been found to be cost effective in randomized controlled studies (Smith *et al.*, 1986; Smith *et al.*, 1995). Management includes the following:

- Establish the diagnosis from review of the patient's records.
- One general practitioner (or other named person) should be responsible for the development of the long term relationship.
- Arrange regular, spaced visits (do not see the patient on demand).
- Attempt to demonstrate links between mind and bodily complaints, for example introduce the possibility that psychological factors may have caused relevance.
- Minimize the use of psychotropic/analgesic drugs.
- Enlist the help of family or others and as 'therapeutic allies'.
- 'Damage limitation' is a more realistic goal than aiming for a cure.
- Support should be arranged for the general practitioner.

# Further reading

Groves JE. Taking care of the hateful patient. *New England Journal of Medicine,* 1978; **298**(16): 883–7.

Main TF. The Ailment. *British Journal of Medical Psychology,* 1957; **30**(3): 129–45.

Sharpe M, Mayou R, Seagroatt V, *et al.* Why do doctors find some patients difficult to help? *Quarterly Journal of Medicine,* 1994; **87:** 187–93.

Smith GR, Monson RA, Ray D. Psychiatric consultation in somatization disorder: a randomized controlled study. *New England Journal of Medicine,* 1986; **314:** 1407–13.

Smith GR, Rost KR, Kashner M. A trial of the effect of a standardized psychiatric consultation on health outcomes and costs in somatizing patients. *Archives of General Psychiatry,* 1995; **52:** 238–43.

Winnicott DW. Hate in the counter-transference. *International Journal of Psychoanalysis,* 1949; **XXX**(2): 69–74.

# Related topics of interest

# DRUG DEVELOPMENT

**Development of a 'new chemical entity'**

This could come from a variety of sources. The earliest drugs were isolated from plants used in traditional remedies. Unexpected effects which occur during the development of a drug can lead to discoveries. Many drugs have been developed as a result of the synthesis of thousands of compounds, followed by screening these for biological activity in animals. Investigation of the metabolites of active drugs can also be fruitful. More recently, targeted molecular design has been possible as a result of discoveries in neuropharmacology.

**Preclinical development**

Animal pharmacology confirms the mechanism of action, explores effects on other organ systems and investigates interactions with other drugs. It provides pharmocokinetic data to determine the route of administration and dose range, and for the design of toxicology studies.

Animal toxicology is required by statute, and drugs must be tested for acute (up to 14 doses), subchronic (up to 6 months) and chronic dosing (up to 24 months) to determine their safety in all organ systems. Usually two mammalian species are used.

Pharmaceutical investigation prior to clinical trials attempts to define effective and stable formulations of the drug.

**Clinical development**

This stage includes all studies which provide evidence of efficacy and safety in man. The studies are controlled by statute and the regulatory authorities (Medicines Control Agency), they usually take 5–10 years and cost approximately £100 million. The studies are divided into three phases:

- *Phase I*. Normal volunteers (approximately 100) provide pharmacokinetic, metabolic and pharmacodynamic data.
- *Phase II*. Patients (up to 500) are used to confirm phase I data, provide some evidence of efficacy and suggest a likely dose range.
- *Phase III*. Patients (1000–3000) are used in clinical trials to obtain evidence of efficacy and safety. A clinical trials certificate (CTC) or clinical trials exemption certificate (CTX) is required to conduct these trials.

At this point all available data is submitted to the regulatory authority (Medicines Control Agency) for a product licence.

- *Phase IV.* Post Marketing Surveillance (PMS). (Using many thousand patients). Provides evidence of long-term safety. Each newly licensed drug in the UK is subject to intensive PMS during the first 2 years and is identified in the British National Formulary to aid doctors' recognition of its status. Sources of data at this stage include ongoing clinical trials by the drug company and clinical trials by clinical pharmacologists, spontaneous reporting of adverse reactions by doctors using the 'yellow card' system and others.
- *Phase V.* Ongoing trials to evaluate efficacy and safety relative to other treatments.

**Drug safety**

When evaluating drug safety the following factors must be taken into account:

- The risk of serious adverse events. This includes effects of the drug which are fatal, life-threatening, lead to hospitalization or to prolonged disability. Risk is most meaningfully expressed as a percentage derived from the number of patients affected, divided by the number exposed to the drug.
- Potential benefits.
- Clinical context in which the drug will be used.

Evidence about serious risks which is gathered during the premarketing phase of drug development will result in cessation of development or limited availability and/or marketing. There will also be appropriate information on the data sheet to ensure it is used in clinical situations in which any risk is acceptable. Rare but serious effects are unlikely to have been demonstrated by the time a product reaches phase IV, and safety trials at this stage must pay attention to the following factors:

- *Sample size.* A cohort of 10 000 patients is the arbitrary standard in PMS. This has sufficient power to demonstrate an event which occurs more frequently than 1 in 3333 patients.
- *Patient selection.* Criteria for selection into a trial determine how applicable it is in the general prescribing situation. Patients may be selected to give information in a particular relevant population, such as the elderly in antihypertensive drugs.
- *Observational studies* can be useful to obtain information about safety in ordinary prescribing practice but are open to many sources of bias. The use of prescription event

monitoring (a method in which adverse events are expressed as a function of the number of prescriptions of the drug) or analysis of data from general practice computer records can allow observational study which is free from influence on the prescribing doctor.

# Further reading

Grahame-Smith DG, Aronson JK. Drug development: the pharmaceutical industry and the regulatory authorities. In: *Oxford Textbook of Clinical Pharmacology and Drug Therapy.* Oxford: Oxford University Press, 1984; Chap. 14.

Harry J. Discovery and development of a new drug. *Prescribers' Journal,* 1991; **31**: 221–6.

Waller P. Clinical trials to assess drug safety. *Prescribers' Journal,* 1991; **31**: 243–9.

# Related topic of interest

Research methods (p. 287)

# EATING DISORDERS – AETIOLOGY

**Definitions (ICD-10)**

*1. Anorexia nervosa (AN).*
(a) Body weight 15% below expected or BMI (weight kg/height m²) 17.5 or less.
(b) Weight loss due to food restriction and one or more of the following; self-induced vomiting, purging, excessive exercise, use of appetite suppressants or diuretics.
(c) Overvalued idea of dread of fatness.
(d) Amenorrhoea in women or loss of sexual interest and potency in men.
(e) There may also be elevated growth hormone, elevated cortisol, changes in thyroid hormone metabolism and abnormal insulin secretion.
(f) If prepubertal, pubertal events may be delayed or arrested.

*2. Bulimia nervosa (BN).*
(a) Preoccupation with eating and craving for food leading to episodes of overeating, consuming large amounts of food in a short time.
(b) Attempts to counteract 'fattening effects' by self-induced vomiting, purgative abuse, alternating periods of starvation, appetite suppressants, thyroid preparations, diuretics.
(c) Morbid fear of fatness.

**Epidemiology**

A Danish case register study covering 1977–1986 including all psychiatric in-patients (including children), patients admitted to general hospitals, and out-patients at psychiatric and child psychiatric departments found an annual incidence of AN of 11 per 100 000 females aged 15–24 years and 5.5 per 100 000 females for BN (Joergensen, 1992). The incidence figures in these studies are up to 10-fold less than estimated from a comprehensive population study in the USA (Lucas *et al.*, 1991).

**Aetiology**

*1. Genetic.* There is an increased incidence of eating disorders in the sisters of probands. The following figures are taken from two family studies:

|     | First-degree relative | General population |
| --- | --- | --- |
| AN  | 4.0% | 0% |
| BN  | 2.6% | 1.1% |
| BN  | 10% | 3.5% |

(a) Twin studies in AN provide evidence which is more specific for a genetic cause.

|  | Monozygotic(MZ) | Dizygotic (DZ) |
|---|---|---|
| Concordance | 56% | 5% |

Twin studies in BN do not suggest different rates between MZ and DZ twins.

(b) Suggestions as to what exactly is transmitted genetically include:
- Personality characteristics such as avoidant (harm avoidance, low novelty seeking; see Personality – assessment and classification, p. 214) or compulsive traits.
- Delay in psychosexual development.

(c) Psychiatric illness:
- Increased incidence of affective disorders in families of those with eating disorders.
- Increased incidence of substance abuse in first-degree relatives: 12–19% of fathers and 5% of mothers have been reported as having an alcohol problem.
- The same study reported a higher lifetime incidence of obsessive-compulsive disorder (OCD) and psychosexual problems in the mothers of AN probands.
- No increased incidence of schizophrenia.

*2. Social.*
(a) Eating disorders primarily occur in westernized societies with their social pressures on young women to be slim and emphasis on personal attractiveness. However, non-white girls in transition from a traditional to a westernized culture are also at high risk.
(b) Although much data supports higher prevalence in high social class, this bias can disappear when population-based studies of prevalence are carried out. Presentation to specialist clinics may mediate the apparent social class data.

*3. Family.*
(a) Family functioning in eating disorders has been studied from a 'structural' perspective, a 'systemic' perspective, with regard to expressed emotion (EE) and from more empirical and eclectic perspectives (see Psychological treatment – family therapies, p. 267). The

findings are often difficult to interpret because of difficulties in patient selection and observer bias amongst others (see Research methods, p. 287). However, the following are more general and consistent findings:

- Families are more distressed and dysfunctional than control families, this is more marked for BN than AN. Standard scales have measured and found:
  — less cohesion
  — more conflict
  — more disorganization
  — less support
  — less expression of feelings
  — less disclosure
  — less trust.

(b) A family observational study found different patterns of abnormality in AN as opposed to BN families. AN families tend to be more nurturing and comforting but less attentive to the patient's statements, whereas BN families had more evidence of hostile enmeshment. Both tend to use ambiguous or contradictory communications.

(c) A controlled comparison of families of BN and non-eating-disordered women found older parents at the time of patient's birth, less attention and affection from patients, more parental disharmony and more repressive sexual attitudes in the BN families. No differences in family size, composition, gender ratio or parental divorce rate were found.

(d) A case-control study which interviewed recent-onset anorexics and their mothers found more family problems in the AN group compared with the control group. Family problems included death of a first-degree relative, mental or physical disorder in close family, major parental secrets, parental disagreements, overly strict discipline and poor problem solving.

(e) Families with eating disorders scored low on EE, with AN scores lower than BN. Higher parental EE may be associated with poor prognosis, especially with family therapy.

(f) One study found an increased rate of being adopted in patients referred with eating disorders than in the general population. These patients had higher levels of behavioural disturbance and lower academic achievement than non-adopted matched controls.

*4. Psychological.* Bruch considered early mother–child interactions to be important in aetiology. The child does not develop normal differentiation between bodily sensations, such as hunger and satiety, and psychological states, such as anxiety or depression, because the mother's responses have been to disregard the child's needs or to deal inappropriately with them. As a consequence, the integrated self which recognizes its own needs and wants is not achieved, and this becomes a particularly pertinent abnormality at adolescence.

(a) High rates of sexual abuse are reported by those with eating disorders. The rates do not differ from other psychiatric disorders or from some studies in the general population.

(b) Low self-esteem, perfectionism and 'black-and-white thinking' can lead to the use of appearance, weight and work performance to judge self-worth.

(c) Inability to cope with adolescence, in particular the development of adult sexuality and definition of individuality.

*5. Endocrine.*

(a) The amenorrhoea of AN is accompanied by low levels of luteinizing hormone (LH) and low or normal follicle stimulating hormone (FSH), with a blunted response to hypothalamic releasing factors. Levels rise with increasing weight and eventually the midcycle peak of LH, which is the normal prelude to ovulation, occurs. However this event may lag behind the restoration of an apparently high enough weight and this may be because of persistently abnormal fat/lean ratios.

(b) Circadian rhythm shows an immature pattern with low weight in AN. This also may be delayed in returning to normal after weight restoration.

(c) Hypothalamo-pituitary-thyroid axis shows changes consistent with a normal response to energy intake restriction. Again full recovery may be delayed beyond weight restoration

(d) Hypothalamo-pituitary-adrenal axis similarly shows changes attributable to starvation.

(e) Growth-hormone levels are elevated in 50% of those with AN and fall when the energy intake is increased prior to weight restoration.

It is generally accepted that anorexia is not due to an underlying primary endocrine abnormality but physiological processes can act as perpetuating factors.

# Further reading

Bloch S, Hafner J, Harari E, Szmukler GI. Family aspects of eating disorders. In: *The Family in Clinical Psychiatry*. Oxford: Oxford University Press, 1994.

Garfinkel PE, Garner DM. *Anorexia Nervosa: a multidimensional perspective*. New York: Brunner/Mazel, 1982.

Holden NL. Adoption and eating disorders: a high risk group? *British Journal of Psychiatry*, 1991; **158:** 829–33.

Joergensen J. The epidemiology of eating disorders in Fyn County, Denmark, 1977–1986. *Acta Psychiatrica Scandinavica*, 1992; **85:** 30–4.

Lucas AR, Beard CM, O'Fallon WN, Kurland LT. 50-year trends in the incidence of anorexia nervosa in Rochester, Minnesota: A population-based study. *American Journal of Psychiatry*, 1991; **148:** 917–22.

Szmukler G. Eating disorders. *Current Opinion in Psychiatry*, 1993; **6:** 195–200.

# Related topics of interest

# EATING DISORDERS – OUTCOME AND MEDICAL COMPLICATIONS

**Outcome studies**

Eating disorders are often long lasting but rarely seem to change into other diagnoses, although Axis I and II co-morbidity is common. Anorexia nervosa may progress to bulimia nervosa but rarely vice versa.

In a 5-year outcome study of 60 adolescent in-patients with eating disorders (80% had AN), 10% had AN, 4% had AN and BN, 18% had 'partial syndromes' and 68% had recovered (Steinhausen and Seidel, 1993).

In a 10-year follow up of 50 patients with BN a full recovery was made by 52% with only 9% continuing to meet DSM-IIIR criteria for BN. None had developed AN (Collings and King, 1994).

**Medical complications**

This section describes the medical complications and recommended investigations.

*1. Cardiac.*

(a) Bradycardia of less than 60 beats per minute occurs in 87% of those with AN.

(b) Blood pressure of less than 90/60 mmHg in 85% leads to dizziness and syncope.

(c) Tachycardia and arrythmias are secondary to electrolyte disturbances.

(d) Electrocardiogram (ECG) abnormalities occur, often reflecting electrolyte abnormalities. Many are benign and reversible but Q–T prolongation interval in particular is related to sudden death.

(e) Congestive cardiac failure (CCF) is a terminal event but may also be a consequence of re-feeding.

*2. Gastrointestinal.*

(a) Erosion of enamel and dentine due to vomiting or consumption of large amounts of citrus fruit.

(b) Parotid enlargement is benign, it is most common in BN (25%) but also occurs in AN.

(c) Oesophagitis, erosions and ulcers occur as a result of vomiting.

(d) Oesophageal rupture follows vomiting after bingeing.

(e) Gastric dilatation is uncommon but may occur after re-feeding. Gastric complications are unusual but delayed gastric emptying is common and usually misinterpreted by the patient as being fat.

(f) Duodenal dilatation (50% barium meal examinations).

(g) Constipation due to inadequate food.

(h) Stimulant laxative abuse leads to alternating diarrhoea and constipation, nausea, steatorrhoea, protein-losing enteropathy and malabsorption.

(i) Little evidence of liver disease linked directly to anorexia.

*3. Renal.* These complications occur in up to 70% in AN and include:

(a) Decreased glomerular filtration rate and concentrating capacity.

(b) Increased urea.

(c) Pitting oedema which may be mild but is most severe in massive purgation and chronic laxative abuse leading to hypoproteinaemia and cardiovascular collapse.

(d) Hypokalaemic nephropathy.

(e) Electrolyte abnormalities:
  - Hypokalaemia.
  - Hyponatraemia.
  - Hypochloraemia.
  - Hypocalcaemia.
  - Hypochloraemic metabolic alkalosis.
  - Hyperphosphataemia can result from frequent vomiting and restricting food intake leads to depleted body stores of phosphate. Hypophosphataemia may be a result of refeeding.
  - Hypomagnesaemia in up to 25% can exacerbate other abnormalities and leads to increased risk of renal calculi.

*4. Haematological.*

(a) Anaemia and thrombocytopenia in a third of those with AN.

(b) Leucopenia in two-thirds of those with AN.

(c) Pancytopenia occurs in severe AN.

(d) Acanthocytosis.

(e) Reduced erythrocyte sedimentation rate (ESR).

(f) Bone marrow may be hypoplastic with fat depletion and is usually reversed by refeeding.

*5. Skeletal.*

(a) Bony maturation is retarded during active anorexic illness and development of bones may stop when weight loss is severe.

(b) Osteoporosis has been demonstrated within 2 years of the onset of AN. It is probably due to oestrogen deficiency, malnutrition and excess cortisol secretion.

(c) High-level exercise increases bone density but exercise when bone density is low increases the risk of fracture, and pathological fractures can result.

6. *Endocrinological.*

(a) Menstruation ceases before weight loss in 16% of patients and persists after restoration of body weight in up to half.

(b) Hypothalamic hypogonadism. Low basal luteinizing hormone (LH) and follicle stimulating hormone (FSH) lead to low ovarian production of serum oestrogens.

(c) Testosterone levels are normal in women but low in men.

(d) Hypercortisolaemia with normal adrenocorticotrophic hormone (ACTH). Metabolic clearance of cortisol is decreased and non-suppression by dexamethasone is common, occurring in 70–100%.

(e) Growth hormone (GH) is elevated with a reduced response to insulin-induced hypoglycaemia.

(f) Anti-diuretic hormone (ADH) release is reduced leading to nephrogenic diabetes insipidus in up to 40%.

(g) Thyroid status. Triiodothyronine levels are often 50% of normal level but since free thyroxine levels tend to be normal no replacement is indicated.

7. *Metabolic.*

(a) Low basal metabolic rate.
(b) Hypercholesterolaemia.
(c) Glucose tolerance test is abnormal.
(d) Temperature regulation is impaired.
(e) Total sleep time is reduced and sleep more disrupted than normal.

8. *Dermatological.*

(a) Dry skin.
(b) Lanugo hair.
(c) Carotinodermia.
(d) Purpura.
(e) Bruising.
(f) Calluses on hands.

**Investigations**

1. *On presentation:*
(a) Blood pressure, erect and supine.

(b) Electrocardiogram (ECG).

(c) Urea.

(d) Electrolytes (K, Na, PO$_4$, Ca, Mg).

(e) Creatinine.

(f) Urinalysis.

(g) Bone density.

(h) Triiodothyronine, thyroxine, thyroid stimulating hormone.

(i) Full blood count (FBC).

*2. Monitor (in underweight patients 75% or less of minimum):*

(a) Blood pressure, erect and supine.

(b) ECG.

(c) Urine output.

(d) Urea and electrolytes – 3 monthly.

(e) Creatinine clearance – annually.

(f) FBC and platelets – 3 monthly (with further investigations if granulocyte count <2000/mm$^3$).

(g) Liver function tests – 3 monthly.

(h) Glucose – 3 monthly.

(i) Thyroid function – 6 monthly.

(j) Bone density – annually.

## Further reading

Collings S, King M. Ten year follow up of 50 patients with bulimia nervosa. *British Journal of Psychiatry*, 1994; **164:** 80–7.

Palmer RL, Robertson DN. Outcome in anorexia nervosa and bulimia nervosa. *Current Opinion in Psychiatry*, 1995; **8:** 90–2.

Sharp CW, Freeman CPL. The medical complications of anorexia nervosa. *British Journal of Psychiatry*,1993; **162:** 452–62.

Steinhausen HC, Seidel R. Outcome in adolescent eating disorders. *International Journal of Eating Disorders*, 1993; **14:** 487–96.

## Related topics of interest

Eating disorders – aetiology (p. 118)

Eating disorders – treatment (p. 127)

Psychiatric disorders – neuroendocrine changes (p. 250)

# EATING DISORDERS – TREATMENT

There are more treatment trials for bulimia nervosa (BN) than for anorexia nervosa (AN). There is no evidence yet that treatment/intervention affects long-term outcome in AN. A recent review found a great deal of variability in outcome measures, and the existing literature does not allow prescription of a 'treatment of choice' – this may not be surprising in a disorder with multiple predisposing and perpetuating factors. However the following treatment principles have been agreed by therapists from most theoretical backgrounds.

- A multicomponent treatment programme.
- The reversal of starvation symptoms (ie. those symptoms which are common to any individual who has starved – food preoccupation, eating rituals, binges, social withdrawal, lability of mood, depression, poor concentration, irritability, stealing food, loss of energy, sleep disturbance and obsessional symptoms).
- Open, honest and collaborative relationship with the patient.
- Psychotherapies to be aimed at the predisposing, precipitating and maintaining factors of the disorder in any one individual, taking into account all of the problems that person may have.

## Treatments

**In-patient treatments**

*1. Weight restoration.* Target weights can be difficult for patients to agree to and they need reassurance that weight gain will not be too rapid. They may more readily agree to weight gain aimed at reversing symptoms of starvation which are often unpleasant.

*2. Behavioural techniques with informed consent.* For example, the gradual introduction of privileges in response to weight gain by patient.

*3. Anxiety management techniques.* These may be used to reduce distress, especially at meal time.

*4. Nursing management.* This should be firm, sensitive, supportive, non-judgemental and trusting. In some situations the nurse will take over responsibility for eating, sitting with patients while eating and afterwards if necessary to prevent vomiting. In general nowadays it is considered more appropriate for the patient to take control of his or her eating behaviour.

*5. Generally accepted indications are:*
(a) Rapid weight loss.

(b) Suicide risk.

(c) Dangerous medical complications.

(d) Weight below 65% expected. However there is also evidence that in a low-weight group, weight can be more satisfactorily gained and retained by means of a specialist day-patient programme than in-patient care. This area of research is important when one considers the difficulties of admitting a patient with anorexia under the Mental Health Act.

(e) Failure of response to out-patient treatment.

(f) Individual psychotherapy. The following approaches are used:
- Cognitive behaviour therapy (CBT). CBT is the most well validated treatment for BN, with improvements enduring for at least the first year after treatment.
- Behaviour therapy (BT) is also effective, though probably less so than CBT.
- Interpersonal therapy (IPT) is also effective in reducing overeating and depressive symptoms, though less effective overall than CBT.
- Psychodynamic psychotherapy.

**Out-patient treatments**

*1. Out-patient family therapy.* This is generally used for patients under 18 or when the family is important in maintaining the disorder and willing to be involved in therapy.

*2. Out-patient marital therapy.* This is used when the patient's relationship is an important maintaining factor and when the spouse or partner is willing to be involved.

*3. Drugs.*

(a) Benzodiazepines can be used in the short term to help with the anxiety associated with eating.

(b) Chlorpromazine is not generally recommended nowadays due to side-effects and lack of efficacy.

(c) Antidepressants. Placebo control studies of tricyclic antidepressants fail to show benefit with active drug. Selective serotonin re-uptake inhibitors (SSRIs) are promising but their efficacy is not proven. Reduced levels of homovanillic acid (HVA) and 5-hydroxyindoleacetic acid (5-HIAA) have been found in low-weight individuals. Antidepressants are usually prescribed when there is a syndrome of depression, but the ability of the starvation itself to produce depression should be taken into account in the assessment.

# Further reading

Freeman CP, Newton JR. Anorexia nervosa: what treatments are most effective? In: Hawton K, Cowen P (eds) *Pratical Problems in Clinical Psychiatry*. Oxford: Oxford University Press, 1992; 77–92.

Treasure J. Anorexia nervosa and bulimia nervosa. *Current Opinion in Psychiatry*, 1992; **5:** 228–33.

# Related topics of interest

# ELECTROCONVULSIVE THERAPY (ECT)

**Evidence for efficacy and indications**

*1. Depressive illness.* There are multiple studies comparing the efficacy of ECT with various antidepressants and placebos. An overall meta-analysis of 153 studies showed improvement in 72% receiving ECT, 65% for tricyclics, 50% for monoamine-oxidase inhibitors (MAOIs) and 23% for placebo. The Medical Research Council trial (1965) produced figures of 71% (ECT), imipramine (52%), phenelzine (30%) and placebo (39%). Further trials have shown a clear effect for real versus sham ECT. ECT plus imipramine produces fewer relapses at six months but there is no evidence for a synergistic treatment effect.

Studies have also attempted to establish factors which might predict a good or bad response to ECT. As a general rule, features of severe major depression, especially psychomotor retardation and delusions predict a better response to ECT. By contrast, neurotic traits, hypochondriacal symptoms and poor personality factors predict a poor response, although these factors may also predict a poor response to antidepressant treatments in general.

*2. Mania.* ECT is effective in mania, although it is generally reserved for those resistant to drug treatment.

*3. Acute schizophrenia.* The use of ECT in schizophrenia is more controversial but there is some evidence that ECT plus phenothiazines is more effective than phenothiazines alone, and in particular leads to a quicker improvement in psychotic symptoms. Clinical observation suggests that catatonia and stupor are particular indications for the use of ECT in schizophrenia. It is not effective for negative symptoms or chronic positive symptoms.

*4. Puerperal psychosis.* There are no controlled trials but evidence suggests that ECT is effective. It may also be used in schizoaffective disorder.

*5. Other disorders.* In Parkinson's disease there is some evidence that ECT is effective, even in the absence of affective symptoms.

**Physiological changes**

- EEG. This shows delta and theta activity and returns to normal generally within 3 months of the end of treatment.
- Cardiovascular. Initial bradycardia followed by tachycardia both of which are attenuated by atropine (vagal

blockade). There are also associated blood pressure changes.

- The permeability of the blood–brain barrier is increased.

**Mode of action**

- The passing of electricity (especially amount) and seizure (length) are necessary for therapeutic effect.
- Neurotransmitters and hormones. There are many effects but the specific therapeutic action is unclear. There is an increase in secretion of vasopressin (posterior pituitary), prolactin, adrenocorticotrophic hormone (ACTH), and beta-endorphin (anterior pituitary); but not thyroid-stimulating hormone (TSH) or growth hormone (GH) (anterior pituitary). There are various monoamine changes after electrically induced seizures (ECS) in animal tests. 5-hydroxytryptamine (5-HT). Increase in $5\text{-HT}_2$ receptors (opposite effect to antidepressants) and the same changes in $5\text{-HT}_1$ as antidepressants. Noradrenaline. Reduced $\beta$-receptors, increased noradrenaline turnover, reduced $\alpha_2$ receptors (similar to antidepressants). Dopamine. No change in receptors but an increase in dopamine-mediated behaviour. It is likely that the major effect is through 5-HT and noradrenaline.

**Morbidity, mortality and side-effects**

*1. Mortality.* This is 1 in 22 000 treatments (i.e. very low) and is principally due to the anaesthetic, especially if there is pre-existing physical illness.

*2. Memory.*

- Short-term retrograde amnesia can occur.
- Retrograde amnesia for remote events can occur but is difficult to test. It occurs more often with bilateral ECT.
- Short-term anterograde amnesia is common but short-lived.
- Memory impairment is generally related to the dose of electricity.

*3. Other side-effects.* Headache, confusion and muscle aches and pains.

*4. Contraindications.* ECT should not be given if there is raised intracranial pressure, cerebral haemorrhage, or cerebral aneurysm, although these are not absolute contraindications. Relative contraindications include recent myocardial infarction, aortic aneurysm and acute respiratory infection (i.e. anaesthetic risks).

5. *Interaction with drugs.* MAOIs need not necessarily be stopped if there are good clinical reasons for continuing, but the anaesthetist should be informed. Benzodiazepines should be omitted before ECT and care taken with lithium and the selective serotonin reuptake inhibitors (SSRIs).

**Administration** (Royal College of Psychiatrists, 1989)

*1. Before ECT.* A full explanation should be given and consent should include that explanation has been given and that the patient agrees.

(a) If the patient is informal and gives valid consent, then ECT can proceed.

(b) If the patient is detained under a treatment order and gives valid consent, complete form 38 (section 58(3)(a)) and proceed.

(c) If ECT is urgent but the patient is refusing:
   - If the patient is informal, ECT would be given under common law.
   - If under a treatment order, ECT would be given under section 62, meanwhile a second opinion is sought through the MHAC (section 58(3)(b) and 58(4)).

(d) If the patient is incapable of giving informed consent, and is detained:
   - If the patient is refusing ECT, then a second opinion should be requested through MHAC as above.
   - If the patient is agreeing to ECT, and is detained, then the procedure is generally as for other consenting, detained patients as above but there is debate about whether it might actually be in the patient's best interest to treat as if consenting, having sought a colleague's second opinion and relatives' views.

Full physical examination and medical history should be obtained, and tests carried out as appropriate to the anaesthetic risks.

*2. During ECT.* It is recommended that a senior member of the medical staff take an interest in ECT and train juniors. There should be a suite of at least three rooms, and access to emergency equipment.

A short-acting anaesthetic (methohexitone (Brietal)) is given with muscle relaxant (suxamethonium chloride) and atropine (to dry secretions and reduce post-ECT rise in blood pressure and pulse (or glycopyrrolate for the former)).

Oxygenation is also important.

*3. Prescribing treatment.*

- Unilateral or bilateral. Bilateral treatment is more potent and induces faster recovery but has greater side-effects. Therefore bilateral ECT is the treatment of choice unless side-effects are a problem or speed of action is less important.
- Dose and titration. The current is delivered as a series of brief direct current pulses. The seizure threshold varies with age, sex and treatment.
- Detecting fit. This is generally done by observation, but if in doubt the electroencephalogram (EEG) can be monitored, or the cuff method used.
- If there is no fit, check everything, including the electrode contact. Hyperoxygenation may help. Repeat the stimulation once at a higher level. Check medication that may be raising the seizure threshold. An adequate fit is longer than 25 seconds.
- Number and frequency of treatments. ECT is routinely given twice-weekly, and usually 4–8 treatments are given, or up to 10–12. The patient should be reviewed after each treatment. Most relapses will occur within two weeks after stopping treatment, and the improvement should be maintained with medication.
- Maintenance ECT. There are no properly controlled clinical trials, but there may be a lower relapse rate.

# Further reading

Morgan G, Butler S. *Seminars in Basic Neurosciences*. London: Gaskell, 1994.
Royal College of Psychiatrists: Research Committee: ECT sub-committee. *The practical administration of electroconvulsive therapy (ECT)*. London: Gaskell, 1989.

# Related topics of interest

# ELECTROENCEPHALOGRAM (EEG)

The EEG is safe and without discomfort to the patient, and is accordingly used when organic psychiatric disorders are suspected. Certain marked limitations in its diagnostic usefulness must however be borne in mind.

The normal EEG has a well developed alpha rhythm, maximal in the occipital and parietal regions, which attenuates on opening the eyes and disappears when they are closed again.

**EEG patterns**

*1. Normal range of activity.*
(a)  Amplitude 5–150 microvolts.
(b)  Frequency 1–40 Hz.

*2. Wave patterns.*
(a)  Delta, less than 4 Hz:
   - May be regular or irregular.
   - Diffusely distributed across the cortex in children and when asleep.
   - Abnormal in an adult who is awake.
(b)  Theta, 4–7 Hz:
   - Occurs transiently in 15% of normal subjects.
(c)  Alpha, 8–13 Hz:
   - Prominent over occipital cortex.
   - Accentuated by eye closure.
   - Attenuated by attention.
   - Asymmetry of 1 Hz between the hemispheres is pathological.
   - Frequency slows in old age.
(d)  Beta, more than 14 Hz:
   - Frontocentral position.
   - Enhanced by anxiety.
(e)  Mu, 7–11 Hz:
   - Over precentral areas.
   - Attenuated by contralateral limb movement.
(f)  Lambda, single sharp waves:
   - Occipital region.
   - Associated with visual scanning.
(g)  K complexes, slow waves with short episodes of fast activity:
   - Occur over the vertex in response to sound.

*3. Common abnormalities.*
(a)  Reduced amount or amplitude of normal frequencies. The reduction may be generalized or localized.
(b)  Increased slow wave frequencies.

(c) Abnormal wave forms:
  - Spikes of greater than 80 milliseconds.
  - Sharp waves of between 80 and 200 milliseconds.
  - Spike and slow wave complexes.

**EEG recording techniques**

(a) 40 electrodes are applied to the scalp in standard positions and conventionally recording is done from 8 or 16 channels.
(b) Standard recording includes:
  - Several minutes at rest.
  - Overbreathing.
  - Flashing lights.
(c) The recording procedure often includes periods of photic stimulation, sleep and hyperventilation in order to provoke abnormalities.
(d) Sleep deprivation and recording during sleep can also both provoke recordings which would otherwise be missed.
(e) Video recordings/event recorders can be used to correlate clinical episodes with EEG activity.
(f) Telemetric procedures can give recordings at a distance.
(g) Deep foci of abnormal electrical activity can be missed with standard recording because the recording is of the most superficial few millimetres of the brain. Electrodes inserted via nasopharynx or sphenoidal needles help extend the areas of the brain that can be recorded.
(h) Artefacts can be produced by:
  - Eye movement.
  - Cardiac arrhythmias.
  - Local muscle contraction.

**The EEG in sleep**

*Stage I:*

- Low voltage desynchronized activity.
- Low voltage regular activity in frequency range 4–6 Hz.

*Stage II:*

- Sleep spindles with frequency 13–15 Hz and high voltage K complexes.

*Stage III:*

- High voltage delta activity.

*Stage IV:*

- Delta activity is more than 60% of the record.

- REM sleep usually occurs for 15–30% of sleep time:
  - Low voltage asynchronous fast waves.
  - Rapid conjugate fast waves.
  - Irregular respiration.
  - Tachycardia.
  - Increased blood pressure.
  - Increased cerebral blood flow.
  - Increased gastric motility.
  - Absent tendon reflexes.
  - Penile erection.
  - Vivid dreams.

**The use of the EEG in diagnosis**

*1. EEG is useful in:*
(a)  Making diagnosis of epilepsy.
(b)  Defining seizure type.
(c)  Prognosis if precipitants can be identified.
(d)  Evaluation of treatment.

*2. A normal EEG.*
This does not exclude epilepsy.

*3. Abnormalities in specific conditions:*
(a)  Organic psychoses:
  - Decreased frequency of alpha rhythm.
  - Increased frequency of delta and theta.
  - More fast activity is characteristic of delerium tremens.
(b)  Metabolic abnormalities such as hepatic coma:
  - Widespread slowing of the trace.
(c)  Alzheimer's disease (AD):
  - Widespread slowing of the trace.
  - Diffuse theta and delta wave activity with slowing of alpha rhythms.
  - Less than 5% of histologically confirmed AD have a normal EEG.
(d)  Huntington's chorea:
  - Characteristic diffuse flat trace with an absence of rhythmical activity in all areas.
  - Amplitude less than 25 microvolts.
  - Appearance is not however specific, since it is also found in some normal subjects.
(e)  Creutzfeld–Jacob disease:
  - EEG always abnormal in this condition.
  - Bilateral slow periodic spike-wave discharges which may be accompanied by myoclonic jerks.

- Increased slow wave activity and diminution of alpha activity.
(f) Focal lesions which may be tumours or other structural abnormalities:
  - Asymmetrical traces.
(g) Temporal lobe epilepsy:
  - Spike foci occur in 90% when investigated with a sleep EEG in addition to routine waking recording.
(h) Functional stupor:
  - Preserved normal rhythms may be helpful in differential diagnosis (see Stuporose patients, p. 334).
(i) HIV:
  - Diffuse slowing.
(j) Multi-infarct dementia (MID):
  - The EEG is less helpful in diagnosis than in AD.
  - Asymmetry may be seen if infarcts are large and near the brain surface.
(k) Pick's disease:
  - Alpha activity is less deranged than in AD.
  - At least half have normal EEG.
(l) Psychopathic personality disorder:
  - Generalized theta wave activity in 31–58% of psychopaths.
  - Increased frequency of positive spike phenomenon bursts of activity with positive polarity at 6–8 and 14–16 Hz have been recorded over the temporal lobe in impulsive and aggressive psychopaths.
  - Also increased frequency of abnormal slow wave activity in temporal lobes.
  - Age-related changes:
    — Gradual slowing of alpha rhythm frequency from mean of at least 10 to 8 Hz by the age of 80.
    — Low voltage fast beta activity increases between age 20 and 60 and persists until after age 80.
    — Slow diffuse theta activity is rare under age 75.
    — Focal delta activity in the anterior temporal region occurs in 30–40% of those over 60.
    — Despite these age-related changes, the EEG is not a very helpful screening test in the elderly.

**Effect of drugs on the EEG**

*1. Neuroleptics.*

- Increased delta.
- Increased theta.

2. *Barbiturates.*

- Increased beta.
- Increased theta.

3. *Benzodiazepines.*

- Increased beta.
- Increased theta.

4. *Tricyclic antidepressants.*

- Increased beta.
- Increased delta.
- Increased theta.

5. *Carbamazepine.*

- Increased slow wave sleep.

6. *Phenytoin.*

- Alpha activity slows in early phase of toxicity.

7. *Alcohol.*

- Increased alpha activity.

## Further reading

Lishman WA. Organic Psychiatry. *The Psychological Consequences of Organic Disorder*, 2nd Edn. Oxford: Blackwell Science Ltd; 1987.

## Related topics of interest

Epilepsy (p. 139)
Sleep disorders – assessment and management (p. 315)
Sleep disorders – syndromes (p. 319)

# EPILEPSY

**Epidemiology of epilepsy**

- The prevalence in the general population is between 3 and 20 per 1000.
- Between 3 and 6 per 100 are on treatment for epilepsy or have had a fit in the past 2 years.
- The incidence rates are greatest in childhood, fall in early adult life but rise with old age.
- The onset is before 5 years in 25% of cases.

**Classification**

Epilepsy is classified both by the type of seizure and by the type of epilepsy. Since there is some overlap in the information, only the classification of the epilepsies is described here:

*1. Generalized epilepsies.* Seizure discharge is generalized from the onset and usually, but not always, leads to sudden unconsciousness. Types of seizure include absence attacks, myoclonic, tonic, clonic, tonic-clonic and atonic. The current aetiological hypothesis states that the cortex is in a mild state of hyperexcitability and localized spike and wave discharges can develop in response to normal patterns of cortical electrical activity (see Electroencephalogram (EEG), p. 134). Generalized epilepsy may be primary or secondary to acquired brain disease.

*2. Partial epilepsies.* Seizure discharge originates in a circumscribed area of cortex or subcortical structures. It may remain local or may generalize. The clinical manifestation of the local discharge is determined by its location and is often termed 'an aura', for example, Jacksonian March, paraesthesiae, autonomic sensations, psychic sensations such as fear, *dejà vu*, sensations of taste and smell. When it is generated in a silent area of the brain, such as the frontal cortex, no aura will be present; this occurs in 20% of patients with temporal lobe epilepsy.

**Epilepsy leading to psychiatric presentation**

*1. Pre-ictal events.* Irritability or dysphoria commonly occur in this phase.

*2. Intra-ictal events.* An epileptic seizure, especially when the focus is in the temporal lobe, may mimic psychiatric conditions. The onset is sudden and the duration short. The episode may be associated with alteration in consciousness. Phenomena include:

(a) Violent outbursts.

(b) Disturbed behaviour.

(c) Automatic behaviour.

(d) Mood change.

(e) Hallucinations or illusions; auditory or visual.

(f) Development of secondary delusions in response to epileptic psychic events.

(g) Forced thinking – ideas or delusions.

(h) Memory; *dejà* or *jamais vu*.

Alteration in consciousness itself may be associated with more prolonged complex behaviours, often of a disturbed nature.

Status epilepticus can be divided into:

(a) Absence status, which may result in impairment of consciousness, and may be slight or marked and up to several days in duration.

(b) Complex partial status of temporal lobe origin, which is a rare condition that causes clouded consciousness, anxiety, hallucinations and automatism, and may also last for several days.

*3. Post-ictal events.*

(a) Automatic behaviour.

(b) An acute confusional state following a seizure may give rise to states resembling:
- Fugue or other dissociative state.
- Intoxication.
- Disturbed behaviour.
- Psychosis.

*4. Late events.*

(a) *Short-lived episodes*, resembling affective or schizophrenic illnesses, may follow frequent fits, or in some instances be terminated by a generalized convulsion and preceded by reduced seizure frequency.

(b) *Chronic episodes.* A 'schizophrenia-like psychosis of epilepsy' (SLPE) has been described by Slater in 1963. It occurs after many years of epilepsy. Two-thirds have a temporal lobe focus. It may be distinguished phenomenologically from schizophrenia by less personality and social deterioration and by a lack of a family history of schizophrenia. The content of the delusions is often persecutory or mystical. However, more recent investigations using the Present State Examination (PSE) found no phenomenological difference between psychotic patients with epilepsy and those without. SLPE is now thought to be an inter-ictal as well as a chronic phenomenon, but is distinct from the brief confusional episodes of ictal and post-ictal psychoses. In addition, the temporal lobe abnormalities have acquired a significance in their own right in schizophrenia itself.

**Psychiatric disorders leading to epileptic presentation**

Pseudoseizures are apparent epileptic seizures occurring without any underlying electrical activity. They can occur in those with no epilepsy and in those who also have genuine seizures.

Certain psychological states can exacerbate established epilepsy, for example, the hyperventilation associated with panic disorder could trigger a seizure in a vulnerable individual.

Epileptic presentation may be a feature of:

- Conversion disorder.
- Factitious disorder.
- Malingering (see Medically unexplained symptoms, p. 180).

**Interactions between psychiatric and epileptic disorders**

(a) There is an increased frequency of psychiatric disorder in adults and children with epilepsy. Children with epilepsy have more psychiatric abnormality than children with non-brain-related chronic illness, while in adults the proportion is equal.

(b) Those with epilepsy have suicide rates five times that of the general population.

(c) Unselected populations of patients with epilepsy do not have increased levels of violent behaviour.

(d) An epileptic personality is no longer thought to exist.

(e) Epilepsy can have effects on psychological and social adjustment, especially so when present from childhood when it may result in missed school, restricted activity and stigmatization, or even discrimination from peers and those in authority.

(f) Handicaps can result also from physical trauma to the brain or body.

(g) Anxiety and learned helplessness can result from the experience of unpredictable sudden disruption to consciousness and activity.

(h) Anticonvulsant drugs can reduce cognitive function and emotional control leading to behaviour difficulty and mood disorder.
- Phenytoin may have an adverse effect on intellectual

performance.

- Phenobarbitone, which is now rarely used, especially causes irritability and hyperkinetic behaviour.

(i) The cause of the epilepsy may of course also lead directly to a lowered IQ.

(j) In some cases epilepsy is associated with poor impulse control.

(k) Family attitudes may be overprotective.

(l) Psychological development within the person may include features such as:

- Low self-esteem.
- Learned helplessness.
- External locus of control.
- Dependent attitudes.
- Limited social skills.
- Limited social orbit.
- Depression.
- Paranoid attitudes.

(m) The course of an epileptic condition may be influenced by psychological factors.

- Seizure frequency can be increased by being tense, depressed or tired.
- Compliance with medication can be affected by functional illness, dementia or psychological adjustment.
- Medication for psychiatric disorders such as tricyclic antidepressants and neuroleptics can lower the seizure threshold.

(n) Investigations when epilepsy is considered in the differential diagnosis are as follows:

- History:
  — Details of episode(s) from patient and witness.
  — Birth details.
  — Febrile or teething convulsions?
  — Blackouts as a child?
  — Head injury, including duration of any loss of consciousness or post-traumatic seizures.
  — Intracranial infection.
  — Family history.
  — Substance misuse.
- Examination:
  — Skin; neurofibromatosis/tuberose sclerosis.
  — Hypotension.
  — Pulse rate and rhythm.

- Heart sounds.
- Liver/spleen for evidence of alcohol damage or glycogen storage disease.
- Limb asymmetry.
- Cranial bruits.
- Smell (anosmia).
- Optic discs.
- Visual fields.
- Limb weakness.
- Reflex asymmetry.
- Plantar responses.
- Electroencephalogram (EEG); normal, sleep, 24-hour event recorder (see Electroencephalogram (EEG), p. 134).
- Computerized tomography or magnetic resonance imaging.

# Further reading

Fenton GW. Epilepsy. In: Lader MH (ed.) *Handbook of Psychiatry*, Vol 2. *Mental disorders and somatic illness*. Cambridge: Cambridge University Press, 1983.

Fenton GW. Epilepsy and psychiatric disorder. In: Kendell RE, Zeally AK (eds) *Companion to Psychiatric Studies*. Edinburgh: Churchill Livingstone, 1988; chap. 15.

Mace CJ. Epilepsy and schizophrenia. *British Journal of Psychiatry*, 1993; **163:** 439–45.

Marsden CD, Fowler TJ. *Clinical Neurology*. London: Edward Arnold/Hodder and Stoughton, 1989.

Ovsiew F. Neuropsychiatry of epilepsy. *Current Opinion in Psychiatry*, 1994; **7:** 79–82.

# Related topics of interest

# ETHICS

**Introduction**

It may be argued that an ethical approach would come naturally to those practising psychiatry: by serving the best interests of their patients, psychiatrists would perform their function without encountering ethical difficulties. A psychiatrist who considered at length the ethics of each clinical decision would be likely to become paralysed in practice.

The following aspects of psychiatry indicate the need for consideration of ethical issues:

(a) The role of assessing the mental state of another person.

(b) The need to make a judgement to deprive a person of his/her liberty.

(c) The balance between individual and social responsibilities.

(d) Poor agreement about what constitutes psychiatric disorder, for example, homosexuality, or any disorder where the diagnostic criteria are arbitrary.

The following developments have encouraged debate about the ethical principles which underlie our work:

(a) Medical consumer awareness has increased. Patients, pressure groups and community health councils promote a more egalitarian relationship with those who deliver health care and closer scrutiny of clinical psychiatric activities.

(b) The psychiatric civil liberties movement. Laing argued that mental illness is a painful reaction to extreme social pressure. Szasz describes psychiatrists as social engineers. He argues that treatment should never be coerced. Mental illness should not carry removal of responsibility for personal actions.

(c) The nature of mental illness and its treatment may lead to a perception of 'prisoner and powerless victim'.

(d) Human rights organizations, such as Amnesty International, have highlighted the plight of prisoners in repressive regimes where psychiatric labels were given to political dissenters.

(e) Increased dialogue between psychiatry and other professions – notably philosophy (in particular moral philosophy) – but also sociology, psychology and theology.

(f) The advent of modern treatments which are effective, but in some cases controversial, make such consideration more complex. Before such treatments ethical considerations would have centred on the conditions of living and restriction of liberty of those suffering from mental disorders. In addition to these factors we must now consider those we wish to treat against their will. The efficacy of certain treatment has been questioned and psychiatrists have been forced to pay greater attention to issues of informed consent. In some regions this has led to extreme restrictions on the use of some treatments, such as electroconvulsive therapy (ECT) in California. In these conditions another ethical dilemma may appear, that of the psychiatrist unable to treat a severely disordered patient by reason of legal restriction. With knowledge of the effectiveness of treatment comes consideration of the ethical position of denying or failing to provide treatments. (The right to treatment can become an ethical issue when one works in a state-funded service in which facilities do not exist for treatment.)

Recognition of the importance of ethics in psychiatry came at the World Psychiatric Association Congress of 1977, in which a set of guidelines for practising psychiatrists was accepted.

**Consent to treatment**

Informed consent is required for medical procedures in most situations.

Treatment of a psychiatric disorder may be given against the expressed wishes of the patient, or in cases where the patient is unable to give informed consent, under the provisions of the Mental Health Act (MHA) 1983.

Any medical treatment may be given without consent under the common law. The underlying common law principle is the duty of any citizen to intervene in an emergency to prevent serious harm to another. Psychiatric situations in which the common law would apply include the following:

(a)  An unconscious patient who is at risk of death or serious harm without treatment, unless there is clear evidence that the patient would not want that treatment.

(b)  The prevention of behaviour causing serious danger to self or others. Treatment would include emergency sedation to prevent violence.

(c)  A patient who is incompetent. Such patients would include those with learning disability, organic brain disorder and severe depression.

**Ethics of involuntary hospitalization**

Protest about involuntary hospitalization arose in the context of vast incarceration in asylums on the outside of communities and as a result of mistreatment; for example, hospitalization of people for religious views, or the practice of inhumane experiments. Libertarian arguments suggest that one should not deprive another of his/her liberty. However, the libertarian philosopher J.S. Mill in *On Liberty* specifically excluded those 'not in the maturity of their faculties' or 'in a state to require being taken care of by others'. There is an alternative argument which considers the mentally ill person not to be truly free. Ethical considerations also apply to voluntary hospitalization, which may itself be a complex and ambiguous procedure. Coercion may be brought to bear by legal processes, the family and the employer, as well as the doctor.

**The ethics of suicide**

The value of life can be considered to be the highest ethical value of all. Unlike most medical situations, the doctor and patient differ fundamentally about the end which is desired.

Proponents of rational suicide put quality of life above life itself, and may consider suicide to be rational in the following situations:

● To avoid shame.
● When terminally ill to avoid pain.
● To avoid immorality.
● To reduce risk to others.
● To avoid violation of divine commands.

*1. Intervention* with a suicidal patient may have the following moral dimensions:
(a) Taking the patient's decision as irrational, impulsive or distorted by mental illness.
(b) On the assumption that his/her decision is reversible, certain steps, which are also reversible, are taken to prolong his/her life.
(c) Paternalism: forcing the patient to act rationally as an expression of care for his/her real interests.
(d) Care for the patient's family, who usually ask for intervention.
(e) The price: forcing the patient to act against his/her will, prolongation of mental and physical misery, serious loss of liberty.
(f) Underlying assumption; the instinctive drive to save other people's lives plus the professional duty and practice of other doctors to do so.

2. *Non-intervention* may have the following moral dimensions:

(a) Taking the patient's decision as authentic, deliberate, clear headed and rational.

(b) On the assumption that the decision is irreversible, no steps are taken, thus irreversibly allowing the patient to commit suicide.

(c) Respect for the other person's autonomy and liberty to kill him/herself, as to take any other decision, even if it seems irrational to us.

(d) Taking the person's side rather than that of the family, giving priority to his/her freedom over the family's interests.

(e) The price: missed opportunities, the infinite loss involved in death, possibility of the most 'tragic mistake'.

(f) Underlying assumption; *'nothing in life is as much under the direct jurisdiction of each individual as are his own person and life'*. (Schopenhauer).

**Ethical principles**

Moral philosophy is a discipline in which one attempts to show how value judgements are arrived at. It involves concepts such as good, bad, right, wrong, should, ought, desirable, justice, duty and obligation.

*1. Utilitarian position.* Emphasis on the consequences of acts. Consideration of a balance between good and harm.

*2. Absolutist position.* Certain acts are intrinsically wrong, independent of their consequences. Moral judgements have universal applicability.

# Further reading

Bloch S, Chodoff P (eds). *Psychiatric Ethics,* 2nd Edn. Oxford: Oxford University Press, 1991.

Cope R. Mental health legislation. In: Chiswick D, Cope R (eds) *Seminars in Practical Forensic Psychiatry.* London: Gaskell, 1995; 272–309.

# Related topics of interest

Legal process (p. 175)
Suicide – prevention (p. 343)

# GENDER IDENTITY PROBLEMS

**Definitions**

*1. Fetishistic transvestite.* Man wears female clothes as fetish objects. Clothes are arousing and wearing them usually leads to masturbation. Women do not exhibit fetishistic behaviour.

*2. Double role transvestite.* Usually a male who spends part of his life as a normal heterosexual male and part dressing and 'passing' as a woman. There is no desire to change sex permanently.

*3. Homosexual transvestite.* Man or woman who cross-dresses with less intention of actually being taken for the opposite sex. May be as a caricature rather than a serious impersonation.

*4. Trans-sexual.* Man or woman who believes himself or herself to be the opposite sex and has a strong desire to be accepted as such. Cross-dressing is part of expressing the preferred gender identity. The trans-sexual is likely to seek medical help with gender reassignment.

The above 'types' can be expressed at different times by a single individual who may pass from one situation to another, commonly during early adult life. For example, repeated fetishistic cross-dressing may be followed by the development of a trans-sexual identity, while other trans-sexuals may report their feelings as a stable state from adolescence. Male child trans-sexualism is rare, however.

The aetiology of these conditions is poorly understood. Conditioning of penile erection may be relevant in fetishistic situations. No overall theory is described here, since individual case theory leads to hypotheses which are not effectively testable.

**Management**

*1. Fetishistic transvestism.* The emphasis is on strengthening the existing sexual relationship, if any. Positive behavioural techniques aim at weakening the link between sexual excitement and the fetishistic object. Aversion therapy (see Psychological treatment – behaviour therapy, p. 258) has been reported to be effective in weakening the link, and may occasionally be part of a treatment strategy.

2. *Trans-sexualism.* The strength of feelings may vary, but gender reassignment is usually requested rather than help in coming to terms with the situation. Requests are more commonly for reassignment from male to female rather than in the opposite direction. The selection of suitable candidates is crucial.

*Note:* Assessment before embarking on the following course of management needs to exclude organic and functional conditions which could result in the belief that one is the wrong sex.

*Organic:*

- Kleinfelter's syndrome.
- Pseudohermaphrodite (have indeterminate genitalia).

Investigations would include physical examination of external genitalia and secondary sex characteristics, genetic screening, serum follicle stimulating hormone, luteinizing hormone and testosterone.

*Functional:*

- Schizophrenia.
- Delusional disorder.
- Affective disorder.
- Antisocial personality disorder.

If these differential diagnoses are ruled out, then definitive surgery follows a prolonged period (usually up to 2 years) of assessment of the individual's ability to function physically and psychologically as a woman.

(a) The initial stage involves psychosocial change. Help with appearance such as electrolysis, make-up, dressing and social interaction will be provided initially. Specific help may be given to learn feminine gestures, speech delivery, body posture and walking.

(b) Hormone therapy may then be introduced to induce secondary sexual characteristics. The patient needs to be aware of the health risks of oestrogen, which include thrombosis and an increased risk of breast cancer.

(c) If the individual makes a good adjustment and demonstrates a realistic and robust approach then surgery may go ahead, at least a year after beginning to live as a woman.

(d) Professional help will be needed for practical issues, such as changing name, and altering documentation, such as driving licence and passport. In the UK an individual remains legally male and so marriage would only be possible with a female.

## Further reading

Bancroft J. Sexual disorders, In: Kendell RE, Zealley AK (eds) *Companion to Psychiatric Studies,* 4th Edn. Edinburgh: Churchill Livingstone, 1988.
Snaith P. Gender reassignment today. *British Medical Journal,* 1987; **295:** 454.

## Related topic of interest

Psychological treatment – behaviour therapy (p. 258)
Sexual disorders (p. 309)

# HEAD INJURY

Head injuries cause *primary* damage principally by shearing of nerve fibres from rotational movements, and *secondary* damage from *intracranial factors*:

- Haematomas.
- Brain swelling
- Infection.
- Subarachnoid haemorrhage.

Also from *extracranial factors*:

- Respiratory failure.
- Hypotension.

The consequences of a head injury are the result of damage to the brain, of emotional reactions to cognitive and physical disabilities, and of the interaction with changes in mood/personality.

**Post-traumatic amnesia (PTA)**

This is the period between injury and return of continuous memory for everyday events. It is a good predictor of the prognosis in terms of functioning and is also related to the severity of the head injury, but individual variations occur. The effect varies with age, and the relationship is different for penetrating injuries.

| PTA | Injury | | Return to work |
|---|---|---|---|
| PTA < 1 hour | Mild injury | | 1 month |
| PTA 1–24 hours | Moderate injury | | 2 months |
| PTA 1–7 days | Severe injury ⎤ | Lasting cognitive | 4 months |
| PTA > 7 days | Very severe injury ⎦ | impairment likely | 1 year + |

The Glasgow coma scale and Glasgow outcome scale are used to predict and measure outcome. The majority of the total recovery occurs by six months; of those who have made a good recovery at 12 months two-thirds have achieved this by three months, and 90% by six months. This applies to basic brain mechanisms but more complex functions continue to improve over years.

**Epilepsy**

The overall risk of seizures (after the initial seven days after injury) is 5%. Slightly more than half those who develop epilepsy have fits within one year, and epilepsy is more likely if there are seizures within the first week of injury. There is a higher incidence with penetrating wounds. Epilepsy developing in the first year is directly related to the level of psychiatric disability.

**Cognitive functions**

After closed head injury there are various effects. Performance IQ is affected more than verbal IQ. Memory, especially short-term memory (STM) is affected. The majority of recovery happens by 6–9 months, and verbal memory returns more slowly than simple learning. There is a general relationship between the severity of the injury and the cognitive disability. In terms of language, there is frequently an expressive/non-fluent aphasia, but communication in general is often impaired even when the aphasia has resolved.

**Changes in personality and behaviour**

These changes cause the majority of problems.

*1. Organic personality syndrome.* This is a change in personality or exaggeration of a previous trait as a result of an organic factor. Instability of mood, aggression, impaired social judgement, apathy and paranoia are common. Aggressive behaviour may be the exaggeration of a previous propensity; or episodes may be the equivalent of epilepsy (but without loss of consciousness) which can be treated with carbamazepine and behaviour treatment; or may be the result of partial complex seizures (again treat with carbamazepine). Disinhibition may exhibit as sexual disinhibition and precautions may need to be taken such as contraception/cyproterone acetate, with behavioural techniques and possibly carbamazepine. Loss of drive is very difficult to deal with and has a detrimental effect on rehabilitation.

*2. Organic affective syndrome.* Mood changes are often the result of disinhibition, or as a reaction to consequences of injury, rather than as a direct result of the trauma. Counselling is often helpful, with anti-depressants as appropriate. Hypomania can also occur.

*3. Organic delusional syndrome and hallucinosis.* Symptoms of this are often seen during periods of altered consciousness, but, more rarely, it may be seen in clear consciousness. It is self-limiting.

*4. Amnestic syndrome.* This occurs with bilateral temporal damage. There is total loss of recall except for events before the injury. Patients often have insight so it is very distressing. It may be helped to a degree by environmental cueing and repetition.

**Post-traumatic neuroses**

- Anxiety and depression are common and often respond to counselling and psychological techniques.
- Conversion/hysterical states are more likely with milder injuries. The symptoms may be related to actual disabilities.
- Obsessional states. Patients often show obsessional traits which may represent organic orderliness or a response to disruption.
- Alcoholism. This may predate the injury or may be a consequence of it, and head-injured patients are less tolerant to the effects of alcohol.
- Suicide. This accounts for 14% of all deaths, and is usually related to social problems and depression.
- Post-traumatic stress disorder (PTSD) can occur in 10% of road traffic accident victims. It is more likely to occur if the patient retains consciousness and therefore remembers the trauma.

**Post-concussional syndrome**

This is an area of debate particularly about the contribution of physiological and psychological factors. Even with minor head injuries there may be physiological changes which are short-lived but may contribute to later problems. Post-concussional syndrome is characterized by a variety of diverse symptoms: headache, dizziness, fatigue, anxiety, insomnia, sensitivity to noise, difficulty concentrating, irritability, subjective mental impairment and depression. The differential diagnosis should include chronic subdural haematoma and epilepsy. Post-concussional syndrome is probably a consequence of both physiological and psychogenic factors; the former are more important soon after injury, the latter if symptoms persist beyond a year (Lishman, 1988).

Factors relevant to the development and prognosis of post-concussional symptoms include:

- Pre-traumatic: age, cerebral arteriosclerosis, alcoholism, premorbid psychiatric aspects — illness, personality and genetic predisposition, and pre-existing psychosocial issues.
- Peri-traumatic: brain damage — temporary or permanent — other physical damage, emotional impact and meaning, circumstances of accident, iatrogenic factors.
- Post-traumatic: intellectual impairment, physical impairments and scarring, epilepsy, emotional sequelae, psychosocial sequelae, compensation and litigation.

| | |
|---|---|
| **Boxing** | Repeated head injuries have a cumulative effect ('punch drunk' syndrome). This can lead to neurological, intellectual and personality sequelae characteristic of 'dementia pugilistica' (see Dementia – behavioural abnormalities, p. 94). |
| **Management of the sequelae of head injury** | • Assess physical problems and contribution of organic factors.<br>• Assess psychological symptoms and their basis. Use counselling/psychological treatments, and psychotropic medication as appropriate.<br>• Rehabilitation should address physical, social and psychological aspects. It is particularly important to provide support to the family as there is now more awareness of the effects on those closest to the patient. HEADWAY is an organization that provides support and advice to sufferers, and their families and carers. |
| **Prognosis of psychological problems following head injury** | Poor prognostic factors include severe injury, left-sided injury, inadequate compensation or unresolved litigation, personality change and older age. |

## Further reading

Bond MR, Reid J. In: Kendell RE, Zealley AK (eds) *Companion to Psychiatric Studies,* 5th Edn. 1993; 312–20.

Lishman WA. Physiogenesis and psychogenesis in the 'post-concussional syndrome'. *British Journal of Psychiatry*, 1988; **153**: 460–9.

Sumners D. Traumatic Brain Injury. *Current Opinion in Psychiatry*, 1994; **7**: 83–6.

## Related topics of interest

# HIV

**Prevalence**

It is estimated that over the next 10 years the number of cases of AIDS will be between 16 000 and 40 000 in England and Wales.

**Neuropathology**

The neuropathology of primary HIV central nervous system (CNS) infection is complex, and the following have been described at post-mortem:

- HIV encephalitis.
- HIV leukoencephalopathy.
- Vacuolar myelopathy.
- Vacuolar leukoencephalopathy.
- Lymphocytic meningitis.
- Diffuse poliodystrophy.
- Cerebral vasculitis.

**Neuropsychiatric syndromes**

These are caused by organic conditions which result either from direct infection by the HIV virus itself or from opportunistic infections. They include:

1.  *Directly related to HIV virus.*
    (a) There is no unequivocal evidence that asymptomatic HIV-positive individuals have decreased neuropsychological function compared with normals. As a group there is probably no overall difference from age-matched normals, but some population groups do have deficits and the significance of this continues to be researched.
    (b) Aseptic meningitis is transient and occurs at the time of seroconversion.
    (c) AIDS–dementia complex has an uncertain prevalence, with estimates ranging from 6.5–38%. This variation is partly explained by a lack of consistent terminology and inclusion criteria in early studies. This situation has been clarified since the adoption of ICD-10 criteria for dementia (see Dementia – assessment, p. 89). The criteria for dementia in AIDS patients are modified: a milder decline in memory is needed, motor abnormalities should not be explicable by other manifestations of HIV infection, the minimum duration is reduced to 1 month, there should be laboratory evidence of HIV infection, and other CNS processes, for example, tumour should be ruled out. Characteristic symptoms are decreased memory and concentration,

apathy, psychomotor retardation, minor motor abnormalities progressing to global intellectual impairment and major neurological signs. Prognosis is generally poor, probably because it occurs in a late stage of AIDS. The condition may be helped by antiretroviral therapy such as zidovudine.

(d) Psychotic illness (affective or schizophrenia-like presentation) may be coincidental in this age range or may have an organic cause, in which case it could be secondary to HIV infection, drug treatment or drug misuse.

2. *Opportunistic infections.*

(a) Cytomegalovirus: encephalitis, ventriculitis and choroid plexus inflammation.

(b) Herpes simplex virus: ascending myelitis and encephalitis.

(c) Varicella-zoster: peripheral nervous system involvement and occasional encephalitis.

(d) Papova virus: progressive multifocal leukoencephalopathy, a demyelinating disease of the white matter.

(e) Cryptococcus: meningitis and meningoencephalitis caused by this fungus occur in 2.5–7% of AIDS patients.

(f) Candidiasis: abscess and meningitis.

(g) Toxoplasmosis: focal abscesses due to this parasite are common, occurring in 8–48% of AIDS patients.

3. *Vascular disorders:* cerebrovascular haemorrhage and infarction.

4. *Cranial tumours:* lymphomas – non-Hodgkin and highly malignant B-cell lymphomas (Kaposi's sarcoma is rare in the CNS).

**Psychosocial disorders**

1. *Adjustment disorder.*

(a) Occurs with information about HIV seropositivity or at times of deterioration of the disease.

(b) Pre- and post-test counselling by properly equipped individuals can be important in minimizing catastrophic reactions.

(c) Symptoms fluctuate with physical health and social situation.

2. *Depressive disorder.*
(a) Also more common at times of bad news or setbacks, with less psychological ill health at times of improved physical health.
(b) Major depression is much more common later in
. disease.

3. *Neurotic disorder.* This may present in the same situations as depression.

4. *Suicide risk.*
(a) In AIDS the risk of suicide is increased by 16–36 times compared with the general population, and most studies indicate that these deaths are not in end-stage disease.
(b) Whether these rates are raised at the time of receiving news of seropositivity or in symptomatically well HIV-positive patients is not currently known.

5. *Substance misuse.*
(a) May be a coping strategy in response to the multiple physical, social and psychological aspects of the disease.
(b) May relate to premorbid risk-taking behaviour.
(c) Support groups may be of some benefit.

6. *Morbid fear of infection.* When this occurs despite negative tests and appropriate reassurance, it is secondary to hypochondriasis, depression or delusional disorder.

**Ethical considerations**

1. *HIV status and confidentiality.* A common dilemma is the difficulty of balancing the rights to privacy of an individual with the greater good. A General Medical Council ruling (1988) permits disclosure of medical information where public interest is greater than the doctor's duty to maintain confidentiality. This would authorize a doctor to inform the sexual partner of a patient with HIV when the patient is unwilling or unable to do so. A neurocognitively impaired patient may not have insight that his/her behaviour is risky to others. In this situation there would be a duty to inform those at risk, but in many situations they would not be known to the doctor and the judgement about the extent of a patient's cognitive impairment and consequent lack of insight can be difficult to make.

2. *HIV-infected health-care provider.* Risk of transmission is estimated at 1 per 100 000 medical interventions.

Professional organizations recommend that infected professionals should refrain from clinical activity in which there is any identifiable risk.

*3. Medical decision making.* Issues of the 'right to die', withholding of medical treatment, suicide, assisted suicide and euthanasia are all germane to patients with HIV, and case law continues to be made in this area.

**HIV and general psychiatry**

*1. Consideration* of the possibility of HIV-related disorder should be part of routine psychiatric practice. Specific predictive characteristics should be present before considering its exclusion as high priority, that is, detailed consideration of the individual's risk factors, specific presentation and development of psychiatric presentation.

*2. Determination* of HIV status should occur with the patient's consent when the whole clinical picture suggests that this is a relevant differential diagnosis. Testing without the patient's consent should only take place in rare clinical situations, where it is important for the safety and treatment of the patient and protection of others that HIV status is known.

*3. Disclosure* of status to others without the patient's consent should likewise occur only when not to do so would cause serious risk to others. It should probably occur only after consulting one's medical defence society.

## Further reading

Beckett A. Ethical issues in the psychiatry of HIV disease. *International Review of Psychiatry,* 1991; **3**: 417–28.

Catalan J. HIV and AIDS-related psychiatric disorder: what can the psychiatrist do? *Dilemmas and Difficulties in the Management of Psychiatric Patients.* Oxford: Oxford University Press, 1990; 205–17.

Catalan J. HIV-associated dementia: review of some conceptual and terminological problems. *International Review of Psychiatry,* 1991; **3**: 321–30.

Everall IP, Lantos PL. The neuropathology of HIV: a review of the first 10 years. *International Review of Psychiatry,* 1991; **3**: 307–20.

General Medical Council. *HIV Infection and AIDS: the ethical considerations.* London: General Medical Council, 1988.

## Related topics of interest

# HYPERVENTILATION

The importance of hyperventilation lies in its protean manifestations, which can result in a patient being seen in almost any part of a general hospital or psychiatric service. If the appropriate diagnosis is established early, then inappropriate investigations can be avoided, underlying causes sought and appropriate treatment begun.

Hyperventilation is a physiological term implying breathing in excess of metabolic requirements, as reflected in carbon dioxide production. There are few symptoms strongly suggestive of hypocapnia and hyperventilation. Tetany is rare, but atypical or non-ischaemic chest pain and dyspnoea are common presentations, the latter often manifesting as 'air hunger' or inability to take a satisfactory breath. In general the symptoms are related either to reduction in blood flow (vasoconstriction) induced by hypocapnia, nervous hyperirritability associated with alkalosis or mechanical factors related to abnormality of chest wall movement. The table below shows common modes of presentation with suggested pathophysiological mechanisms.

| Symptom/system | Mechanism of symptom production |
|---|---|
| Cardiac | |
| Chest pain (pseudoangina) | Intercostal spasm/fatigue |
| Angina | Coronary spasm/vasoconstriction |
| Palpitations | Paroxysmal dysrhythmia |
| Neurological | |
| Dizziness, syncope | Cerebral vasoconstriction |
| Unilateral symptoms (clumsiness, paraesthesia) | Alkalosis affects peripheral nerves |
| Tetany (uncommon) | |
| Respiratory | |
| Air hunger, sighing | ? Enhanced proprioception |
| Gastrointestinal | |
| Dry mouth | Mouth-breathing |
| Flatulence /distention | Aerophagy |
| Retrosternal pain (pseudoangina) | ?Increased oesophageal contractility |
| Psychiatric | |
| Poor concentration | All secondary to cerebral vasoconstriction |
| Forgetful | |
| Psychosensory experiences, e.g. | |
| Hallucinations | |
| Euphoria | |
| Depersonalization | |
| General | |
| Weak, listless | Increased sympathetic activity, hypokalaemia |

**Diagnosis**

The diagnosis may be obvious, with the patient clearly hyperventilating, and complaining of difficulty in breathing, whilst physical examination reveals nothing untoward. Lung function tests may be normal, or if there is any abnormality it may be out of proportion to the degree of breathlessness (as in some patients with asthma). In a patient not currently symptomatic, a hyperventilation provocation test may be carried out. This involves vigorous voluntary hyperventilation (with the physician demonstrating) for a minute in an attempt to reproduce the symptoms.

Sometimes, however, patients may hyperventilate chronically, albeit to a minor degree, which nevertheless produces unpleasant long-term symptoms. Useful investigations include blood biochemistry, which will show a low bicarbonate concentration in acute (but not chronic) hyperventilation, and possibly hypokalaemia (due to potassium ions being excreted by the kidneys as they retain bicarbonate). One definitive investigation is of arterial blood gases (but note that pain or the anticipation of this may cause hyperventilation, so the arteriopuncture must be done quickly and efficiently to avoid the chance of a spurious false-positive result). Non-invasive sampling of end-tidal $p$CO$_2$ using a nostril catheter is preferable.

**Causative factors**

A diagnosis of hyperventilation by itself is not sufficient, and the underlying cause should always be sought.

Physical causes include:

- Previously undiagnosed mild asthma.
- Pulmonary embolism.
- Other acute or chronic pulmonary disease.
- Drugs, such as aspirin, alcohol withdrawal or neuroleptic-induced dyskinesia.

Psychiatric causes include:

- Anxiety or panic disorder.
- Hypochondriasis (which may be worsened by the symptoms of hyperventilation).
- Depression.
- Simulated illness or factitious disorder.

**Treatment**

Treatment should be directed primarily at any underlying physical or psychiatric cause. If no underlying cause is discovered, then patients should be encouraged to view their symptoms as generated by anxiety, or stress, and to seek ways to relieve this. Cognitive approaches may be useful for hypochondriacal concerns, and anxiety management and relaxation training may help hyperventilation itself.

## Further reading

Gardner WN, Bass C. Hyperventilation in clinical practice. *British Journal of Hospital Medicine,* 1989; **41:** 73–81.

## Related topics of interest

Anxiety and panic (p. 39)
Medically unexplained symptoms (p. 180)
Psychological treatment – cognitive therapy (p. 261)

# ILLNESS BEHAVIOUR AND ASSOCIATED CONCEPTS

Illness behaviour was originally defined as 'the ways in which given symptoms may be differentially perceived, evaluated and acted (or not acted) upon' (Mechanic, 1962). Ensuing research has helped to place illness-related behaviours into their social and cultural context.

More recently, Pilowsky (1986) has defined abnormal illness behaviour as 'the persistence of a maladaptive mode of experiencing, perceiving, evaluating and responding to one's own health status despite the fact that a doctor has provided a lucid and accurate appraisal of the situation and management to be followed (if any) with opportunities for discussion, negotiation and clarification, based on adequate assessment of all relevant biological, psychological, social and cultural factors.

In clinical practice inappropriate illness behaviour can be recognized as illness behaviour (beliefs, symptoms, behaviour, disability) that is out of proportion to the underlying physical disease (if any), and related more to associated psychosocial disturbances than to any relevant organic disease.

Patients with abnormal illness behaviour tend to be somatically focused and illness-affirming, and many will have neurotic or somatoform disorders (see Medically unexplained symptoms, p. 180).

**Determinants of consultation in primary care**

Symptom severity plays an important part, but so do *sociodemographic factors*. Women report more acute illnesses and are greater users of health-care services than men of a similar age, but this may be due to consultations connected with pregnancy, gynaecological disorders and breast disease (accounts for 79% of the reported female excess in utilization between ages 15 and 24 and 31% excess between ages 45 and 64 years).

*1. Life stresses,* such as moving house and living with aircraft noise, are associated with increased consultation, although much of this correlation can be explained by the association between stress and disorders of mood (see below).

*2. Cultural factors* are also important. In one study North American patients of Jewish and Italian extraction tended to respond in a more emotional manner than 'Old Americans' (i.e. those with ancestral origins linked to the earlier, largely British settlers). The latter were more stoical in their expression of discomfort, while patients of Irish origin tended to deny pain. Jewish patients were also more concerned with the implications for their future health, while the Italians had less desire to know why the pain arose and what implications it might have for the future.

*3. Different family atmospheres and cultures* influenced these attitudes: Jewish and Italian patients grow up in a family atmosphere of caution in relation to illness, whereas the Old American families emphasize the need to take pain 'like a man', and not to cry or demonstrate behaviour which, in that culture, might connote moral weakness.

Prospective studies have shown that emotional stress is a significant factor in predicting the utilization of general medical services, even when other key variables such as past physical health and severity of symptoms are controlled. There is also a close association between physical and psychiatric disorder:

- Psychiatric disorder can arise as a reaction to physical discomfort.
- Both psychiatric and physical illness may occur independently.
- Neurotic illness may increase the risk of later physical illness.
- Psychiatric disorder can mistakenly be perceived as physical disorder by some patients.

*4. Lay beliefs and attitudes* can also exert pressures. For example, self-help groups for patients with myalgic encephalomyelitis (ME) have become widely established, and the ME Association is now Britain's fastest growing charity. Political interest in the disorder has even resulted in legislation to mandate official research in the USA. It is apparent that many patients who are labelled (by themselves, their families and the medical profession) as suffering from ME may actually have an emotional illness. The consequence of this labelling is often to deny the sufferer appropriate psychological treatment (see Chronic fatigue syndrome, p. 59).

**Factors that promote the chronicity of symptoms**

Psychiatric disorders, particularly those involving anxiety and depression, can contribute to the persistence of somatic symptoms. Markedly abnormal illness beliefs, especially if they are shared by other family members, are also important. In non-surgical medical conditions the rating of psychological distress while the patient is in hospital is a better predictor of outcome than the clinician's assessment of prognosis. High levels of distress make an important contribution to recovery, independently of the nature of the physical disorder involved (Craig and Boardman, 1990).

**Determinants of consultation in tertiary care**

In patients with chronic pain (especially those who attend problem back clinics) the management is often determined more by the patient's distress and demands for help than by the severity of the physical disease (see Chronic pain, p. 62).

Clinical observation of illness behaviour can be illustrated by a pain drawing (see figure below). The way in which the pain is drawn is strongly influenced by distress.

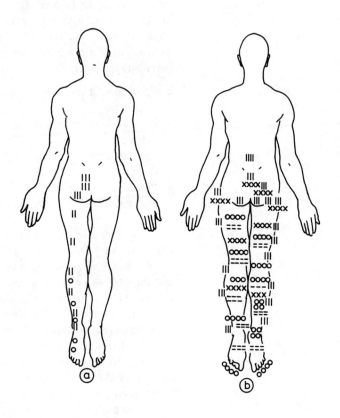

Pain drawing. Patient (a) describes the physical pattern of S1 sciatica from a disc prolapse. Patient (b) with simple backache, is communicating distress. Many patients do both to varying degrees. (‖ = pain; 0 = pins and needles; X = ache; === numbness.) Reproduced with permission from The British Medical Journal from Waddell G, Bircher M, Finlayson D, Main CJ. Symptoms and signs: physical disease or illness behaviour? *British Medical Journal*, 1984; **289**: 739–41.

Similarly, inappropriate descriptions of symptoms and inappropriate responses to physical examination in chronic backache have been shown to be clearly separable from the standard symptoms and signs of physical disease, and to be closely related to distress (see the table below). In general, patients showing a large amount of inappropriate illness behaviour receive significantly more treatment.

Illness behaviour is important in practice, because if it is not recognized it may lead to inappropriate treatment. This may be dangerous, as misdirected treatment, for example invasive surgery, may not only fail but actually reinforce and aggravate the illness behaviour (Waddell *et al.*, 1984, Porter, 1995).

|  | Physical disease | Inappropriate illness behaviour |
|---|---|---|
| **Symptoms** | | |
| Pain | Localized | Tailbone pain / Whole-leg pain |
| Numbness | Dermatomal | Whole-leg numbness |
| Weakness | Myotomal | Whole leg giving way |
| Time pattern | Variable | No intervals free of pain |
| Response to treatment | Variable benefit | Intolerance of treatment / Emergency admissions |
| **Signs** | | |
| Tenderness | Localized | Superficial, widespread, non-anatomical |
| Simulated rotation | No pain | Pain |
| Simulated axial loading | No pain | Pain |
| Raising straight leg | No change on distraction | Improves with distraction |
| Sensory | Dermatomal | Regional |
| Motor | Myotomal | Regional |
| General reaction | Appropriate pain | Over-reaction (crying out, facial expression, muscle tension, sweating, collapsing) |

**Management**

In the long run advances in management will be based on primary prevention through educational and community-health programmes, and through secondary prevention by advances in the education of doctors and other health-care professionals.

Management is usually based on strategies derived from learning theory and cognitive therapy (modifying patients' beliefs and assumptions). Treatment starts with reassurance – based on physical examination and relevant investigation – about the absence of serious organic pathology, and explanation concerning the ways that somatic symptoms may be associated with stressful experience. This is followed by:

- Differential reinforcement whereby undesirable behaviours, such as repetitive somatic complaints and inappropriate disability, are given minimal attention and more appropriate ways of coping with stressful events are positively reinforced.
- Rapid changes can be obtained in a controlled environment provided that staff are consistent in their approach.
- Involvement with close family members and other key figures in the patient's environment is essential, and long-term follow-up is regarded as necessary for at least 2 years.
- It is also essential to inform and incorporate into the management plan other medical personnel, particularly the GP, in order to maintain a consistent approach.

## Further reading

Benjamin S. Illness behaviour and neurosis. *Current Opinion in Psychiatry*, 1988; 142–9.
Craig TK, Boardman AP. Somatization in primary care settings. In: Bass C (ed.) *Somatization: Physical Symptoms and Psychological Illness*. Oxford: Blackwell Science Ltd, 1990; 73–103.
Mechanic D. *Journal of Chronic Disease,* 1962; **15:** 189–94.
Pilowsky I. Abnormal illness behaviour. *Psychotherapy and Psychosomatics*, 1986; **46:** 76–84.
Porter RW. *Back Injury and Litigation*. Oxford: BIOS Scientific Publishers, 1995.
Waddell G, Bircher M, Finlayson D, Main CJ. Symptoms and signs: physical disease or illness behaviour. *British Medical Journal,* 1984; **289:** 739–41.

## Related topics of interest

# INTOXICATED PATIENTS

Intoxication refers to the acute mental and physical effects (the latter are largely beyond the scope of this book, although they are mentioned where relevant) of ingesting alcohol or other psychoactive substances. Most intoxicants are self-administered, but when given by others without the consent of the subject may be *poisoning*, with forensic implications.

**Common intoxicants**

*1. Alcohol.*
(a) Commoner in males.
(b) Commonest cause overall.
(c) Very small proportion of episodes present to psychiatrists.

*2. Deliberate self-harm* (see Self mutilation, p. 306).
(a) 'Overdose', commonest in young females.
(b) Analgesics, prescribed drugs, especially psychoactive, often combined with alcohol.

*3. Illegal drugs.*
(a) Opiates: older age group predominantly.
(b) Polydrug abuse, especially hallucinogens, prescribed medications including benzodiazepines, inhalants: younger subjects.

**Reasons for presentation**

This may be due to the behaviour of the person (see below) or due to other factors, for example, a homeless alcoholic may be referred because his usual hostel happens to be full or because of a change in local police policy regarding the degree of disturbed behaviour of intoxicated persons which can be tolerated on the street.

**Who should assess?**

Most of these problems, which can be very difficult, present 'out of hours' to junior members of staff, who should not hesitate to seek the assistance of a senior colleague.

**Safe assessment**

All the standard factors (accompanied by colleagues, nearest to door, panic button, staff available for restraint if necessary, etc.) need to be considered in order to allow the assessment to take place with minimum risk to the assessor and others.

**Assessment: history**

History from the patient or others usually forms the basis of the diagnosis. Caution is required if the subject is unconscious or if the degree of intoxication seems to be out of proportion to consumption.

**Assessment: physical**

*1. Level of consciousness.*
This determines the immediate management. Semi- or unconscious patients require medical admission; for example, to prevent aspiration in the vomiting drunk with no gag reflex.

*2. Other factors?*
Physicians must carry out a full assessment (trauma/inflammatory/metabolic, etc.) before accepting intoxication as the sole cause as further problems frequently coexist; for example, head injury, hypoglycaemia.

*3. Physical signs.*
(a)  Alcohol: characteristic smell.
(b)  Injectors: needle tracks.
(c)  Opiates: pinpoint pupils.
(d)  Inhalants: smell of solvents, perioral rash.

*4. Special investigations.*
(a)  Breathalyser underused.
(b)  Alcoholic may be intoxicated with little obvious sign.

**Assessment: psychiatric**

During intoxication, the patient shows signs of an acute organic reaction, namely a greater or lesser reduction in levels of consciousness and global cognitive impairment, with marked abnormalities often present in emotional arousal, mood and behaviour: these resolve entirely with sobriety.

Thus, the cardinal point is that proper assessment cannot be carried out during intoxication. Requests for psychiatric examination of an intoxicated person are properly dealt with by deferring examination until the patient is sober. Supervision of the subject during this period should, if necessary, be provided by the referrer. Disturbed behaviour of an intoxicated person is not, generally speaking, reason for psychiatric in-patient admission.

# Common clinical problems

As always, old notes and telephone contact with informants, including previous carers, are an integral part of the assessment, and can save much time and trouble.

**The alcoholic**

The alcoholic frequently presents while intoxicated. He/she may request, or indeed demand, immediate psychiatric admission/ detoxification/rehabilitation. Appropriate management is to offer to re-assess when the patient is reasonably sober.

**The suicidal patient**

The suicidal patient who presents whilst intoxicated can be one of the most difficult problems in clinical psychiatry, particularly if there is no one to look after him/her until he/she is sober.

Most hospitals have a small, floating population of patients who present repeatedly, intoxicated and threatening suicide, with previous (often multiple) psychiatric admissions and/or a history of self-harm. Personality disorder is common, and such patients have frequently failed to benefit from several attempts at psychiatric treatment. Such patients are not likely to benefit from in-patient admission, but can be offered out-patient follow-up. However, there is a high risk of suicide, and the wise psychiatrist will discuss his/her management plan with colleagues before discharging the patient.

The mentally ill frequently attempt to self-medicate with alcohol, so a new presentation with, for example, a clear history of depression beforehand, should be assessed and managed according to the immediate risk of suicide (see Suicidal patients, p. 337). This is one of the few occasions when it is reasonable to consider the admission of an intoxicated patient to a psychiatric bed.

**Psychotic patients**

Patients with a known history of chronic psychosis not infrequently present whilst intoxicated. Management is largely that of the underlying condition.

Prominent delusions and hallucinations may follow consumption of MDMA ('ecstasy'), amphetamines, LSD and 'magic mushrooms'. These frequently present as acute psychotic reactions. Although they can be classed as intoxications, particularly with MDMA where delirium/physical problems occur, they are usually managed by psychiatric services (e.g. brief in-patient admission and neuroleptic medication).

**Violence**

Unless there is clear evidence of a major, pre-existing mental disorder, the intoxicated person who is violent is not a psychiatric problem. He/she should be dealt with by the police, as appropriate.

# Further reading

Brown TM. *Handbook of Emergency Psychiatry.* Edinburgh: Churchill Livingstone, 1990.

# Related topics of interest

# LEARNING

Associative learning describes the process of learning that events go together. It includes *classical conditioning*, learning that one event follows another, and *operant conditioning*, learning that a particular response by the individual will be followed by a particular consequence.

**Classical conditioning (respondent learning)**

Described by Pavlov in his classic experiments, the unconditioned stimulus (food) which leads to salivation (unconditioned response) is paired with the conditioned stimulus (e.g. light) which does not normally cause salivation. The conditioned stimulus (light) on its own then leads to salivation (now called the conditioned response). This type of learning is responsible for automatic behaviour, as the association does not need to be understood.

- *Reinforcement*. The conditioned association is strengthened by reinforcement, by continued and repeated associations. If reinforcement does not continue, extinction occurs (this is not the same as forgetting). Reinforcement is more effective if the stimuli are closely related in time (time contiguity). Response strength is measured by the number of continued responses during extinction.
- *Generalization* is when similar stimuli to the conditioned stimulus also produce the conditioned response.
- *Discrimination* between different but similar stimuli can be produced by differential reinforcement.
- *Predictability*. The strength of the association is directly related to the predictability of the conditioned stimulus.
- *Blocking*. A previous association can block the development of a new association.

**Operant conditioning (instrumental learning)**

This describes learning that a particular behaviour leads to a particular goal (Skinner). This is learning by 'law of effect' (Thorndike) whereby responses which are followed by positive consequences are selected. In reward training behaviour increases because the consequences are rewarding. The operantly conditioned response (e.g. pressing a food lever) is reinforced by the reward (e.g. food).

Reinforcement changes the likelihood of a response being made. Primary reinforcers act through satisfying a basic drive (food, sex), and secondary (or conditioned) reinforcers act because they have been associated with a primary reinforcer; examples include money and praise.

Reinforcement can be continuous, fixed ratio or interval, or variable interval or ratio. Variable ratio reinforcement is associated with the slowest rate of extinction. Reinforcement can be positive or negative; negative reinforcement involves increasing a particular behaviour because it involves the removal of something unpleasant. This is different from punishment which involves suppressing a response because of its unpleasant consequences. Operant conditioning is most effective when the organism perceives the reinforcement as being under its control.

**Learning and psychiatric disorders**

Behavioural theories of anxiety and phobias employ the principles of conditioning. A combination of classical and operant conditioning can explain the origin of phobias, with the addition of the concept of preparedness. Pairing of a neutral event/object with a traumatic event (classical conditioning) sets up the phobia and this is reinforced by avoidance (operant conditioning involving avoidance training). Pairing may be directly by experience or learnt vicariously, for example, from parents. Incubation, which describes how the strength of an emotional conditioned response increases with repeated brief exposures to the stimulus, also perpetuates the phobia. Preparedness is a concept whereby certain objects, for example, spiders, the dark, are much more likely to be the subject of phobias because humans are biologically predisposed to react with fear to certain stimuli, and in such circumstances conditioning occurs rapidly and is very resistant to extinction.

**Learning and psychological treatments**

Therapies based on behavioural principles concentrate on the behaviour itself rather than the reasons for it. The goals are circumscribed, and the techniques are evaluated experimentally.

*1. Systematic desensitization.* This involves deconditioning or counter-conditioning by substituting a response which is incompatible with anxiety (i.e. relaxation). Patients learn to relax then, having composed a graded hierarchy, expose themselves (actual or imagined) to these stages in turn whilst staying relaxed.

*2. Positive reinforcement and extinction.* Systematic reinforcement (operant conditioning) is an effective way of modifying behaviour and involves selectively reinforcing desired behaviour with rewards, and ignoring undesirable behaviour.

*3. Shaping (operant conditioning).* This is used when the desired behaviour is rare or absent. It involves reinforcing approximate behaviour and, by doing this in steps, the reinforced behaviour becomes closer to the desired behaviour. It is used, for example for autistic children where rewards can be changed from primary ones, for example, food, to social rewards, for example, praise, attention and privileges.

*4. Autoshaping.* This is a mixture of operant and classical conditioning. The novel behaviour happens spontaneously in response to a secondary reinforcer.

*5. Token economies (operant conditioning)* employ tokens which can be exchanged for privileges and encourage socially appropriate behaviour in chronic, regressed patients (generally hospital based).

*6. Modelling.* This is based on observational learning and is a combination of classical and operant conditioning (Bandura). Symbolic modelling (watching on film) and live modelling with participation (watching a model and also completing feared activities with encouragement) are effective for specific phobias. It is also effective for social skills training because observational learning is especially important in the acquisition of social behaviour and skills. This is particularly so if learnt from someone of high status, competence and social power who has something in common with the observer.

*7. Biofeedback.* This uses operantly conditioned responses to information about heart rate and blood pressure and is effective in stress management in conjunction with relaxation training.

Other behavioural techniques include:

- Behaviour rehearsal or role-playing.
- Self-regulation which includes monitoring and self-reinforcement.
- Self-punishment.
- Control of stimulus conditions.
- Development of incompatible responses to modify behaviour.

# Further reading

Atkinson RL, Atkinson RC, Smith EE, Hilgard ER. *Introduction to Psychology*, 9th Edn. Harcourt, Brace, Jovanovich, 1987; 214–44.

# Related topics of interest

# LEGAL PROCESS

A psychiatrist may have a role in the legal process, particularly of criminal cases, at several stages, and these are considered in turn here.

**Civil sections**

1. *Admission for assessment (or assessment then treatment).* (Section 2, Mental Health Act (MHA) 1983). Application is by an approved social worker (ASW) or nearest relative; recommendations by two doctors, one of whom is Section 12 approved. The grounds are that there is evidence of a mental disorder and there is risk to the patient or others. The period of detention is up to 28 days with the right to a Mental Health Tribunal (MHRT).

2. *Admission for treatment* (Section 3, MHA 1983). Application is by an ASW or nearest relative; recommendations by two doctors, one of whom is Section 12 approved. The grounds are that:

- The patient suffers from mental illness, mental impairment, severe mental impairment or psychopathic disorder requiring treatment in hospital.
- In the case of the latter two conditions that treatment will alleviate or prevent deterioration.
- That there is risk to the patient or others.

The period of detention is up to 6 months (renewable), with the right to MHRTs.

3. *Admission for assessment in an emergency* (Section 4, MHA 1983). Application is by an ASW or nearest relative; one recommendation by a doctor who preferably knows the patient. The grounds are as for Section 2, and the period of detention is for 72 hours. It is rarely used.

4. *Detention of patients already in hospital* (Section 5(2), MHA 1983). Application is by the doctor in charge or their nominated deputy. Detention is for 72 hours, or until assessment for Section 2 or Section 3 can be carried out.

5. *Nurse's holding power* (Section 5(4), MHA). Detention of a patient already in hospital for up to 6 hours by a registered mental nurse, until a doctor can assess for detention under Section 5(2).

6. *Warrant to find and remove mentally disordered persons* (Section 135, MHA 1983). Requested by an ASW from a

magistrate. The warrant is issued to a police officer, who is then accompanied by an ASW and a doctor.

*7. Removal to a place of safety of mentally disordered persons from a public place* (Section 136, MHA 1983). Carried out by a police officer.

**Psychiatric intervention before conviction**

*1. Remand.*
(a) *Remand to hospital for assessment* (Section 35, Mental Health Act (MHA), 1983) is available on the basis of one medical opinion. A hospital bed must be available. The defendant must agree and accept treatment voluntarily.
(b) *Remand to hospital for treatment* (Section 36, MHA 1983) provides for compulsory treatment and requires two medical recommendations. It does not include psychopathic disorder.
(c) *Remand on bail for out-patient psychiatric assessment.* The defendant may be allowed to remain in the community before a trial and attend psychiatric out-patient sessions for assessment.
(d) *Remand in custody for psychiatric opinion.* The defendant is kept in custody pending the trial. This is a quick method of dealing with the case, which most courts may employ if there is a delay in obtaining a psychiatric opinion or a bed.
(e) *Court diversion schemes* have existed since 1990 to increase the availability of psychiatric opinion to the court to reduce unnecessary remands in custody. National provision of these schemes is patchy; in 1992 only a quarter of purchasing health authorities had a policy for such provision.

*2. Fitness to plead.*
This depends on the defendant's mental state at the time of trial, and is distinct from fitness to appear in court. Unfitness to plead is determined by a jury on medical evidence and is subject to appeal. The defendant must be able to:

- Understand the charge.
- Instruct a lawyer.
- Challenge a juror.
- Plead to the charge.
- Understand the offence.

Unfitness to plead most commonly results from severe mental illness or learning disability. The defendant may return to trial at a later date if he/she subsequently becomes fit to plead. Alternatively, a 'trial of facts' may take place. The disposal of the defendant is then at the judge's discretion. Options include hospital admission with or without a restriction order, guardianship order, probation with a condition of treatment and absolute discharge.

3. *Psychiatric defences.*

(a) *Insanity defence.* This depends on impaired reasoning due to disease of the mind at the time of committing the act. Thus psychiatric assessment must determine whether there was a disease of the mind present and whether it resulted in the defendant's reasoning being defective. Sentencing occurs at the discretion of the judge. Disposal options are the same as for a conviction on the facts after a finding of unfitness to plead.

(b) *Diminished responsibility.* This applies only to murder. It reduces the crime from murder to manslaughter. The defendant is judged on the basis of medical evidence to have been suffering from an '. . . abnormality of mind . . . as substantially impaired his mental responsibility for his acts'. Included in this category have been those with schizophrenia, other psychoses, depression, personality disorder, premenstrual tension, transient situational disturbance and homosexual panic.

(c) *The survivor of a suicide pact* will be convicted of manslaughter rather than murder.

(d) *Infanticide.* This is the killing by a mother (by action or omission) of her child under the age of 1 year, at a time when the balance of her mind was disturbed by the effect of having given birth to the child or by the effect of lactation. A lesser degree of abnormality of mind is required than when a diminished responsibility verdict is sought. In practice, women with severe mental illness who kill are usually found guilty on grounds of diminished responsibility.

(e) *Legal automatism.* If the mind does not have the capacity to have a guilty intent (*mens rea*) at the time of the act, then the defence of automatism may be used. This describes unconscious automatic behaviour, and is different from clinically defined automatic behaviour (e.g. temporal lobe epilepsy).

(f) *Sane automatism.* The event is unlikely to recur, and is said to be due to 'external' events, for example, confusional state, concussion, reflex actions following a shock (e.g. bee sting), dissociative states, night terrors, hypoglycaemia. The defendant is free to leave the court.

(g) *Insane automatism*. This is judged as being likely to recur and to be due to an 'internal' cause. Results in admission under hospital and restriction orders, for example, brain disease, tumour, epilepsy, sleep-walking.

The lists do not indicate a logical physical basis to the distinction between sane and insane automatism.

*4. Substance misuse*

(a) Insanity caused by intoxication (drug-induced psychosis) or dependence (delirium tremens) results in the possibility of a defence of insanity as for any other cause. Long-term sequelae of alcohol or drug use resulting in brain damage/dementia may lead to a defence of diminished responsibility.

(b) Intoxication which prevents the capacity of guilty intent can be a defence in certain crimes: murder, wounding with intent, burglary with intent to steal, handling stolen goods. It would not apply to manslaughter, malicious wounding, assault occasioning actual bodily harm, common assault or rape, since the type of intent is held under law to be different in these two lists.

(c) Intoxication simply resulting in disinhibition is no defence.

*5. Amnesia.* If this is not associated with a specific psychiatric disorder, for example psychosis or head injury, it is not accepted as a medical defence.

**Psychiatric disposals after conviction**

*1. Hospital order (Section 37(2), MHA 1983).* Disposals for the offence include a prison sentence. This order is not applicable to murder. The magistrates court can make a hospital order (Section 37(3)) without a conviction. A recommendation is required from two doctors that the offender suffers from mental disorder and is appropriately detained in hospital for treatment. A hospital bed should be available within 28 days of sentencing. The duration of detention is for 6 months and the order is renewable.

*2. Interim hospital order (Section 38, MHA 1983).* This has similar conditions to Section 37. The order lasts for 12 weeks and is renewable. Its purpose is to assess response to treatment but it is little used in practice.

3. *Guardianship order (Section 37(1), MHA 1983).* The procedure is like that of Section 37.2. Its purpose is to secure care and attention, rather than treatment, for the offender. The local authority social services or an approved person must be willing to receive the offender into their care.

4. *Restriction order (Section 41, MHA 1983).* The patient on Section 37(2) may not be granted leave or be transferred to another hospital without the consent of the Home Secretary. Discharge from a restriction order is absolute or conditional (the patient remains liable to recall and must be supervised by a doctor and social worker/probation officer. Conditions may be attached to a place of residence).

5. *Probation with a condition of treatment. (Section 9(3), Criminal Justice Act 1991).* The offender requires treatment but does not need to be detained. The provisions of the order will be determined on an individual basis and the offender must agree to them.

# Further reading

Bowden P. Psychiatry and criminal proceedings. In: *Seminars in Practical Forensic Psychiatry.* London: Gaskell, 1995; Chap. 5, 106–34.
Grounds A. The criminal justice system. In: Chiswick D, Cope R (eds) *Seminars in Practical Forensic Psychiatry.* London: Gaskell, 1995; 87–105.

# Related topics of interest

Addiction – physical and psychological aspects (p. 5)
Dangerousness assessment (p. 73)

# MEDICALLY UNEXPLAINED SYMPTOMS

The conditions considered in this topic are dissociative (conversion) disorder, somatization disorder (SD), hypochondriasis, factitious disorder and malingering. A common related topic is chronic fatigue syndrome, referred to as neurasthenia (F48.0) in ICD-10 (see Chronic fatigue syndrome, p.59).

The conditions have in common the presence of physical symptoms which are not explained by a medical cause. It is not uncommon for an individual patient to show clinical features of more than one of the categories.

**The relationship between symptoms and somatization**

People experience bodily sensations and these become symptoms when the person considers them to represent disease.

The decision to consult is determined by a balance between the seriousness with which the symptoms are viewed (illness worry) and the utility of the sick role for that person at that time.

*Disease* is defined in terms of objective biological abnormalities in the structure and/or function of bodily organs and systems (Sharpe *et al.*, 1995).

Somatization is a term used to describe a process and refers to the somatic manifestation of psychological distress. The process of somatization occurs in several of the above conditions, but it is also part of normal behaviour and does not in itself indicate psychopathology.

**Dissociative disorders**

(a) The term 'conversion disorder' is also used to describe these conditions and reflects the mechanism which is thought to result in this presentation. Namely that dangerous, threatening or otherwise unpleasant ideas that the patient has are made tolerable by their conversion into physical symptoms.

(b) Loss or impairment of some bodily function is central. The function affected is often neurological leading to paralysis, convulsions or numbness, but may also be mental leading to psychogenic amnesia, fugue or stupor.

(c) In contrast to the classical 'la belle indifference', patients have been shown to have high levels of anxiety and arousal.

(d) There is often an acute onset in clear relation to stressful life events or difficulties which may be insoluble.

(e) In motor loss secondary physical symptoms, for example muscle wasting and contractures, may develop when the condition is prolonged.

(f) Psychogenic amnesia, fugue and stupor result in sudden short-lived loss of integrative functions of consciousness leading to symptoms including memory loss, wandering and possibly the acquisition of a new personality. Memory impairment unaccompanied by any other cognitive deficits is rarely organic in nature.
- Fugue involves wandering which may be purposeful and difficult to distinguish from malingering.
- Stupor can be differentiated from that due to affective illness by its sudden onset.
- The existence of multiple personalities is highly contentious and most common in the USA, where it often occurs in the context of an intense psychotherapeutic relationship.

**Somatization disorder (SD)**

(a) Before 1980 this was known as Briquet's syndrome and before 1970, as St Louis hysteria.

(b) It consists of chronic (usually at least 2 years' duration in ICD-10) reports of multiple somatic complaints in a variety of organs and bodily parts. Commonly affected organ systems are:
- Gastrointestinal (GI) – pain, belching, regurgitation, vomiting, nausea.
- Skin – itching, burning, tingling, numbness, soreness.
- Neurological.
- Gynaecological.

(c) The behaviour can usually be recognized as beginning in childhood.

(d) There is some evidence that SD runs in families, although the existence of a genetic as opposed to a familial component has not been identified. There is an excess of psychopathic personality and alcoholism in male relatives. It is much more common in, though probably not exclusive to, women.

(e) Estimates of prevalence:

| | |
|---|---|
| Community (Epidemiology Catchment Area (USA)) | 0.38% |
| Medical out-patient clinic (USA) | 9.0% |
| University consulting service (USA) | 6.0% |

(f) Depression and anxiety are common and should be treated in their own right.

(g) Somatoform autonomic dysfunction is a related disorder (included in ICD-10 but not DSM-IV) in which symptoms are recognizable as being caused by autonomic dysfunction. Systems involved are:

- Heart and cardiovascular (non-cardiac chest pain).
- Upper GI (dyspepsia, hiccough).
- Lower GI (irritable bowel syndrome).
- Respiratory (hyperventilation).
- Genitourinary (urinary frequency).

(h) Persistent somatoform pain disorder is also a related condition (see Chronic pain, p. 62).

**Hypochondriacal disorder**

(a) This is characterized by the conviction of the presence of a disease or fear of developing a disease. It is distinguished from SD by preoccupation with the cause of symptoms rather than with the seeking of symptom relief, but overlap with SD has been described.

(b) Hypochondriacal symptoms occur in:

- Hypochondriacal disorder.
- Depressive disorder.
- Delusional disorder (somatic type).
- Panic disorder.

Twenty per cent of people presenting with hypochondriacal symptoms are regarded as having HD. The primary disorder may be less amenable to treatment than those secondary to another condition. A case has been made for a hypochondriacal personality disorder.

(c) Reassurance is a key concept in the management of (non-psychotic) hypochondriacal presentations. The reaction of the doctor at initial consultation about a symptom can be a factor leading to the development of hypochondriacal ideas. Any of the following can help to perpetuate hypochondriacal symptoms:

- Failure to use simple terminology and explanations.
- Conflicting statements within the consultation.
- Conflicting medical opinions.
- Perceived disinterest and hostility.
- Making false predictions.

A doctor can only give effective reassurance after listening to and indeed eliciting the patient's fears and attributions in detail. It may include sympathetic clarification of previous misunderstandings. Later in the treatment the provision of reassurance whenever the patient requests it is unhelpful (Warwick, 1992). Treatment should involve family and other medical or non-statutory agencies who may be involved if it is to be effective.

**Factitious disorders**

(a) Symptoms or signs are consciously feigned or produced. Any bodily system can be involved and so patients may present in any branch of medicine, including psychiatry and surgery. The patient is aware that they are presenting a fictitious history, feigning symptoms or self-inflicting signs. However, they remain unaware of the psychological processes behind their actions.

(b) Epidemiology does not give accurate figures but it is a rare condition.

(c) Aetiological features are thought to include:
  • Parental abuse or abandonment.
  • Early experiences with chronic illness in self or others.
  • Relationship with a physician or other medical worker in the past.
  • Employment in the medical field.
  • Experiences of medical mismanagement.

(d) The underlying psychological processes can be understood as follows:
  • A desire to achieve patient status and thus certain benefits at the same time as relinquishing the demands of good health, such as the expectation of success at work.
  • Playing out their conflicts within the medical field.

(e) There are no systematic studies of treatment. Engaging the patient in treatment is vital. Close liaison between the medical doctor and psychiatrist is essential. Best practice usually involves the presence of both at a supportive interview where the patient is confronted with the cause of the symptoms and offered help (Reich and Gottfried, 1981). Help will involve psychological support, and in some cases physical treatment such as physiotherapy.

(f) Munchhausen's syndrome is a rare and severe form of the condition which occurs usually in men and indicates severe personality dysfunction. The often itinerant nature of their behaviour makes engagement in treatment rare, although the same principles apply; most leave the ward or casualty department once they have been confronted to try their luck elsewhere.

# Further reading

Bass C. Patients with chronic somatization: what can the psychiatrist offer? In: Hawton K, Cowen P (eds) *Practical Problems in Clinical Psychiatry*. Oxford: Oxford University Press, 1992; 105–15.

Freeman CP. Neurotic disorders. In: Kendell RE, Zealley AK (eds) *Companion to Psychiatric Studies*. Edinburgh: Churchill Livingstone, 1988; chap 19.

Reich P, Gottfried LA. Factitious disorders in a teaching hospital. *Annals of Internal Medicine*, 1981; **99:** 240–7.

Sharpe M, Mayon R, Bass C. Concepts, theories, and terminology. In: Mayon R, Bass C, Sharpe M. *Treatment of Functional Somatic Symptoms*. Oxford: Oxford University Press, 1995.

Warwick H. Provision of appropriate and effective reassurance. *International Review of Psychiatry*, 1992; **4:** 76–80.

# Related topics of interest

# MEMORY

Memory is a subject that can sometimes cause confusion, as the basic terms (for example, short-term and long-term memory) are used in slightly different ways by psychologists and psychiatrists. Great advances have been made in the last 20 years in understanding the psychophysiological basis of memory.

A basic division can be made into short-term and long-term memory, and within these, into processes concerned with *encoding, storage* and *retrieval,* each of which can be affected independently of the others (Atkinson *et al.,* 1993).

**The psychological organization of memory and attention**

Information from sense organs is initially encoded and stored in a *short-term store* (STS, otherwise known as the acoustic/visual buffer) where it is subject to very basic processing only. The memory trace in STS is very short-lived (of the order of about a second) and information for further processing is selected by attentional processes. These can be conceived as a single channel filter for each sensory modality, so it is not possible to attend simultaneously to more than one input through each modality (although rapid switching of attention may allow a subject to attend, for example, to two conversations at once). The attentional filters for the modalities function independently, so it is quite possible for people to learn simultaneously to perform visio-spatial and auditory/linguistic tasks (for example, sight-reading music simultaneously whilst repeating a string of words fed into the ears by headphones — 'shadowing'). The very basic processing afforded to all information in the STS allows attention to be switched to potentially significant changes in the environment, which would be missed if the limited attention channel was immediately after perception. It is the STS which allows such phenomena as hearing a clock stop ticking, or hearing one's name in someone else's (unattended) conversation (the 'cocktail party pheno-menon').

Information subject to attentional processing is stored in *short-term memory* (STM) in which it is stored in the form of electrical activity within neurones. STM has a limited capacity (usually about seven 'chunks' of information), and is also referred to as 'working memory', because of its role in conscious thought, where it is used to 'hold things in mind'. There seems to be a separate short-term memory for processing language, so some patients with impaired STM may retain simple sentences normally, and vice versa. Retrieval from STM is relatively error-free and complete (the seven items are usually recalled correctly).

The information in STM decays rapidly (over the order of about a minute), or is displaced by new incoming information. It is lost unless it is transferred to *long-term memory* (LTM), through rehearsal or other forms of consolidation. LTM is initially encoded as electrical traces, which are disrupted, for example, by electroconvulsive therapy (ECT) or epilepsy, then subsequently stored through more permanent changes, probably synapse formation, which can be prevented by inhibitors of protein synthesis.

**Memory and the psychiatric mental state**

The psychiatric term STM is tested by such things as immediate sentence recall or digit span, and attention is tested by serial sevens. LTM is tested by delayed sentence recall, or recall of a name and address after five minutes. Very long-term recall is tested by asking for recent news items, or biographical details.

*1. Explicit and implicit memory.* Studies of brain lesions indicate clearly that there are two major types of memory. Explicit (conscious, declarative or propositional) memory, which is conscious memory for facts and day-to-day events, is separate from implicit (unconscious, procedural, or non-declarative) memory, which encodes concrete visio-spatial structural information and affective valence.

Declarative (conscious) memory is concept based and is stored in symbolic form (as explicit words, images, or symbols which are available to consciousness). It can be improved by rehearsal, 'chunking', or other mnemonic strategies designed to increase the depth of information processing. Non-declarative memory involves presemantic processing, is percept-driven, is not explicitly available to consciousness, and is expressed through performance. It is data driven, and is unaffected by cognitive mnemonic strategies. Non-declarative memory allows cumulative changes in perceptual and response systems, and the development of new skill and habits, motor learning, visio-spatial memory, and simple conditioning (e.g. conditioned fear).

*2. Disorders of explicit memory.* Explicit memory disorders are of several types:

- *Dementia.* Memory impairment is global, with both retention and recall, of recent and remote events, being affected progressively.
- The *amnestic syndrome*, of which two types can be distinguished, involving failure of information storage or

information retrieval. In both, immediate memory is unaffected, so digit span, etc., are normal. Failure of information retrieval is seen in Korsakoff's psychosis, where there is destruction of the mamillary bodies and periventricular grey matter. It is characterized by a dense anterograde amnesia (i.e. from the time of injury forwards), variable retrograde amnesia, lack of insight and confabulation. Disorders of information storage are seen in patients with bilateral damage to medial temporal structures, particularly those around the hippocampus, for example as a result of herpes simplex encephalitis, and the subject usually retains full insight. The classic example of this is Milner's patient H.M. who had a bilateral temporal lobectomy for intractable epilepsy, and has had a complete amnestic state for 30 years. Implicit memory is completely unaffected in amnestic patients.

- *Psychogenic fugue*, in which selective memory loss occurs for significant personal and biographical information, usually in the context of some severe psychosocial stressor. The memory loss is restricted, and there is no impairment of the capacity to form new memories, nor of ability to recall past events of a general nature.

**Neuroanatomical substrates of memory**

*1. Immediate and explicit memory.* Widespread co-ordinated neocortical activity underlies perception and immediate memory, but for this to be transformed into stable long-term memory, the medial temporal lobe memory system (as well as linked areas of the basal forebrain) must be involved. Central to this is the hippocampus (especially area CA2), which probably works by forming conjunctions between otherwise cortically unrelated stimuli. The hippocampal system (including entorhinal, perirhinal and parahippocampal cortex) thus forms an 'index' for memory. Its role is in rapidly learning new information, available to consciousness, but this role is temporary. More permanent memory, developing over a period of weeks, presumably as a result of new synapse formation, is independent of the medial temporal lobe. Thus people with Korsakoff's psychosis have only a partial retrograde amnesia, very remote memory remaining intact.

*2. Implicit memory.* This is processed and stored in different areas, particularly the amygdala, and a cortico-striatal system including the sensory cortical areas, and the caudate and putamen.

# Further reading

Atkinson RL, Atkinson RG, Smith EE, Bem DJ. *Introduction to Psychology*, 11th Edn. Orlando: Harcourt Brace Jovanovitch College Publishers, 1993; 289–316.

Squire LR, Zola Morgan S. The medial temporal lobe memory system. *Science,* 1991; **253:** 13806.

# Related topics of interest

# MENTAL HANDICAP – AUTISM

A discussion of the features of autism should also include descriptions of Asperger's syndrome, Rett's syndrome and disintegrative disorder.

**Autism**

*1. Definition.* The modern concept of autism derives from Kanner's description in the 1940s. This is a disorder characterized by delayed and abnormal development of social relationships and language. The other principle features are resistance to change, mannerisms, unusual attachment to objects and acute emotional reactions. ICD-10 requires that these abnormalities be apparent before the age of three years, DSM-III-R has onset in infancy or childhood. The features may be present from birth or appear after a period of normal development.

*2. Features.* These can be divided into behavioural and intellectual abnormalities, and associated physical disorders.

(a) *Behavioural abnormalities.* The most prominent feature is abnormality of social interactions and relationships. The child may be abnormal from birth, being less responsive, not enjoying physical contact and avoiding eye contact. At two to three years the child will prefer its own company and not seek out its parents for comfort. With age other abnormalities appear, for example not playing with other children. In puberty the individual has abnormal relationships with a lack of awareness for other people's opinions or feelings. Friendships with peers are uncommon.

Both verbal and non-verbal communication are abnormal. Comprehension and expression are delayed and very significantly delayed in almost half of autistic individuals. When speech does develop there are particular abnormalities such as echolalia and neologisms. The echolalia may be responsible for pronomial reversal ('you want' instead of 'I want'). Language is often very sporadic. Non-verbal communication is also affected, for example the absence of gestures. There is also little imaginative play or thought, probably related to the absence of symbolic thought in autism.

Mannerisms are common, and characteristically are twirling, walking on tiptoe or flapping the hands. There may be mannerisms of speech. Autistic children often have stereotyped rituals to their life which, if disturbed, cause great distress, and sometimes challenging behaviour. They often become attached to strange objects like tins, rather than the usual cuddly toys. Emotional outbursts are common, for example of anger, excitement or anxiety. These are precipitated by what would normally be seen as minor events.

Autistic children may also have problems with sleeping, and with soiling and wetting.

(b) *Intellectual.* IQ is assessed by measuring non-verbal development because of the abnormalities of language. IQ is below 70 in 70% and below 50 in 50%. However 5% have an IQ over 100. Autistic children find tasks involving symbolic thought or empathy difficult. They may have areas of particular ability, although it is rare for this to be more than above average. When developed to an unusual degree the ability is often mathematical or depends on memory skills.

(c) *Physical.* Epilepsy occurs in about 15%, in adolescence, although it is often mild. Interestingly, about one-fifth of autistic children deteriorate cognitively around puberty. Autism is associated with a range of physical disorders (see Aetiology, below).

*3. Epidemiology.*

Autism occurs in approximately 20 per 10 000 according to recent studies. The sex ratio is greater for males, 4:1. It occurs across the social classes and in all countries studied.

*4. Aetiology.*

There is controversy about the underlying cognitive deficit, but this may include difficulty perceiving facial expression and lack of symbolic thought, which then lead to the other clinical features. It is now clearer that there is some degree of brain dysfunction underlying autism (rather than it being a psychological reaction).

- *Genetic factors.* Autism is familial (a rate of 2% in siblings) with greater concordance in monozygotic than dizygotic twins (35% to 0%). Chromosomal abnormalities, particularly fragile X, contribute to a small proportion of cases.
- *Physical factors.* There is an excess of a range of physical conditions related to pregnancy and childbirth. Specific disorders include rubella, syphilis, phenylkelonuria,

tuberose sclerosis, fragile X and disorders of unknown aetiology, for example, infantile spasms. No consistent neuroanatomical or biochemical abnormality has yet been established.

- *Family/parents.* Previous theories that autism is caused by abnormal parental or family behaviour have been discredited. Fathers of autistic children have a higher prevalence of schizoid personality traits but this is likely to be genetically determined. Conversely autistic children can have a profound effect on their families, principally because of their abnormalities in relationships.

*5. Management.* The diagnosis is made clinically, but further investigations should be carried out to investigate associated central nervous system (CNS) abnormalities and exclude other pervasive developmental disorders, early schizophrenia and emotional disorder in a child with learning disabilities. These investigations should include chromosomal culture, electroencephalogram (EEG) and computerized tomography (CT) or magnetic resonance imaging (MRI).

Treatment is generally symptomatic and involves support, education and reassurance for the family, and behavioural and educational management for the child. Effective management can make a significant difference to the outcome. Pharmacological interventions that are currently being evaluated include fenfluramine, lithium, haloperidol and naltrexone. There is no specific treatment for the underlying deficits.

*6. Outcome.* This is generally poor with the majority being dependent as adults, although a small proportion (15%) achieve a degree of independence and may have a job. Prognosis is related to intelligence, and is adversely affected by epilepsy and behavioural problems. However children do generally continue to develop through childhood, and the family and educational input is very important in the overall outcome.

**Asperger's syndrome**

Individuals with Asperger's syndrome are distant, aloof and lacking in empathy. They are rigid, sensitive to criticism and have unusual, often solitary, interests. In general, the picture is similar to autism but without the cognitive impairment. The outcome in adult life is variable, but even with fully independent living there are often problems with anxiety, depression and obsessional symptoms. Recent studies have indicated that Asperger's syndrome is at least three times as common as autism.

It is probably best to view this syndrome as part of the autism spectrum, as high-functioning autism. In particular they appear to be genetically related as there are reports of families containing individuals both with autism and Asperger's syndrome. There are similarities with schizoid personality disorder but research indicates that they are different entities. This view is supported by evidence that Asperger's syndrome patients often have a history of abnormalities in infancy, and also that schizoid personality disorder predisposes to schizophrenia, whereas there is no association between Asperger's syndrome and schizophrenia.

**Rett's syndrome**

This is a syndrome found in girls who develop relatively normally until the age of about two years and then develop autistic features, loss of purposeful hand movements, and abnormal movements and muscle tone. The abnormal movements are characteristically hand washing or wringing. The same deterioration can occur without the autistic characteristics.

**Disintegrative disorder**

In this disorder, cognitive function deteriorates after a period of normal development, usually longer than two years. The prognosis is similar to or worse than autism and may or may not be progressive. Most cases are idiopathic.

## Further reading

Berney TP. Autism. *Current Opinion in Psychiatry*, 1995; **8:** 286–9.
Frith U. *Autism and Asperger Syndrome*. Cambridge: Cambridge University Press, 1991.
Gillberg C. Autism and pervasive developmental disorders. *Journal of Child Psychology and Psychiatry*, 1990; **31:** 99–119.
Graham P. *Child psychiatry: a developmental approach,* 2nd Edn. Oxford: Oxford Medical Publications, 1991.
Kanner L. Autistic disturbance of affective contact. *Nervous Child*, 1943; **2:** 217–50.

## Related topics of interest

# MENTAL HANDICAP – CHALLENGING BEHAVIOUR

**Definition and prevalence**

Challenging behaviour has been defined as 'behaviour of such an intensity, frequency or duration that the physical safety of the person or others is placed in serious jeopardy, or behaviour which is likely to seriously limit or deny access to and use of ordinary community facilities'. This emphasizes the way in which behaviour may challenge the system of care. The most common forms of challenging behaviour are: aggression, damage to the environment, self-injury and non-compliance. Many surveys have estimated the overall prevalence of such behaviours to be about 40% in people with mild mental handicap and 50% in those with moderate or severe mental handicap. Self-injury is particularly common in people with sensory impairments, whilst sleep problems, aggression and self-injury are associated with communication problems. Challenging behaviour is more common in those with progressively more severe mental handicap and there is no significant decline in the proportion displaying such behaviours as age increases. Other than the overall level of handicap, challenging behaviours and psychiatric disorders are the most common reasons for breakdown of community placements.

**Aetiology**

This is often multifactorial and biological, psychological and social factors should be considered. Medical illnesses are more common in people with a mental handicap and they may be difficult to diagnose in the presence of limited language to report symptoms. Dental caries, constipation and various infections are all common in this population and may cause pain which is acted out as challenging behaviour. Many mental handicap syndromes are associated with specific medical complications. Behavioural phenotypes whereby behavioural abnormalities arise as a more or less direct expression of the genotype may be relevant, and examples include self-injurious behaviour in Lesch–Nyhan and Prader–Willi syndromes.

Psychiatric disorder is about four times as common in children and adults with mental handicap as in the general population. The full range of psychiatric disorders encountered in the general population may be seen, and it is important to look for other symptoms of such syndromes in people who find describing internal states very difficult or impossible. People with mental handicap may be subject to social disadvantage for a variety of reasons which may be important in the aetiology of challenging behaviour, either alone or in combination with the above factors (see Mental handicap – social issues, p. 200).

**Assessment**

This should be multidisciplinary. At all times, causes and effects of mental handicap and causes and effects of challenging behaviour should be considered. A comprehensive history should be taken and mental state examination is often performed across several settings, as it may be difficult to gain full compliance. Physical examination should concentrate on signs of general health problems and the neurological system. Medical investigations may be specific to the suspected aetiology of the mental handicap as well as general health screening.

Neuroimaging and electroencephalogram (EEG) studies may be indicated – the latter especially as prodromal, pre-, peri- or post-ictal events can occasionally present as challenging behaviour. Psychological investigations may include background information from formal psychometry, adaptive behaviour or criterion-referenced tests. These will give a picture of relative strengths and weaknesses which may inform clinical management. More specifically, some form of behavioural assessment including direct observations will be undertaken. Careful consideration of antecedents, specific behaviours and consequences over time will allow a 'functional analysis' which refers to the determination of the function of the various stimuli impinging upon the individual as a precursor to planning treatment.

**Treatment**

Underlying physical illness or psychiatric disorder should be treated accordingly. The aim is to provide positive and rewarding behaviours and experiences – not just to abolish challenging behaviour. Broad social issues may need to be addressed, especially residential placement or educational provision. Behavioural techniques are the mainstay of treatment for most challenging behaviours. These may include: stimulus control, differential reinforcement of other behaviours (including shaping, backward chaining, or use of the Premack principle), extinction, time out or response cost.

There is a lack of large-scale systematic studies of psycho-dynamic psychotherapy for challenging behaviour in mental handicap. Supportive family therapy is often helpful and valued. Medication may be used in the significant group of people who do not respond to other treatments and in whom the anxiolytic and anti-agitation properties of antipsychotics may allow symptomatic relief and the resumption of other treatments. Haloperidol, thioridazine, chlorpromazine and zuclopenthixol have been shown to reduce assaults, self-injurious behaviours, hyperactivity and stereotypes. It should be noted that new learning may be promoted at lower doses but diminished at higher doses of such medication. Opioid blockers such as naltrexone have been successfully used in the treatment of severe self-injurious behaviours, where such mediating mechanisms, are suspected. Stimulant medication such as dexamphetamine sulphate may prove helpful in reducing hyperactivity associated with challenging behaviour in mild mental handicap but less so in severe cases, and responses and side-effects are often idiosyncratic. Lithium and carbamazepine are sometimes used in the management of aggressive behaviours but large-scale studies in mental handicap are lacking.

## Further reading

Aman MG, Singh NN (eds). *Psychopharmacology and the Developmental Disabilities.* New York: Springer Verlag, 1988.
Scott S. Mental retardation. In: Rutter M, Taylor E, Hersov L (eds) *Child and Adolescent Psychiatry. Modern approaches.* Oxford: Blackwell Science Ltd, 1994.
Yule W, Carr J. *Behaviour Modification for People with Mental Handicaps,* 2nd Edn. New York: Croom Helm, 1987.

## Related topics of interest

Mental handicap – autism (p. 189)
Mental handicap – social issues (p. 200)
Psychological treatment – behaviour therapy (p. 258)

# MENTAL HANDICAP – GENETIC CAUSES

## Chromosome abnormalities

**Chromosomes**

There are normally 46 chromosomes: 22 pairs of autosomes, and two sex chromosomes. This is conventionally described as 46XY or 46XX. Chromosome abnormalities include a change in amount of material (trisomy, triploidy, unbalanced translocation or deletion), or in the structure of a chromosome (inversion or ring formation) or in the position of chromosomal material (balanced translocation). The mosaic form of a disorder is where only some of the cells have the abnormality. Chromosome abnormalities account for a large number of individuals with mental handicap.

**Syndromes**

Nomenclature: q = long arm, p = short arm; + = trisomy, - = deletion.

*1. Autosomes.*

- 4p- syndrome (Wolf–Hirschhorn syndrome). Multiple physical abnormalities, seizures and mental retardation.
- 5p- (Cri du chat, Lejeune syndrome). Cat-like crying, facial abnormalities and severe mental retardation. It is more common in females.
- 13+ (Patau syndrome). Severe mental and physical defects. Individuals rarely survive infancy (except for the mosaic form).
- 15p- (Prader-Willi syndrome). Obesity, excessive eating and mental retardation.
- 18+ syndrome (Edwards syndrome). Severe mental retardation and facial abnormalities. Individuals rarely survive infancy.
- 18p- (de Grouchy syndrome). Facial abnormalities and a variable degree of mental retardation.
- 21+ syndrome (Down's syndrome). 5% of cases are due to translocation. It occurs in 1 per 600 live births (increases with maternal age, to, for example, 1 in 50 if the mother is over 45 years old). The risk of further Down's syndrome children depends on the causal chromosome abnormality (and is a very significant risk for translocations). Down's syndrome accounts for about one-third of cases of severe mental retardation but the

degree of mental retardation ranges from moderate to severe. Individuals have characteristic facial features; one-third have single palmar crease; two-thirds have significant deafness, cardiac and gastrointestinal abnormalities. Epilepsy occurs in 12% over 40 years. Alzheimer's dementia develops in 95% over 40 years.

- 22+ syndrome. Facial and skeletal abnormalities with mental retardation.
- Triploidy. Low birth weight, webbed fingers and mental retardation.

2. *Sex chromosomes.*

- XO (Turner syndrome). Occurs at a rate of 1 in 2500 live births. IQ is generally at the lower end of normal. Individuals often have a webbed neck, poor secondary sexual characteristics, heart, kidney and hearing defects. Characterized by the absence of a Barr body (inactivated X chromosome; the number of Barr bodies is one less than the number of X chromosomes).
- XXX, (XXXX, XXXXX) 1 in 800 live births. There is little abnormality with one extra X chromosome, but this increases with the number of extra X chromosomes.
- XXY (Klinefelter syndrome). Individuals are male, lack secondary sexual characteristics and are infertile. It occurs in 1 out of 500 live births. They have normal to low intelligence, behavioural problems and psychiatric disorders. The XXXY and XXXXY karyotypes are associated with increasing mental handicap with extra X chromosomes. Barr body(ies) are present.
- XYY. Occurs in 1 out of 700 live births. Individuals are male, tall and generally show behavioural problems rather than mental retardation. The XXYY karyotype is associated with facial abnormalities and mental retardation or normal intelligence.
- Fragile X (Martin–Bell–Renpenning syndrome). This accounts for up to 5% of severe mental retardation in males. It is found in 1 in 800 live births. Fragile sites on the X chromosome are revealed when cells are cultured with folic acid. This syndrome is characterized by a large jaw and large testes, and is also associated with autism. Female carriers may have mild mental handicap.

# Other genetic causes of mental retardation

**Autosomal dominant**

*1. Tuberous sclerosis.* Occurs in 1 in 20–40 000 live births. It accounts for almost 1% of those with significant mental handicap. Mental handicap is evident in 40%, and epilepsy and adenoma sebaceum (butterfly rash) are characteristic. There is a high spontaneous mutation rate, and variable penetrance.

*2. von Recklinghausen's disease/Neurofibromatosis.* This is characterized by tumours on central and peripheral nerves, skin lesions and variable mental handicap (one-third have mild handicap).

**Autosomal recessive (many inborn errors of metabolism)**

*1. Protein metabolism* (hereditary aminoacidurias). These are rare as a group except for phenylketonuria. Phenylketonuria (PKU) is the most common cause of mental retardation after Down's syndrome and fragile X (accounts for 1% of moderate to severe mental retardation). PKU occurs in 1 in 5000 to 20 000 live births and is due to absence of phenylalanine hydroxylase activity (converts phenylalanine to tyrosine). Because of its prevalence, routine testing of newborns is carried out (Guthrie test). A low phenylalanine diet can avert handicap if started as soon as possible and continued at least through to the teen years. Apart from mental retardation, children with this disorder have fair hair and blue eyes.

*2. Carbohydrate metabolism.* Galactosaemia occurs in 1 in 30 000 live births. Mental retardation can be averted by a low galactose diet.

*3. Mucopolysaccharidoses.* Hurler's syndrome (gargoylism) is characterized by severe deteriorating mental retardation and physical abnormalities. Hunter's syndrome (X-linked) is more benign.

*4. Fat metabolism.* Cerebromacular degeneration (Tay–Sachs disease) is characterized by a cherry red macula and is particularly found in Jewish populations. Niemann–Pick disease is the result of an abnormality of storage of sphingomyelin, often with epilepsy. It is more common in Jewish people. Progressive leucodystrophies result in progressive physical and mental deterioration with death in infancy.

**5. *Mineral abnormalities*.** Hepatolenticular degeneration (Wilson's disease) is a disorder of copper metabolism which is progressive, with deteriorating physical and mental functioning. Kayser–Fleischer rings are due to deposition of copper in the cornea.

**Sex-linked**

*1. Lesch–Nyhan syndrome*. This is due to deficiency of hypoxanthineguanine phosphoribosyl transferase (HGPRT), which leads to hyperuricaemia. It is characterized by choreoathetosis, and self-mutilation is common.

*2. Thalassaemia/mental retardation syndrome*.

*3. Fragile X* (see above).

**Other**

*1. Sturge–Weber syndrome*. This is not inherited, but may be due to spontaneous mutations. It is characterized by capillary haemangiomata in the trigeminal nerve distribution, variable mental handicap (50%) and epilepsy.

## Further reading

Gilbert P. *The A-Z Reference Book of Syndromes and Inherited Disorders*. London: Chapman and Hall, 1993.
Worthington A. *Glossary of Mental Handicap and Associated Physical Disorders*. Manchester: Manchester Free Press, 1985.

## Related topics of interest

Mental handicap – autism (p. 189)
Mental handicap – challenging behaviour (p. 193)
Mental handicap – social issues (p. 200)
Psychiatric disorders – genetics (p. 241)

# MENTAL HANDICAP – SOCIAL ISSUES

All major classificatory systems emphasize the contribution of social competence as well as intelligence quotient to the concept of mental handicap. This is to distinguish those who can lead a near normal life from those who require extra help to do so. It should be remembered that both environmental and genetic contributions are important in the aetiology of mild mental handicap, and that this group of people are more likely to be subject to various forms of social disadvantage, including: financial adversity, social isolation and housing problems.

**A brief history of mental handicap**

How societies care for people with mental handicap in many ways reflects the nature of their humanitarian concerns. Historically, some cultures have regarded mental handicap as a manifestation of evil, whilst others have revered it as a form of holy message necessitating special care. In England, there has been a legal distinction between those with mental handicap and those with mental disorder since the Middle Ages. In 1601, the Poor Law began a system of relief by Parishes leading to the foundation of workhouses, where people with mental handicap were housed along with a variety of social misfits and unfortunates.

The nineteenth century saw a proliferation of asylums, and the first specifically for mental handicap was Parkhouse in Highgate (1847). The 1876 Elementary Education Act legislated for some education for all children, and by the turn of the century Binet's standard tests of intelligence provided a quantitative method of separating children who were regarded as ineducable so that they could go on to receive special training instead.

The turn of the nineteenth century was a time of increased societal intolerance and faulty concepts of genetics flourished. The latter included Morel's doctrine of 'degeneration', whereby successive generations were thought to display neurosis, psychosis and then mental handicap. This was fertile ground for the Eugenics movement which advocated the wholesale segregation of people with a mental handicap.

The 1913 Mental Deficiency Act categorized people with mental handicap, in order of increasing IQ, as: idiots, imbeciles, feeble-minded and moral defectives. It can be seen that terms in this field have had a limited 'shelf-life' because of acquiring pejorative meanings. The Act led to admissions by legal process for all and the numbers in institutions rose sharply. Many were admitted for social transgressions including vagrancy, minor offences or having illegitimate children, rather than their level of handicap *per se*. The total care of such individuals was thought to be the rightful province of the health authorities. The number of beds in such hospitals rose from that time until 1959 (peak = approximately 70 000), since when there has been a steady decline.

The 1959 Mental Health Act redefined terms and referred to degrees of mental subnormality as well as providing for informal admissions. The 1960s and early 1970s were marred by a series of scandals concerning poor quality of care and abuse in large institutions. This led to the 1971 Government White Paper 'Better Services for the Mentally Handicapped', which provided the impetus for increasing community-based care.

The 1970 Education Act removed the stigma of ineducability and the 1981 Education Act expanded this and referred to 'special educational needs' as well as 'special educational provision', thus paving the way to increasing integration into mainstream educational services.

The past 20 years have seen an increase in social services, voluntary and private sector provision of day-time occupation and residential placements. Much care is now provided by multidisciplinary community mental handicap teams, mostly comprising health 'providers' but working alongside 'purchasers', who tend to be from a social work background (care managers).

The 1989 Children Act reinforced the need for a range of supportive provisions to allow community living as opposed to long-term hospital placements. Since the 1960s much care has been based on the principles of 'normalization' and 'social role valorization', whereby provision is based on individual needs and a range of services which are as close to those enjoyed by the general population as possible. This may require support and specialist services where necessary to promote better quality of life. The recent Mansell Report and subsequent correspondence from the authors addressed many of these issues and attempted to clarify the lead role of specialist mental handicap psychiatrists in the care of people with mental handicap and psychiatric disorders. Local authorities remain the lead agency for social care.

**Social factors in the aetiology of psychiatric disorders**

The following is a checklist of factors which may be relevant to the predisposition to, the precipitation of, or the maintenance of psychiatric and behaviour disorders in people with mental handicap:

1. Adverse childhood experiences due to developmental delay (includes problems in bonding and in establishing appropriate discipline by carers).

2. Experience of losses/separation. Maternal deprivation may arise from repeated in-patient admissions and bereavements may not be explained.

3. Reaction by peers to intellectual impairment, physical stigmatization or the label of mental handicap.

4. Difficulties in differentiating fact from fantasy.

5. Educational failure.

6. Diminished autonomy may lead to lack of choice and decisions being made on the grounds of administrative convenience.

7. Difficulty for the individual and those around them in coming to terms with sexuality (often not talked about).

8. General communication difficulties.

9. Services are rather patchy – some needy people may not come to specialist attention in good time, and assessment and treatment of clinical problems require considerable expertise.

## Further reading

Berrios GE, Freeman H. *150 years of British Psychiatry 1841–1991*. London: Gaskell Press, 1991.
Corbett JA. The development of services for the mentally handicapped: a historical and national review. In: Apley J (ed). *The Care of the Handicapped Child*. London: Heinemann, 1978.

## Related topics of interest

# MENTAL ILLNESS IN THE PUERPERIUM

Women are more likely to be admitted to a psychiatric hospital in the 2 weeks following childbirth than at any other time in the 2 years preceding and the 2 years following childbirth. The incidence of psychosis peaks on the third postpartum day and falls to baseline levels at 9 months postpartum. This is also a time when mild to moderate depression which is chronic and disabling may remain unrecognized and untreated.

**Postnatal depression**

The incidence of depressive illness within 6 weeks of childbirth is 10–15%. An additional 6–17% have depressive symptoms which do not reach the criteria for a depressive episode. This incidence is increased compared with control women but period prevalence may be the same, due to the chronic nature of this illness.

*1. Clinical features.* Depressed mood, varying from day to day. Alternative presenting features are changed behaviour, preoccupation with physical symptoms or worry about physical illness. Sleep disturbance is characteristic but may be wrongly ascribed to the baby wakening. Other features are anxiety about the baby, fear of harming the baby, guilt, irritability, feelings of inadequacy as a mother, loss of libido, phobic symptoms and suicidal thoughts. Onset is insidious and starts at least a week after delivery.

*2. Predisposing factors.* Psychosocial factors include loss of or unsatisfactory relationship with own mother in childhood, poor marital relationship, lack of social support, previous psychiatric illness (including depression in early pregnancy) and emotional lability in first postpartum week (including 'maternity blues'). Specific biological factors have not been reliably implicated in this form of depression.

*3. Treatment.* Recognition is important, and ideally by primary health workers. Initial steps consist of educating the mother about her condition (i.e. she is not unusual, recovery is likely) and mobilizing social support. This support may be from family, professional or voluntary sources. Specific counselling, cognitive behaviour therapy or group therapy may be indicated. For more severe or persistent symptoms, or in a woman with a history of depression which responds to drugs, medication should be used as for any depressive illness. Admission is indicated for a woman who is suicidal or severely depressed (see Puerperal psychosis below).

Prevention is likely to come from education of primary health workers to detect those most at risk. This may be facilitated by the use of rating scales; for example, the Edinburgh Post Natal Depression Scale. Antenatal counselling is of proven benefit and prophylactic medication is indicated for those with a history of bipolar affective disorder/schizophrenia to reduce the risk of relapse, which is increased at this time.

**Puerperal psychosis**

The incidence following childbirth is 0.2%. It is usually classifiable as an affective/schizophrenic/organic psychosis. Affective psychosis is the most common. However, it may not be classifiable according to conventional criteria and there is an ICD-10 category, F53, for 'mental and behavioural disorders associated with the puerperium not elsewhere classified'.

*1. Clinical features.* Onset is most commonly on the third day and is characterized by confusion. Symptom groupings are less clearcut than in non-puerperal psychosis; schizophreniform periods occur in an otherwise affective psychosis and prominent affective symptoms can colour a schizophrenic psychosis. If presentation is major depression, delusions, disorientation and hallucination are more common than in non-puerperial women. Delusions concerning the baby may lead to infanticidal/suicidal thoughts.

*2. Predisposing factors.* A personal or family history of psychosis is most important. Psychosocial factors include unmarried status, primiparity, Caesarean section, perinatal death and substance misuse. Biological factors suggested by timing include falls in oestrogen and progesterone, changes in adrenal steroids, low luteinizing hormone and neuropeptide in breast milk which crosses the blood–brain barrier, but none are well substantiated.

*3. Treatment.* Admission is usually indicated. Ideally the mother and baby are admitted to a specialized unit, unless the mother is too disturbed to have any contact with the baby. A general psychiatric ward with special arrangements may be acceptable but may not be a safe environment for a baby. Intensive community support (pioneered in

Nottingham) may be a good option. Drug treatment is as appropriate to clinical presentation (see below). Electro-convulsive therapy is indicated if the mother is suicidal, severely disturbed, not eating or drinking or not responding to medication. Attention must also be paid to the physical complications of the puerperium; for example, deep vein thrombosis (DVT). Behavioural programmes and supportive psycho-therapy have a role. There is a 20% relapse rate with further childbirth, and a 50% relapse rate throughout lifetime.

**Maternity blues**

This affects 50% of women during the 10 days after childbirth, with onset in the third to fifth day, and duration up to 48 hours.

*1. Clinical features.* Anxiety, depression, tearfulness, emotional lability, poor concentration, irritability, apparent confusion.

*2. Causative factors.* No proven hormonal differences from 'non-blue' women, but may have increased urinary free cyclic AMP, reduced plasma tryptophan, modification of alpha-2 adrenoceptors.

No specific treatment is indicated.

**Drugs in the puerperium**

Guidance on the use of drugs in the pueperium is regularly updated in Appendix 5 of the British National Formulary (BNF).

# Further reading

British National Formulary. No. 28 (September 1994) Appendix 5.
Cox JL. Psychiatric disorders of childbirth. In: Kendell RE, Zealley AK (eds) *Companion to Psychiatric Studies,* 5th Edn. London: Churchill Livingstone; 555–63.
Cox JL, Holden JM, Sagovsky R. Detection of post natal depression: development of the Edinburgh Post Natal Depression Scale. *British Journal of Psychiatry*, 1987; **150:** 782.
Grahame-Smith DG, Aronson JK. *Oxford Textbook of Clinical Pharmacology and Drug Therapy.* Oxford: Oxford University Press, 1984; Chap. 9.
Holden J, Sagovsky R, Cox JL. Counselling in a GP setting; a controlled study of health visitor intervention in the treatment of post natal depression. *British Medical Journal*, 1989; **298:** 223.
Pitt B. Depression following childbirth. *Hospital Update,* 1991; February: 133–9.

# NEUROSIS DIVISIBLE?

A number of the problems of psychiatric nosology beset those attempting to classify and subdivide neurotic disorders. Particularly troublesome for neurosis are:

(a) The stability of neurotic diagnoses over time is very low (except obsessive-compulsive disorder): less than 40% attract the same diagnosis 5 years after initial presentation (cf 75% for schizophrenia)(Kendell, 1974).

(b) The overlap of symptoms within neurotic syndromes: for example, panic and anxiety are frequently associated, as are depression and anxiety. This is known as 'co-morbidity'.

(c) The high incidence of neurotic symptoms within normal populations, as well as those with other illnesses and personality disorders.

(d) Problems with the definition of 'neurotic' (the term can be an illness descriptor, a personality dimension, a personality type, a way of behaving or simply a pejorative label).

**Classification**

As a result of these nosological problems, ICD-10 uses the term only as a vague descriptor, and gives less emphasis to the loose division between neurotic and psychotic which was in ICD-9. The term does not even appear in the index of DSM-IV.

In ICD-10, 'Neurotic, stress-related and somatoform disorders' includes most neurotic categories (neurotic depression being classified with mood disorders), and there are seven subdivisions:

• F40 Phobic anxiety disorders: 'Anxiety is evoked only, or predominantly, by certain well-defined situations or objects (external to the individual) which are not currently dangerous'. For example, agoraphobia, social and specific phobias.

• F41 Other anxiety disorders: 'Manifestations of anxiety ... not restricted to any particular environmental situation'. For example, panic disorder, generalized anxiety disorder, mixed anxiety and depressive disorder.

• F42 Obsessive-compulsive disorder: '..recurrent obsessional thoughts or compulsive acts' (see Psychiatric disorders – life events, p. 246).

• F43 Reaction to severe stress, and adjustment disorders: '... arise always as a direct consequence of the acute severe stress or continued trauma'.

• F44 Dissociative (conversion) disorders: '... a partial or complete loss of the normal integration between memories of the past, awareness of identity and immediate sensations, and control of bodily movements' (see Medically unexplained symptoms, p. 180).

- F45 Somatoform disorders: '... repeated presentation of physical symptoms, together with persistent requests for medical investigations, in spite of repeat negative findings and reassurances by doctors that the symptoms have no physical basis' (see Medically unexplained symptoms, p. 180).
- F48 Other neurotic disorders: (neurasthenia, depersonalization-derealization syndrome).

DSM-IV divides neurotic disorders into three groups:

- *Anxiety* disorders.
- *Somatoform* disorders.
- *Dissociative* disorders.

**Overlap and co-morbidity**

The problem of accurately distinguishing different neurotic disorders has been criticized from several quarters. Using latent-trait analysis on a general practice population, Goldberg *et al.* (1987) showed that depressive and anxiety disorders are more accurately described as lying on a continuum than as separate entities, with an orthogonal dimension related to the severity of illness. The continuum theory is not supported by family studies, which show both anxiety and depression 'breeding true' (Cloninger, 1990).

The stability of the diagnoses over time is poor, and Vollrath and Angst (1989), looking at the Zurich cohort, found no patients with a diagnosis of pure panic disorder retained at follow-up 7 years later: those who continued to have a psychiatric diagnosis reported either depression or mixed panic and depression. There is some suggestion that the mixed group (i.e. those with co-morbid panic and depression) have a more severe illness (nearly a third will have a lifetime history of suicide attempts), with a worse response to treatment and lower recovery rates (see Anxiety and panic, p. 39).

The association of mixed anxiety and depressive symptoms, as well as panic and agoraphobia, with anankastic or passive-dependent personality traits has been termed the 'general neurotic syndrome' by Tyrer (1985, 1992). A third of patients in the Nottingham study of neurotic disorder were thought to suffer from this syndrome, and they also constituted a group with significantly poorer prognosis. It is hypothesized that the general neurotic syndrome is an inherited personality diathesis increasing vulnerability to noxious events, and particularly to depression and anxiety in response to these, and hindering recovery. Cloninger (1986) came to a similar conclusion, highlighting individuals high in the temperamental trait of harm avoidance as those at increased risk of both anxiety and depressive disorders.

The co-morbidity with personality disorder also influences the effectiveness of different treatment modalities, with personality-disordered patients responding better to drug treatments (particularly antidepressants). In those patients without co-morbid personality disorder, psychological treatments such as cognitive behaviour therapy (CBT) or self-help programmes are more effective (Tyrer *et al.*, 1993).

## Further reading

Cloninger CR. A unified biosocial theory of personality and its role in the development of anxiety states. *Psychiatric Developments*, 1986; **2**: 83–120.

Cloninger CR. Co-morbidity of anxiety and depression. *Journal of Clinical Psychopharmacology,* 1990; **10**: Supplement, 435–65.

Goldberg DP, Bridges K, Duncan-Jones P, Grayson D. Dimensions of neuroses seen in primary care settings. *Psychological Medicine*, 1987; **17**: 461–70.

Kendell RE. The stability of psychiatric diagnoses. *British Journal of Psychiatry,* 1974; **124**: 352–6.

Tyrer P. Neurosis divisible? *Lancet,* 1985; **i**: 685–8.

Tyrer P.The general neurotic syndrome: a coaxial diagnosis of anxiety, depression and personality disorder. *Acta Psychiatrica Scandinavica*, 1992; **85**: 201–6.

Tyrer P, Seivewright N, Ferguson B, Murphy S, Johnson AL. The Nottingham study of neurotic disorder. Effect of personality status on response to drug treatment, cognitive therapy and self-help over two years. *British Journal of Psychiatry,* 1993; **162**: 219–26.

Vollrath M, Angst J. Outcome of panic and depression in a seven year follow-up: results of the Zurich study. *Acta Psychiatrica Scandinavica*, 1989; **80**: 591–6.

## Related topics of interest

# OBSESSIVE-COMPULSIVE DISORDER (OCD)

**Epidemiology**

Until recently, this was thought to be a rare disorder, with a prevalence of approximately 0.05% in the general population. However, recent studies have shown it to be more common (Epidemiological Catchment Area Study: prevalence 1.9–3.1%). Rates are similar across different cultures and there is an equal male and female prevalence. The peak of onset is in early adulthood, but it can start in childhood or adolescence. Patients are commonly affected by other psychiatric disorders: the lifetime prevalence of depressive disorder is 67%. Other common disorders include alcohol misuse, simple phobia, panic disorder and eating disorder.

**Clinical picture**

The disorder is characterized by obsessions and compulsions.

*1. Obsessions* can occur in several forms:

- *Obsessional thoughts:* repeated intrusive words/phrases (e.g. obscenities ) or worries (e.g. about contamination).
- *Obsessional ruminations:* more complicated sequences of thoughts (e.g. meaning of existence).
- *Obsessional doubts:* uncertainties about a previous action (e.g. turning the gas off).
- *Obsessional impulses:* urges to carry out actions (often violent or socially unacceptable).

Common themes seen in obsessions include dirt and contamination, aggressive actions, orderliness, illness, sex, religion.

*2. Compulsions.* Repeated, stereotyped and seemingly purposeful actions which the person feels compelled to carry out, but often resists, recognizing that they are irrational. Most are associated with obsessions and in the short term reduce the anxiety associated with the obsession. Common themes include checking, cleaning and counting. The majority have both obsessions and compulsions, but rarely, obsessions occur alone. Obsessions and compulsions have the following features in common:

- They are persistent and intrusive.
- They are ego-dystonic, for example they are experienced as being foreign to the person's experience.

- They are recognized as absurd and irrational.
- There is usually a strong desire to resist them (although a minority show little or no resistance).

There are four common patterns of presentation:

- Obsessional thoughts of contamination accompanied by compulsive hand washing and/or avoidance of objects.
- Obsessional doubts accompanied by compulsive checking.
- Obsessional thoughts alone of, for example, aggressive or sexual acts.
- Need for symmetry or precision accompanied by obsessional slowness.

Depressive symptoms are present in 50%.

**Aetiology**

*1. Biological.*
(a) *Neurotransmitters.* Research evidence supports the possibility that there is a dysregulation in serotonin (5-hydroxytryptamine (5-HT)) function:
- 5-hydroxyindoleacetic acid (5-HIAA) levels in the CSF may be reduced.
- mCPP (a 5-HT agonist) may exacerbate symptoms.
- Metergoline (a 5-HT antagonist) may ameliorate symptoms.
- Drugs that result in an increase in serotinergic transmission are the most effective in ameliorating symptoms (e.g. SSRIs and clomipramine).

However this does not necessarily mean that reduced 5-HT neurotransmission is the cause of OCD.
(b) *Brain imaging.*
- *Functional brain imaging:* PET (positron emission tomography) shows increased activity in the frontal lobes, basal ganglia (especially caudate) and cingulum of patients with OCD. Pharmacological and behavioural treatments are reported to reverse these abnormalities.
- *Structural brain imaging:* CT (computer tomography) and MRI (magnetic resonance imaging) scans show smaller caudates bilaterally.
(c) *Genetics.* There is a significant genetic component and family studies show an increase in OCD in relatives of sufferers. In twin studies, monozygotic (MZ) concordance is slightly higher than dizygotic (DZ) (but few studies have been performed).

(d) *Electroencephalogram (EEG) studies.* There is an increase in non-specific abnormalities. The sleep EEG shows similar abnormalities to depression (e.g. reduced rapid eye movement (REM) sleep).

(e) *Neuroendocrine tests.* One-third show non-suppression on the dexam-ethasone suppression test and also decreased growth hormone (GH) after clonidine infusion.

*2. Psychosocial factors.*

(a) *Personality.* The majority of patients with OCD do not have premorbid obsessional personality traits.

(b) *Psychodynamic factors.* Three major defence mechanisms are said to be operating in OCD:

- *Isolation.* Under ordinary circumstances, a person is conscious both of the affect and the imagery of an emotion-laden idea. When isolation occurs the affect is separated from the idea and is pushed out of consciousness, and the person is aware only of the affectless idea.

- *Undoing.* A compulsive act that is performed in an attempt to prevent or undo the consequences that the patient irrationally fears from the frightening obsessional thought or impulse.

- *Reaction formation.* Involves behaviour and consciously experienced attitudes that are exactly the opposite of the underlying impulses.

According to classic psychodynamic theory, OCD is a regression from the oedipal to the anal phase of development.

**Differential diagnosis**

*1. Depressive disorder.* Obsessional symptoms and depressive symptoms often occur together. Low mood often occurs secondary to long-standing OCD. Conversely, 30% of severe depressives develop obsessional symptoms which subside when the depression is treated. The rate of attempted suicide in this latter group is 1/6 that of uncomplicated depression. However, OCD is not simply a complication of depression. In particular the anti-obsessional effects of selective serotonin reuptake inhibitors (SSRIs) are not dependent on the initial level of depression.

*2. Phobia.* Phobias and OCD have similarities in that the fears are recognized by the patient to be irrational. However, phobics tend to avoid the object that they fear, whereas OCD sufferers tend to seek it out. Phobics tend to have a direct fear of the object or situation, whereas OCD sufferers tend to fear the imagined consequences.

*3. Obsessive personality/obsessional compulsive personality disorder.* These do not have a simple one to one relationship with OCD. This type of personality is over represented in those with OCD but a significant proportion do not have these traits. Although people with these traits may develop OCD they are more likely to develop a depressive disorder.

*4. Schizophrenia.* This is occasionally difficult to distinguish from OCD if the thoughts or actions have a peculiar content.

*5. Gilles de la Tourette syndrome.* There is an increase in obsessional symptoms in this disorder. There is an increase in OCD and in Tourettes in relatives of these patients. Conversely, 20% of OCD patients have tics (see Tourettes and related conditions, p. 347).

**Course and prognosis**

Onset may be acute or gradual. Patients are embarrassed about their difficulties and there is often a delay of 5 to 10 years before presentation to psychiatrists. 20–30% show significant improvement, 40–50% have moderate improvement, and 20–40% do not improve or worsen. Approximately one-third of OCD patients have major depressive disorder, and suicide is a risk, although lower than in uncomplicated depression.

*1. Factors indicating a poorer prognosis:*

- Lack of resistance to compulsions.
- Childhood onset.
- Coexisting depressive disorder.
- Delusional beliefs or overvalued ideas.
- Personality disorder.

*2. Factors indicating a good prognosis:*

- Good social and occupational adjustment.
- A clear precipitating event.
- Episodic symptoms.
  Obsessional content does not seem to relate to prognosis.

**Treatment**

*1. Pharmacological.* Many trials have shown that drug therapy is effective. The efficacy in trials is enhanced by the fact that the placebo response rate in OCD is low, at about 5% (usually 30–40% in trials of antidepressants or anxiolytics). The main drugs used are serotonin selective. Initial effects may be seen at 4–6 weeks, although 8–16 weeks is usually needed to gain the maximum therapeutic effect.

(a) *Clomipramine.* This is a serotonin selective tricyclic antidepressant that is also used for treating depressive disorder. Other less specific tricyclics are not as effective in OCD. Its efficacy in OCD is supported by many clinical trials. It is started at a dose of 25–50 mg and increased gradually up to a usual dose of 150 mg/day.

(b) *Selective serotonin reuptake inhibitors (SSRIs).* Fluoxetine and other SSRIs are effective. In trials, doses of up to 80 mg of fluoxetine have been required. Although side-effects such as restlessness, headaches, insomnia and nausea are commonly reported, in general the SSRIs are better tolerated than clomipramine and are therefore sometimes used as first line drugs. However, a recent meta analysis suggests that clomipramine may be more effective in severe cases.

*2. Behaviour therapy.* This is thought to be as effective as drug therapy although there have been few direct comparisons. Its effects may last longer. The main approaches used are exposure and response prevention. Modelling by the therapist of 'fearless' behaviour is also used. The technique of thought stopping can be used to reduce obsessional thoughts.

Psychodynamic psychotherapy has not been shown to be of benefit. Supportive psychotherapy including explanation and reassurance is important in all cases both for patient and for the family.

*3. Psychosurgery.* This is performed rarely and only in extremely treatment resistant patients.

# Further reading

Greist JH, Jefferson JW, Kobak KA, Katzelnick DJ, Serlin RC. Efficacy and tolerability of serotonin transport inhibitors in obsessive-compulsive disorder. A meta-analysis. *Archives of General Psychiatry,* 1995; **52:** 53–60.

# Related topics of interest

Tourettes and related conditions (p. 347)
Psychological treatment – behaviour therapy (p. 258)

# PERSONALITY – ASSESSMENT AND CLASSIFICATION

Personality may be defined as a cluster of habitual patterns of thinking, feeling and reacting. It is a combination of basic inherited temperamental traits, learned behaviours, and cognitive schemata (broadly defined as beliefs and assumptions). The definition of personality disorder, 'maladaptive patterns of behaviour, present since childhood or early adolescence and causing significant distress to the person, or to others, or to the whole society' (ICD-10), implicitly defines personality simply as a pattern of behaviour. This is rather simplistic, but entirely in keeping with the tendency of current diagnostic systems to avoid suggesting putative underlying mechanisms.

## Assessment of personality

Current and pre-morbid personality is assessed as part of the psychiatric history. An attempt should be made to discover both how the person views himself/herself when he/she is well, and whether this has changed. Questions relating to how others see them may help people who are reticent about describing themselves.

## Classification of personality

Both ICD-10 and DSM-IV adopt a categorical approach to classification of personality. In DSM-IV it is coded on a separate axis 2 from mental disorder (axis 1). Disappointingly, given the evidence that personality is an independent predictor of illness course and prognosis, even the multiaxial version of ICD-10 fails to separate it out. There are serious problems with the all-or-nothing nature of categorical personality classifications, because some people with distinctly abnormal personalities may not fulfil the requisite criteria, and they also fail to take into account the high degree of overlap between the categories. DSM-IV recognizes this to some extent by grouping the different types of personality disorder into three clusters, each containing similar types of personality.

- Cluster A: 'odd or eccentric'.
- Cluster B: 'dramatic, emotional or erratic'.
- Cluster C: 'anxious and fearful'.

The overlap between the categories within each cluster is considerably greater than that between categories in different clusters.

## Mode of presentation

In clinical practice, there is considerable variation in the likelihood and mode of presentation of different categories of personality disordered patient (Oldham, 1994).

- 'Cluster A' (odd or eccentric) may be severely disabled by symptoms, but these personality disorders involve either interpersonal mistrust or aversion, and so will not usually present, although they may do so at the urging of a friend, family member, or trusted professional.
- 'Cluster B' (dramatic, emotional or erratic) covers a wide variety of disorders. Their defining characteristic is of a pervasive persistent abnormality in maintaining social relationships, and so 'disease' is common. Histrionic patients may experience a great deal of unhappiness, but may not regard themselves as needing treatment, although they may present requesting psychotherapy, or as a result of depressive disorder. Antisocial personalities are usually seen in a forensic setting, as they are unlikely to present unless the consequences of their actions are sufficiently aversive to force them to acknowledge a problem. Narcissistic personalities do not regard themselves as having a problem; however, they are at risk of depression if their narcissistic defences fail, and are then amenable to psychotherapeutic work, although recovery from depression usually results in their reinstating their defences and refusing further treatment. The most common personality disorder in treatment is the borderline, which causes huge distress to sufferers and others. This is reflected in the relatively much greater volume of literature on this disorder. Cluster B personality disorders are those most often encountered in work with addictions.
- 'Cluster C' (anxious and fearful) patients usually present with fears and difficulties over social relationships, or social anxiety.

## Dimensional classifications of personality

Given that personality is not a unitary concept, has many different components, and is ubiquitous (i.e. everybody has a personality!), there is a case for describing it in dimensional terms, where different facets or factors of personality are compared with the rest of the population. Questionnaires, such as the Cattell 16-PF or the MMPI, use the results of an extensive questionnaire to categorize people in exactly the same way. The traits used in these personality questionnaires are derived from extensive factor analysis of hundreds of different personality traits, many of which are found to co-vary to the extent that they can be viewed as being essentially unitary.

**Classification of temperament**

At a more fundamental level, attempts have been made to reduce the number of dimensions to a minimum (usually two or three). These dimensions are related to three separate systems which interact in the control of emotional behaviour. These are a fight-flight system, a behavioural inhibition system and an approach or behavioural activation system (Gray, 1987). The resulting traits are more like aspects of temperament, in that they describe constitutional psychophysiological states. The best known is probably the Eysenck Personality Questionnaire (EPQ), whose three dimensions are:

- *Introvert–extravert*. This dimension is postulated by Eysenck to be related to the constitutional degree of cortical arousal, and the degree of tonic stimulation of the cortex by the reticular activating system (RAS). Those with relatively inactive RASs, and therefore low constitutional arousal, will seek out stimulation to raise themselves towards a putative optimal level and their behaviour will thus tend to be extraverted.
- *Neurotic–stable*. This is postulated to be due to the reactivity of the autonomic nervous system. Those with highly reactive ANSs show high levels of neuroticism.
- *Psychotic–reality based*. This is a rather weaker dimension, and seems to be related more to cognitive or information-processing style than to any underlying psychophysiology.

These three dimensions are said to be orthogonal to one another, that is, they do not correlate. Very similar personality dimensions are postulated by Jeffrey Gray, whose two axes are *anxiety* and *impulsivity*. Along similar lines, Costa and McRae (1990) have proposed a five-factor model of personality functioning, for which there is empirical support. The factors are N (*neuroticism*), E (*extraversion*), O (*openness to experience*), A (*agreeableness*) and C (*conscientiousness*).

**An integrative psychological model**

More recently a 7-factor modification of Cloninger's (1986) tridimensional scheme has been outlined by Cloninger *et al.* (1993). A distinction is made between dimensions of *temperament* and *character,* depending upon whether they involve preconceptual or concept-based memory. *Temperamental* factors are heritable, manifest early in life, and involve preconceptual or unconscious biases in learning. Four independent dimensions are identified, these are:

- *Harm avoidance* (behavioural inhibitions systems). Phylogenetically the earliest temperamental factor to appear. The capacity to be influenced by and learn from punishment or frustrative non-reward. This is postulated to be related to central 5-hydroxytryptamine (5HT) activity: high 5HT leads to high harm avoidance.
- *Novelty seeking* (behavioural activation systems). The capacity to be excited or stimulated by novel situations. This is thought to be related to the constitutional activity of central dopamine systems: low constitutional dopamine produces high novelty seeking.

- *Reward dependence* (behavioural maintenance subsystems). The need for reward, particularly in the form of social approval. Central noradrenaline pathways are involved, with high reward dependence being correlated with high levels of central noradrenaline.
- *Persistence.* Perseverance despite frustration or fatigue (uncorrelated with other aspects of reward dependence). One of the interesting things about this part of the dimensional classification is that the personality types associated with extremes of any two or three of these dimensions bear resemblance to the categorical personality types in ICD and DSM. For example, sociopathic personality disorder is high novelty seeking, low harm avoidance and low reward dependence; histrionic personality is high novelty seeking, high harm avoidance and high reward dependence. However, whilst it distinguishes between different personality disorders, many well-adapted individuals have extreme temperaments. Differences which seem important are those of *character,* which are based on conscious differences in self-concept. Three dimensions are identified.
  - — *Self-directedness.* "Self determination and willpower" or "the ability of the individual to control, regulate and adapt behaviour to fit the situations in accord with individually chosen goals and values". Internal locus of control, goal directedness, resourcefulness, self-acceptance, and sponaneous unconflicted actions characterize self-directedness. *Low self-directedness is the common characteristic of all categories of personality disorders.*
  - — *Co-operativeness.* The capacity for identification with, and acceptance of, other people. Social tolerance, empathy, helpfulness and compassion characterize individuals high in co-operativeness. *All categories of personality disorder are associated with low co-operativeness.*
  - — *Self-transcendence.* "Identification with everything conceived as essential and consequential parts of a whole". Characterized by: self-forgetful as opposed to self-conscious experience; transpersonal identification (identification with nature) as opposed to self-differen-tiation; and spiritual acceptance as opposed to rational materialism. Psychiatric patients, and those with schizoid personality, are low in transcendence.

The key features of this model are that it intergrates (on a descriptive level, at least) biological and psychological models of personality (see Personality – psychological models, p. 234) and also the effects of both nature and nurture. Few other models can claim to contain Eysenck's concepts of extraversion, Maslow's self-actualizers and the effects of emotional deprivations within such simple schema.

## Further reading

Cloninger CR. A unified biosocial theory of personality and its role in the development of anxiety states. *Psychiatric Development,* 1986; **3**: 167–226.

Cloninger CR, Srauric DM, Przybeck TR. A psychological model of temperament and character. *Archives of General Psychiatry*, 1993; **50:** 975–90.

Costa P, McRae RR. Personality disorders and the five factor model of personality. *Journal of Personality Disorder*, 1990; **4:** 362, 371–81.

Gray JA. Perspectives on anxiety and impulsivity: a commentary. *Journal of Research in Personality,* 1987; **21:** 493–509.

Oldham JM. Personality disorders: Current perspectives. *Journal of the American Medical Association*, 1994; **272:** 1770–6.

## Related topics of interest

Personality – development (p. 223)
Personality – psychological models (p. 234)

# PERSONALITY – BORDERLINE DISORDERS

Since it was first included in DSM III, borderline personality disorder has been a controversial topic which has attracted debate about its nature, causation, and even existence.

**Definition**

As with many controversial entities, there are a number of different definitions of borderline personality disorder (BPD). It is important to distinguish between two main perspectives from which it is described: the psychoanalytical perspective, as opposed to the agnostic, operationalized criteria in DSM-IV and ICD10 (in which it is a sub group of an emotionally unstable personality disorder). The core features are as follows:

- Impulsivity.
- Affective instability.
- Unstable self image, aims and internal (including sexual) preferences.
- Chronic feelings of emptiness.
- Tendency to become involved in intense and unstable relationships.
- Efforts to avoid real or imagined abandonment.

Self-destructive acts or threats, often in response to a fear of abandonment or expectations of assuming increased responsibility, are common. Completed suicide is said to be the outcome in 8–10% of people with this disorder. Transient psychotic like or dissociative states may occur in response to stress.

**Epidemiology**

DSM-IV states that 2% of the general population, 10% of psychiatric out-patients, and 20% of psychiatric in-patients suffer from BPD. This seems a very high estimate, and authors in the UK (e.g. Freeman, 1994) caution that the term is in danger of being used indiscriminately as a synonym for personality disorder, and becoming no more specific than the term 'psychosis'.

**Aetiology**

The weakness of current diagnostic systems is that they take a purely empirical or positivist frame, and so eschew statements regarding putative underlying mechanisms (Walker, 1994). The causes of borderline personality are unknown, but Paris (1994) discusses a stress-diathesis type of model very much in line with current models of psychiatric aetiology. Three groups of factors interact, with psychological and social stressors causing trait amplification of fundamental biological vulnerabilities, as follows:

- *Biologial vulnerability:* probably in the form of basic temperamental traits and core dimensions of personality. In BPD these are impulsivity and affective instability.
- *Psychological:* trauma, especially early sexual abuse, which seems to have occurred in 80% of BPD patients, and has led some to hypothesize that it is a form of post-traumatic stress disorder (PTSD). Early separation from or loss of parents, or abnormal parenting are also important risk factors.
- *Social:* anything which reduces the potential for buffering of psychological problems by extrafamilial influences. In particular, the contemporary problems of rapid social change and loss of social structures, which increase both the pressure on, and the isolation of, the nuclear family. In addition, fluid or disorganized social structures will further impair individuals with BPD as they become independent adults. There is some circumstantial evidence that BPD is increasing in prevalence, and this is presumably because of the rapidity of change and increasing fragmentation of post-modern society.

**Dynamic psychopathology**

In psychodynamic terms, borderline personality organization can be understood as a persistence in the Kleinian paranoid-schizoid position, in which the world is populated by split part objects, which have opposing characteristics of good or evil. The predominant defence mechanism of this stage is projective identification, in which the patient takes an unwanted aspect of the self and ascribes it to another person. The other is then unconsciously pressured to own the projected attribute (Gabbard, 1991). This stage of development is normally followed by the depressive position, in which good and bad part objects are integrated into a whole, and the individual experiences depression and fear at the realization that the object which they hate and wish to destroy is identical with that which they love and cherish. This type of personality organization is clearly extremely maladaptive to an adult, but it may be explained in terms of a learned behaviour, i.e. as a way of coping with severe abuse from a close relative: the unacceptable evil part of the object is split off and projected out into the environment, allowing the child to continue to love the abuser.

| | |
|---|---|
| **Significance of the defence style** | Borderline patients are notoriously difficult to treat. In a therapeutic milieu, they are characterized by behaviour which is seen as 'grossly manipulative', and by their ability to produce serious splitting among staff groups (Shapiro, 1978). This may be viewed as an acting out by a staff group of the patient's internal world. The patient's tendency to alternate between extreme idealization and violent devaluation, or persistent rage, at a therapist, makes them extremely challenging (Gabbard, 1991). |
| **Treatment** | Treatment can be aimed at biological, psychological or social problems, and is covered in detail elsewhere (see Personality – management of disorders, p. 229). |

In the psychotherapeutic field, there are often problems in establishing a rapport and a therapeutic relationship. The extreme transference reactions of these patients may be very difficult for therapists to tolerate, but many authors have emphasized the importance of the therapist holding the transference as in itself a mutative process. On a practical level, these patients respond to clear boundary setting, with a focus on practical treatment measures. It is helpful to offer regular appointments over a long period of time emphasizing that treatment will be of prolonged duration. It should be stressed to the patient that they will be seen in these sessions rather than as the result of self destructive behaviour, which is often used as an attempt to elicit care and deal with feelings of abandonment. A single named key worker, with whom all concerned parties agree to communicate any information regarding the patient, is the most effective way to prevent splitting between professional groups.

# Further reading

Freeman CPL. Personality Disorders. In: Kendell RE, Zealley AK (eds) *Companion to Psychiatric Studies,* 5th Edn, Edinburgh; Churchill Livingstone, 1994; 603–5.

Gabbard GO. Technical approaches to transference hate in the analysis of borderline patients. *International Journal of Psycho-analysis,* 1991; **72:** 625–37.

Gabbard GO. Splitting in hospital treatment. *American Journal of Psychiatry,* 1989; **146:** 444–51.

Paris J. The etiology(sic) of borderline personality disorder: a biopsychosocial approach. *Psychiatry,* 1994; **57:** 316–25.

Shapiro ER. The psychodynamics and developmental psychology of the borderline patient: A review of the literature. *American Journal of Psychiatry,* 1978; **135:** 1305–15.

Walker C. From empiricism to neural networks: philosophical analysis of the basis of psychiatric practice. *Current Opinion in Psychiatry,* 1994; **7:** 411–13.

## Related topics of interest

Personality – development (p. 223)
Personality – management of disorders (p. 229)
Stress reactions (p. 330)

# PERSONALITY – DEVELOPMENT

*(Personality is) the sum total of the actual or potential behaviour patterns of the organism, as determined by heredity and environment; it originates and develops through the functional interaction of the four main sectors into which these behaviour patterns are organised: The cognitive sector (intelligence), the conative sector (character), the affective sector (temperament), and the somatic sector (constitution).* (Hans Eysenck)

**Cognitive development**

The essential feature of cognitive development is that, during childhood, the individual goes through a series of Copernican revolutions described by Piaget as the following four stages of development:

*1. The sensorimotor stage. Age 0–18 months/2 years.*
(a) Developing ability to distinguish between self and outside world (primary decentring).
(b) Development of coordination between vision and prehension.
(c) Development (around 9 months) of 'object permanence'.

*2. Pre-operational (stage of animism and precausal logic). Age 1½–7 years.*
(a) Development of symbolic functions, thinking and reasoning.
(b) Egocentrism: cannot imagine another's point of view; child believes he or she is the centre of the universe.
(c) Animism: child believes all objects are alive and have thoughts, feelings or intent.
(d) Precausal logic. Based on the child's internal model of the world, not observations. Quantities are not conserved.
(e) Authoritarian morality.
(f) Rules of games are sacrosanct. Bad events are punishments for wrongdoing.

*3. Concrete operations. Age 8–12 years.*
(a) Loss of egocentrism, animism and authoritarianism.
(b) A second 'decentring' of thoughts from objects, and objects from the subject.
(c) Child can see other people's points of view.
(d) Can construct logical arguments on the basis of observations (e.g. quantities are now conserved).

(e) Justice rather than obedience is the basis of morality.

(f) Still unable to reason in an abstract way.

*4. Formal operations (stage of abstract or propositional thought). Age 12–15 years.*

(a) Abstract logical operations become possible and the child learns to recognize the difference between form and content and so can reason from the possible, not simply the actual.

(b) Up to one-third of people do not achieve the stage of formal operations in their thinking in adulthood.

## Development of character and temperament

Whilst trait theorists such as Eysenck or Cloninger (1986) see temperament as largely inherited, both of them postulate progressive environmental modulation or alteration of this over time, in the same way that weight training might modify genetic factors determining muscle size. Eysenck theorizes that the development of personality is related to conditioning by environmental experiences, and stimulus generalization from specific events. Introverts and extroverts differ in their ability to be conditioned, and so fundamental temperament traits will determine what the individual learns from his environment. Cloninger (1986) examines the role of anxiety in producing an increase in harm avoidance over time, this in turn producing a reduction in novelty seeking. This certainly corresponds with everyday experience that people do become more cautious as they grow older. Cloninger (1992) also distinguishes temperament from character, the latter relating to conscious aspects of self-image and role in the world (see Personality – management of disorders, p. 229).

In terms of categories of personality disorder, Tyrer divides these into mature and immature types. Immature personality types (e.g. histrionic, sociopathic, asthenic) tend to improve with age, whilst the mature types (e.g. paranoid, schizoid, anankastic) worsen.

## Psychosocial theories of development

Under this heading can be grouped most of the psycho-analytical theories. These view personality development either as a series of stages or barriers to be overcome, or as driven by one overarching drive or aspiration, such as the 'self-actualization' of Maslow.

Freud's theory of development is specifically a psychosexual one, the five stages of development being:

1. *Oral (first year of life)*. The mouth is the focus of Sensual life. Two forms of oral activity, biting and chewing or swallowing, are said to represent the foundation for later character traits of oral incorporation (collecting things or acquiring knowledge) and oral aggression (sarcasm and argumentativeness).

2. *Anal stage (age 1–2 years)*. Focus of Sensual life switches to the anus, and there is a fascination with the ability to produce faeces. Toilet training forces the child to delay gratification. Rebellion against this occurs, and forms the foundation for later traits of anal retentiveness (stinginess and stubbornness) and anal eliminativeness (disorderliness, destructiveness or cruelty).

3. *Phallic stage (age 2–6 years)*. The genitals become the main area of sexual pleasure, and masturbation is common. Children of both sexes develop sexual desires towards the parent of the opposite sex, and the Oedipus complex, with its castration anxiety in the male, and penis envy in the female, develops at this stage. Resolution of the Oedipus complex occurs through identification with the same-sex parent, and the superego matures at this stage. The Oedipus complex is considered by some to be a culture-bound syndrome, determined by a society in which the family is the primary unit of child care, and in which males have considerable advantages over females.

4. *Latency (age 5–12 years)*. Overt sexual activities and desires cease, probably more due to increasing awareness of parental disapproval than actual change in behaviour. The child develops the capacity for sublimation and begins to feel concern for others.

5. *Genital stage (12 years to ? death)*. As puberty re-awakens sexual desires, these are further modified, and the narcissism of earlier stages is modified towards concern for others and altruistic love. The Oedipus complex is modified from vicarious possession of the parent of the opposite sex towards attachment to others of that sex.

Freud's theory is limited in that it sees development (a) entirely in psychosexual terms and (b) as ending in the late teens. His theories were broadened by those of his daughter, Anna Freud, who saw childhood development as a series of developmental lines covering far greater areas than simply sexuality and aggression. Erik Erikson has modified Freud's theory into a general eight-stage psychosocial theory of development covering the period from birth to maturity, for which there is some empirical evidence (Vaillant and Milofsky, 1980). Erikson postulates a series of psychosocial 'crises' (the best known being the 'identity crisis' of adolescence) which require the resolution of certain basic conflicts, for example, between trust and mistrust. Successful resolution of these leads to the development of a 'virtue', in this case 'hope'. Erikson's stages can be compared to those of Piaget and Freud, as shown in the table below.

| Age | Piagetian stage | Freudian/*Jungian* stage | Eriksonian stage/*virtue* |
|---|---|---|---|
| 0–1 years | Sensorimotor | Oral | Trust versus mistrust /*hope* |
| 1–3 years | Pre-operational | Anal | Autonomy versus shame and doubt/*will* |
| 3–5 years | Pre-operational | Phallic-Oedipal | Initiative versus guilt/*purpose* |
| 6 years to puberty | Concrete operations | Latency | Industry versus inferiority/*competence* |
| Adolescence | Formal operations | Puberty | Identity versus identity confusion/*fidelity* |
| Early adulthood | | Genitality | Intimacy versus isolation/*love* (career consolidation versus self-absorption[a]) |
| Middle adulthood | | *Mid-life crisis Shift from 'nature' to 'culture'* | Generativity versus stagnation/*care* (keepers of the meaning versus rigidity[a]) |
| Later adulthood | | *Individuation* | Integrity versus despair/*wisdom* |

[a] Stages tentatively added by Vaillant and Milofsky (1980) as part of the lifecycle.

**Theories of adult development**

Maslow's theory concerns motivational drives, postulating a hierarchy of needs, those which are lower down the hierarchy requiring at least partial satisfaction before higher ones become important. The hierarchy (from bottom up) is:

- *Physiological:* food, drink.
- *Safety:* feeling secure and safe.
- *Belongingness/love:* to affiliate, belong, be accepted.
- *Esteem:* to gain approval and recognition for achievement and competence.
- *Cognitive:* understanding, knowledge.
- *Aesthetic:* beauty, order, symmetry.
- *Self-actualization:* self-fulfilment, achievement of potential.

Whilst some of this may seem to be a statement of the obvious, it may be helpful to view the development of adult personality as being constrained by environmental demands as well as innate potentialities, and Maslow's theory gives some idea of the order in which those potentialities are liable to be expressed.

In addition to Erikson, the other major psychoanalytical theorist of adult development is Carl Jung (Moraglia, 1990). Jung's observations led him to propose a change in temperament towards introversion with age, with increasing integration of contrasexual characteristics (i.e. those stereotypically belonging to the opposite sex, e.g. aggression in women). Within the life journey, there is a significant transitional period (the 'mid-life crisis') between the ages of 35 and 45. During this period, a change occurs in the focus of life activities from 'nature' (individual development, achievement in the outside world, procreation and the care of children) to 'culture'. Culture is seen both in terms of the heritage of a society (Vaillant and Milofsky's (1980) 'keepers of the meaning'), and the individual effort to develop a wider consciousness through individuation and personality development (which bears a striking similarity to the 'self-actualization' of Maslow). Individuation, with the shift of the centre of personality from ego to self, both allows the individual to meet the demands of life more effectively and, finally, by generating 'a consciousness detached from the world', allows him or her to meet death itself.

With the increasing fluidity of the lifecycle, and particularly the relatively long lifespan available to most people in advanced societies free from the deleterious effects of ageing, the mid-life crisis might be expected to become less pronounced, to occur at more diverse ages, and the shift in attitudes to become marked more as a comingling of 'nature' and 'culture' (Moraglia, 1994).

# Further reading

Cloninger CR, Surakic DM, Przybeck TR. A psychological model of temperament and character. *Archives of General Psychiatry*, 1993; **50:** 975–90.

Cloninger CR. A unified biosocial theory of personality and its role in the development of anxiety states. *Psychiatric Developments,* 1986; **3:** 167–226.

Hall CS, Lindzey G. *Introduction to Theories of Personality.* Chichester: John Wiley, 1985.

Moraglia G. CG Jung and the psychology of adult development. *Journal of Analytical Psychology,* 1994; **39:** 55–75.

Vaillant GE, Milofsky E. Natural history of male psychological health: IX. Empirical evidence for Erikson's model of the life cycle. *American Journal of Psychiatry,* 1980; **137:** 1348–59.

# Related topics of interest

Developmental disorders (p. 106)
Learning (p. 171)
Personality – assessment and classification (p. 214)
Personality – management of disorders (p. 229)

# PERSONALITY – MANAGEMENT OF DISORDERS

*People with personality disorders suffer considerably and merit help, even if it cannot always be given in reliable and effective form*
(Tyrer *et al.*, 1991)

**Paradigm shift in treatment of personality disorder**

Over the last ten years opinions about personality disorders, their treatment and treatability have undergone a revolutionary change described by Stone (1993) in terms of 'breakthroughs, conceptualisations, assessment and treatment':

- A shift from a characterological viewpoint (e.g. 'anal character'), towards an integrative neurobiological, biosocial or biopsychosocial model. Adult personality is conceptualized as the outcome of environmental factors acting on biological vulnerabilities, and also of the behaviours learned by the individual to cope with the vicissitudes of both temperament and environment.
- Increasing differentiation and clarification of descriptions and assessment tools for personality disorder.
- A move in treatment methods and focus away from psychodynamic methods aiming to change character structure and towards more focused and structured approaches, with a more active therapist role.
- Developing understanding of the use of drugs in the treatment of personality disorder (Siever and Davis, 1991).
- A growing consensus that pharmacological treatment modalities (Stein, 1992) and psychological approaches (e.g. dynamic, cognitive, supportive and group work) can and should be integrated in the treatment of personality disorders (Soloff, 1994; Rosenberg, 1994). This is especially true in less treatable patients.
- A recognition that the goal of treatment is to facilitate moving from a maladaptive personality disordered functioning to 'personality style' functioning, which is highly adaptive functioning behaviour for that particular personality type.

**Specific treatments**

*1. Biological treatments.* Distinction can be made between the use of biological treatments for the 'axis 1' disorders that often coexist with personality disorder, and the treatment of the disorder itself. In either circumstance, caution needs to be exercised in prescribing potentially toxic treatments to impulsive people who may be at risk of self-harm, but otherwise, the treatment of coexisting disorders is unchanged from normal management. The coexistence of a personality disorder with a mental or physical illness worsens the prognosis and response to treatment of the latter. Understanding the impact of personality disorder on the way in which the individual views the world may be useful in enabling clear communication, and thus optimizing treatment (Oldham, 1994).

In psychobiological terms, personality disorder can be formulated as a dimensional model grounded on the major axis 1 syndromes (Siever and Davis, 1991), and the treatment used for various features of personality disorder is therefore selected by analogy with treatment of corresponding symptoms of axis 1 disorder. In general, results are less clearcut than for the treatment of axis 1 disorders, and many treatments seem to be effective over a broad spectrum of symptoms (i.e. there is less specificity of action). The core psychobiological dimensions are thought to be:

- Cognitive/perceptual organization: disturbed in the psychoses and schizotypal patients, and related to abnormalities of dopamine metabolism
- Impulsivity/aggression: disturbed in impulse control disorders, and across a variety of 'cluster B' personality disorders. Related to abnormalities of serotonin metabolism.
- Affective instability: disturbed in affective disorders, and borderline personality. Related to greater cholinergic responsiveness, and noradrenergic hyper-responsiveness.
- Anxiety/inhibition: disturbed in patients with anxiety disorders, and 'cluster C' (anxious and fearful) patients. The biological basis is uncertain, but may involve noradrenergic or gamma-aminobutyric acid (GABA) function.

2. *Specific physical treatments.*
(a) *Neuroleptics.* Broadly indicated for cognitive/perceptual disturbance. Effective doses are lower than those needed in the control of psychosis, and higher doses seem to be associated with undesirable side-effects, including 'behavioural toxicity' with disturbance, agitation and the precipitation of psychotic symptoms in vulnerable patients (either a histrionic

reaction or an atropine-like psychosis). High potency drugs such as pimozide, flupenthixol, or trifluoperazine are preferred, as they are less sedating, though low doses of thioridazine or chlorpromazine may be helpful in those patients who desire sedating.

Neuroleptics in low dose (e.g. flupenthixol depot, 20 mg monthly) have been shown in the long term (>3 months) to reduce the incidence of self-harm in borderline patients, and also the more general behavioural dyscontrol, of which this is a specific symptom. Improvement in general takes up to three months to appear, and symptoms of a psychotic type (cognitive disturbance, ideas of reference, delusions, psychotic anger and hostility) seem to improve markedly, as do more affective symptoms such as anxiety, phobias, and depression. Low self-image, a psychological symptom, seems also to respond to neuroleptic treatment.

(b) *Mood stabilizers (lithium, carbamazepine, valproate).* Lithium may be useful in the treatment of those with prominent emotional instability, and impulsivity/aggression particularly as manifested by violent behaviour. This effect is not simply due to behavioural inhibition. It is suggested that serum levels need to be somewhat higher (>0.6 mmol/l) than in bipolar patients. In aggressive patients, it seems to introduce what has been termed 'reflective delay' between the impulse to be aggressive and the performance of the act itself. Only a minority of patients respond, and there seem to be a few who become more aggressive. Prediction of response is difficult, though pronounced affective symptoms, and family history of affective disorder and possibly alcoholism may be a feature of responders. Otherwise an empirical trial of 2–3 months' treatment may be needed (Stein, 1992). Similar results have been found for carbamazepine, in doses of 200 mg b.d. or t.d.s., in a wide variety of both mentally ill and personality disordered patients. Behavioural dyscontrol is markedly reduced, and 'reflective delay' becomes possible for impulsive patients. Phenytoin, by contrast, is ineffective in the treatment of behavioural dyscontrol, and so the mode of action of carbamazepine is unlikely to be working through its anticonvulsant properties.

(c) *Antidepressants.* Selective serotonin reuptake inhibitors (SSRIs) have been demonstrated to be useful in patients with impulse control disorders, as have tricyclics. Monoamine-oxidase inhibitors (MAOIs), by stabilizing noradrenergic function, are of value in the treatment of affective instability, e.g. in borderline patients, although their toxicity in overdose may be a problem.

(d) *Benzodiazepines.* Problems exist with tolerance and dependency for this group of drugs, particularly in impulsive patients. They are useful in the short term for control of symptoms of anxiety, and in patients with intermittent explosive disorder, or interictal disorder of temporal lobe epilepsy. Occasional borderline patients may find them valuable (Stein, 1992). Their main drawback is that they may cause rage reactions, so they should be prescribed very rarely.

*3. Psychosocial treatments.* All physical treatments are inadequate alone, and psychotherapy, if only of a supportive nature, is a necessary part of any treatment. In particular, the treatment of personality requires care over a long period of time, and many patients fear abandonment during the process, and may need repeated reassurance that help will be available for as long as they need or can use it. This is not quite an unconditional commitment, as there is a clear expectation that the patient continues to work, and does not simply become dependent upon treatment. Biological and psychological symptoms frequently interact (i.e. many features of personality disorder may be psychological or social adaptations to the biological symptoms of, for example, affective instability or anxiety). For this reason, physical treatments aimed at reducing troublesome symptomatology may themselves aid psychosocial change.

(a) *Cognitive/behavioural/interpersonal.* Behavioural, cognitive and interpersonal approaches have been widely used. They range from simple social skills training and anger management through to much more complex interventions designed to give patients insight into the way others see them, and to identify and modify maladaptive responses to the world (Sperry, 1994). The advantage of these methods is that they reinforce coping mechanisms right from the outset, and provide a clear structure within which patients can frame their problems. They are particularly useful in behaviourally disordered patients.

(b) *Psychodynamic.* Dynamic psychotherapy, often over many years, may be useful for those patients who can control any tendency to act out, and have sufficient coping skills to deal with the regression which occurs during successful analytic treatment. They are particularly helpful with the anxious/inhibited group (Stone, 1993).

(c) *Therapeutic communities (TC).* These can be regarded as the ultimate psychosocial treatment, and may involve residential or day attendance units. Patients are assessed and offered placement, usually for a year to 18 months. A variety of group and individual work encourages subjects to explore their responses to others and rework them. Follow-up studies of those who complete TC placements suggest that they are effective in reducing a variety of indices of distress, such as in-patient stays, visits to medical or other carers, drug taking and criminality.

# Further reading

Oldham JM. Personality disorders: Current perspectives. *Journal of the American Medical Association*, 1994; **272**(22): 1770–6.

Rosenberg R. Borderline states: pharmacotherapy and psychobiology of personality. A discussion of Soloff's article. *Acta Psychiatrica Scandinavica*, 1994; **89**(suppl 379): 50–5 and 56–60.

Siever LJ, Davis KL. A psychobiological perspective on the personality disorders. *American Journal of Psychiatry*, 1991; **148**: 1647–58.

Sperry L. *Handbook of the Diagnosis and Treatment of the DSM-IV Personality Disorders.* New York: Brunner/Mazel, 1994.

Stein G. Drug treatment of personality disorders. *British Journal of Psychiatry,* 1992; **161**: 167–84.

Stone MH. Long-term outcome in personality disorders. *British Journal of Psychiatry,* 1993; **162**: 299–313.

Tyrer P, Casey P, Ferguson B. Personality disorder in perspective. *British Journal of Psychiatry,* 1991; **159**: 463–71.

# Related topics of interest

# PERSONALITY – PSYCHOLOGICAL MODELS

**Psychodynamic models**

Dynamic models focus on the interaction of conscious and unconscious forces via a series of putative mental structures and mechanisms (Brown and Pedder, 1990). *Freud's structural model* of the mind has three components:

- The *Id*: the source of all psychic energy and the original sole mental structure. The Id does not recognize time or space, and uses primary process thinking, where fantasy and reality are indistinguishable. The Id operates on the *pleasure principle*, demanding instant gratification of desires.
- The *Superego*: or ego ideal. An internalized representation of the parent which contains rules and prohibitions over what is allowed within consciousness and which impulses are effectively forbidden.
- The *Ego*: The central balancing force, the Ego has to mediate between the demands of the Id and the prohibitions of the Superego. It is based on the *reality principle* and is the agent of interaction with the real world.

Material which is inaccessible to consciousness is held in the unconscious; that which is accessible, in the conscious, which Freud divides into the *preconscious* (that not currently being attended to but available) and the *conscious* (that currently 'in mind').

Freudian models of personality relate to attempts to satisfy instinctual demands, and the expression of forbidden unconscious desires via the mediation of various defence mechanisms (see Defence mechanisms, p. 76) and to the strength of the various components of the structural model. They are developmental in nature (see Personality – development, p. 223), and current personality traits are seen as the result of past developmental aberrations or accidents.

Carl *Jung's Analytical Psychology*, developed as a result of his famous dream in which he explored the different levels of a house, divides the psyche again into conscious and unconscious. To prevent consciousness becoming flooded with experiences and thoughts, the Ego acts as a gatekeeper (in a very similar manner to the attentional filter postulated by psychologists). That not currently in consciousness is held in the *personal unconscious* (similar to

Freud's preconscious), in which most ideas are readily accessible. Groups of ideas cluster to form a *complex*, which can have enormous emotional significance for the person. Complexes develop as a result both of early experiences, but also from the contents of the *collective unconscious*. This is the 'basement' of the house in his dream, and contains thought patterns or images from our past ancestors, human and non-human. These *primordial images* are predispositions to think of, or compose models of, the world in a certain way. *Archetypes,* of which there are many (e.g. birth, death, the child, the demon, the earth mother, the shadow), are particularly emotionally charged forms of these, and relate to universal experiences during phylogeny. The predisposition to organize mental images in a pre-programmed way as archetypes is analogous to Chomsky's finding that humans have an innate grammar which they apply to the acquisition and organization of language. Archetypes are expressed in consciousness in the form of symbols.

At both unconscious and conscious levels, Jung saw the self as organized into two attitudes:

- *Introversion:* orientation toward subjective experience.
- *Extraversion:* orientation towards objective experience and four functions, two rational (thinking and sensing) and two non-rational: (feeling and intuiting).
  ___ *Thinking:* connecting ideas to understand the world and solve problems.
  ___ *Feeling:* subjective evaluation of ideas or objects.
  ___ *Sensing:* operation of sense organs and perception of the internal milieu.
  ___ *Intuiting:* subliminal, 'sixth sense' perception.

Usually, one of these is the dominant (superior) function, and the others are auxiliary, with the weakest (inferior) being repressed and unconscious.

# Other psychological models

**Radical behaviourism/drive theory**

B.F. Skinner was a radical behaviourist who viewed personality as entirely conditioned: that is as a series of reflex responses to stimuli. Drive theorists like Hull view it as a response to an infinitely expansible series of 'hard wired' drives. Eysenck has suggested that many of the personality differences between introverts and extroverts are related to differences in the ease with which they form conditioned responses, especially to social factors.

**Social learning theory**

As propounded by Seligman or Bandura, this theory views people as essentially rational and views behaviour and personality as learned and conditioned by experience. *'Learned helplessness'* is a powerful model of depression, and Seligman has also done work on *attributional styles*: that is, the ways in which people tend to attribute credit or blame for success or failure. People who become depressed are more likely to attribute failure to factors which are *internal* (to do with oneself) rather than external (e.g. fate); *global* (i.e. generalized across situations) rather than specific to the situation concerned, and *stable* (i.e. unlikely to change over time). This attributional style is also associated with high achievers, presumably because it is highly motivating in the case of success, just as it is unremittingly punishing in the event of failure. Depressed people are also more likely to attribute success to external and situation-specific factors (Seligman *et al.,* 1979). The attributional styles of normal people tend to exhibit the 'self-serving bias', first noted in actors, who tend to blame others for their failures, and take credit for successes on themselves. Depressives, even after recovery, seem to lack this rose-tinted egocentrism in their view of the world: that is, they are more realistic!

Social learning theory is a more believable extension of radical behavioural or drive theory models, and provides the foundation for the cognitive treatments now used with such great success in a wide variety of neurotic problems. (See the introduction in Hawton *et al.,* 1989.)

## Further reading

Brown D, Pedder J. *Introduction to Psychotherapy: an outline of psychodynamic principles and practice,* 2nd Edn. London: Tavistock Publications, 1990.
Hawton K, Salkovskis PM, Kirk J, Clark DM. *Cognitive Behaviour Therapy for Psychiatric Problems: a practical guide.* Oxford: Oxford University Press, 1989.
Seligman MEP, Abramson L, Semmel A, von Baeyer C. Depressive attributional style. *Journal of Abnormal Psychology,* 1979; **88:** 242–7.

## Related topics of interest

Defence mechanisms (p. 76)
Learning (p. 171)
Personality – development (p. 223)

Personality – assessment and classification (p. 214)
Psychological treatment – cognitive therapy (p. 261)

# PREMENSTRUAL SYNDROME (PMS) AND THE MENOPAUSE

**Definition and diagnosis**

- Up to 150 symptoms have been reported as associated with changes in the menstrual cycle. These symptoms are physical, cognitive, emotional, and behavioural.
- Since there are no biological markers of PMS, medical definitions put most emphasis on the timing of the symptoms. Thus, the symptoms should be prominent in the luteal phase of the cycle, relieved by menstruation, and minimal or absent in the follicular phase. Operational definitions rely largely on womens' subjective account of their symptoms. These can be difficult to interpret because severity often varies from month to month. Moreover, women often rate their symptoms more severely in retrospective accounts than they do in concurrent daily diaries. Hence, the standard practice now is to ask women to keep daily ratings of at least two cycles.
- There is controversy as to whether PMS should be a separate category in psychiatric classification. ICD-10 (1992) does not include PMS but DSM-IV includes Premenstrual Dysphasic Disorder in an appendix as a syndrome 'provided for further study'.
- In research and clinical practice the diagnosis of PMS must be distinguished from premenstrual exacerbation of an underlying emotional disorder (e.g. a depressive disorder) and from emotional problems that are not cyclical.

**Epidemiology**

- Over 90% of women experience some psychological symptoms premenstrually, but only approximately 5–10% have symptoms that regularly disrupt their life.
- Psychological symptoms include depressed mood, anxiety, irritability, forgetfulness and loss of libido.
- Physical symptoms include bloating, fatigue, tender breasts, appetite change, abdominal pain, and headaches.

**Aetiology**

- There have been many suggestions as to the aetiology of PMS but there is no convincing evidence that any of these theories is correct.
- There is no convincing evidence of an excess or deficiency of either oestrogen or progesterone in the aetiology of PMS.

| | |
|---|---|
| **Aspects of treatment** | It is difficult to interpret the reported findings because of (a) varying definitions of the syndrome, and (b) placebo effects are large (a 40% response can be expected in the first month in drug treatments of PMS). |
| **Drug treatments** | *1. Hormones.* Extensive anecdotal evidence has led to claims for the efficacy of progesterone and progestogens but randomized double blind placebo controlled trials do not support this view. Other hormones such as danazol, bromocriptine and gonadotrophin-releasing hormone agonists (GnRH agonists) are all expensive and carry a high risk of side-effects. GnRH agonists act by creating a reversible pseudo-menopause (more correctly a pseudo-hypophysectomy) and are of general benefit for most symptoms of PMS. Danazol and bromocriptine have most effect on cyclical breast pain.

*2. Non-hormonal treatments.* Include diuretics (such as spironolactone) for premenstrual bloating and weight gain and mefenamic acid for pain and fatigue. Evening primrose oil has been shown to relieve mastalgia.

*3. Psychotropic drugs.* Those which increase serotonin concentration either by stimulating release or by inhibiting reuptake seem to improve the psychological symptoms associated with PMS. For example, fluoxetine has relatively few side-effects and appears to produce considerable relief of premenstrual symptoms compared with placebo. |
| **Psychological treatments** | Women with physiological premenstrual changes will benefit from counselling, support and reassurance.

More recently cognitive behaviour therapy has been found to be of benefit (Blake *et al.*, 1995). The first step is to establish whether or not the patient is suffering from PMS as defined by diary ratings of premenstrual symptoms. This involves asking a woman to record premenstrual experiences in the previous 2–3 months, as well as past experiences of help seeking, her ideas about the causes of PMS, and her current expectations of treatment. One of the advantages of cognitive therapy is that it is applied both to the symptoms of PMS and to other factors in a woman's life that may be contributing to those symptoms. |
| **The menopause – definition of menopausal status** | The menopause is primarily a physiological event, marked by cessation of the menstrual cycle, experienced by all women who have not undergone earlier disease or surgery. |

The menopause is generally defined by the following menstrual criteria: premenstrual women are regularly menstruating; perimenopausal women have missed 2 or more cycles but have menstruated during the past year; and finally, women who have not menstruated for at least a year are deemed post-menopausal.

**Psychological effects of the menopause – psychological symptoms**

- Studies of menopause in non-clinic samples suggest that for the majority the menopause is not a major stress. Previous depression, social factors such as stressful life events, and attitudes and beliefs about the menopause appear to be more important than menopausal status.
- Also, women who assess their physical health as poor premenstrually are more likely to become depressed as their menopausal status changes.
- Psychological symptoms are the main discriminators between clinic and non-clinic samples of women: clinic samples are significantly more depressed, report more life stress and general symptoms.
- Menopause clinic attenders are also more likely to view the menopause as being not only personally uncontrollable but also associated with physical and emotional problems (approximately half the women who attend gynaecological clinics have psychiatric morbidity, often in association with marital and social problems).
- Decisions to seek medical help may occur when emotional distress occurs with vasomotor symptoms, and when these are experienced in the context of certain beliefs – in particular the belief that the symptoms are due to a current disease process. Thus some women appear to attribute emotional distress to the menopause, which is seen as a disease process responsible for both psychological and physical problems.

**Sexual effects of the menopause**

- There is some evidence that reduction of sexual interest, and of frequency of sexual activity with the partner, and, possibly, orgasm, may accompany the menopause.
- Most women however do not develop frank sexual dysfunction at this time.
- Satisfaction with the sexual relationship is unaffected in the majority of women.
- There is more consistent agreement that vaginal dryness, reduced vaginal lubrication during sexual stimulation, reduced vaginal blood flow and engorgement, and dyspareunia frequently accompany the menopause.

**The effect of HRT on psychological and sexual function**

- There is strong evidence that the addition of testosterone to oestrogen hormone replacement therapy (HRT) can have beneficial effects on reduced sexual desire.
- There is a lack of clear, positive evidence to support the psychological benefits of HRT in depressed menopausal women.

## Further reading

Blake F, Gath D, Salkovskis P. Psychological aspects of premenstrual syndrome: developing a cognitive approach. In: Mayou R, Bass C, Sharpe M (eds) *Treatment of Functional Somatic Symptoms.* Oxford: Oxford University Press, 1995; 271–84.

Hunter M. Gynaecological Complaints In: Bass C (ed.) *Somatization. Physical Symptoms and Psychological Illness.* Oxford: Blackwells Science Ltd, 1990; 235–58.

O'Brien PM. PMS Helping women with premenstrual syndrome. *British Medical Journal,* 1993; **307**: 1471–5.

Pearce J, Hawton K, Blake F. Psychological and sexual symptoms associated with the menopause and the effects of H.R.T. *British Journal of Psychiatry,* 1995; **167**: 163–73.

## Related topic of interest

Sexual disorders (p. 309)

# PSYCHIATRIC DISORDERS – GENETICS

The genetic basis of psychiatric disorders, especially the major psychoses, is well established in quantitative studies. Recent advances in molecular biology have brought about a better understanding of the genetic basis of psychiatric disorders.

**Terminology**

- *Genotype:* the composition of the genetic material.
- *Phenotype:* what we observe.
- *Modes of inheritance* include: single major gene; dominant, recessive or sex-linked, with variable penetrance and expression; or polygenic.
- *Heterogeneity:* describes the situation where the same phenotype (i.e. disorder) is caused by different genes or sets of genes.
- *Alleles* (different versions of one gene) of different genes (loci) may show independent assortment or may be linked.
- *Heritability* is the proportion of the variance due to genetic factors.

**Quantitative genetics**

Various methods can be used to investigate whether and to what extent genes contribute to a disorder.

*1. Family studies.* These compare the rates (as lifetime risk) of a disorder in the relatives of affected individuals with rates in the general population.

*2. Twin studies.* If there is a genetic basis to a disorder, the concordance rates for monozygotic twins should be greater than those of dizygotic twins. Concordance can be defined as probandwise or pairwise. Probandwise concordance is the number of affected co-twins of probands/number of co-twins of probands. The probandwise concordance may differ from pairwise concordance (= number of dually affected twin pairs/number of twin pairs) because twin pairs may be counted twice.

*3. Adoption studies.*

- Adoptee studies compare the rates of a disorder in the offspring of individuals with the disorder adopted into unaffected families, with the rates in control adoptees.
- Adoptee's family studies compare the rates in the biological and adoptive families of adoptees who develop a disorder.

- Cross-fostering studies compare the rates in offspring of affected individuals adopted by unaffected parents, with the rates in offspring of unaffected parents adopted by parents who subsequently develop the disorder.

*4. Linkage.* This is the association between two phenotypes, or genetic markers and a phenotype (i.e. psychiatric disorder). The lod scores (log of probability of linkage) reflect the closeness of linkage at different recombination fractions. Markers can be clinical (e.g. human leucocyte antigen (HLA) typing), or molecular (e.g. restriction fragment length polymorphisms (RFLPs)). Multipoint linkage uses several markers to locate more accurately a locus. The mode of transmission and heterogeneity can be confounding factors.

*5. Association studies.* These investigate the relationship between phenotypes, or a phenotype and genetic markers, in a group of affected individuals compared with a control group.

**Basic principles**

*1. Chromosomes.* The karyotype is the number and type of chromosomes. Mitosis is the simple duplication of the genome, whereas meiosis involves shuffling of the genetic material by recombination (exchange of genetic material between homologous chromosomes). Cytogenetic techniques are used to visualize the chromosomes to detect gross mutations and rearrangements.

*2. Molecular basis.* DNA is the basic genetic material. RNA is then copied (transcribed) from DNA and protein is then made from RNA by translation. Exons are the coding regions of genes and introns are the non-coding regions between exons. Enhancer and promoter sequences influence transcription of the coding regions. Introns contain unique or moderately repetitive or highly repetitive sequences. Their function is unclear but they are useful as markers, for example, in linkage studies. Mutations are alterations in the genetic material, in individual bases or groups of bases, which may or may not lead to a change in the nature of the protein produced.

*3. Genomic phenomena.* Those that are particularly relevant to psychiatry include mutations (see above and Mental handicap – genetic causes, p. 196); changes in particular sequences which have a propensity to being unstable (trinucleotide repeats) and occur in disorders with anticipation (the disorder is more severe and starts earlier in successive generations, for example bipolar disorder); and imprinting which describes biochemical changes in DNA resulting in non-genetic parental influences.

*4. Recombinant DNA technology/the 'new genetics'.* DNA and RNA probes can be used to measure gene expression, characterize the nature of a specific RNA or DNA, detect mutations or be used as markers in linkage studies. Restriction enzymes cut DNA in a sequence-specific manner, which is most useful in producing RFLPs. Southern blotting detects and characterizes DNA; Northern blotting does the same for RNA. Polymerase chain reaction (PCR) is the sequence-specific amplification of DNA or RNA.

*5. Applications.* These techniques can be used to investigate causal mutations, the relationship between DNA markers and disease in linkage and association studies (including the use of candidate genes) and in positional cloning. Gene expression in the central nervous system (CNS) can be studied by Northern blotting and *in situ* hybridization in both human and animal studies.

**Disorders**

*1. Schizophrenia.* The population lifetime risk for schizophrenia is approximately 1%.
(a) Family studies show lifetime risks in relatives of an individual with schizophrenia as follows:
- Siblings 10%.
- Children 12.8 (both parents 46%).
- First-degree relatives 2.8%.
(b) Adoption studies show the following rates:
- Adoptees: 10–18% (depending on diagnosis).
- Adoptees families: 20% of biological relatives compared with 6% of non-biological relatives.
- Cross-fostering: 11% of children of unaffected biological parents compared with 19% of offspring of affected parents.
(c) Twin studies show a probandwise concordance of 46% for monozygotic twins and 14% for dizygotic twins.
(d) Linkage studies have produced inconclusive results. There have been reports of linkage to markers on chromosome 5, but these have not been replicated.

2. *Affective disorders.*
(a) *Family studies.*
- First-degree relatives of unipolar (UP)patients: lifetime risk of UP =11%, lifetime risk of BP = 8%.
- First-degree relatives of bipolar (BP) patients: lifetime risk of UP = 9%, lifetime risk of BP = 0.6%.
- General population: lifetime risk of UP = 3%, lifetime risk of BP = <1%.
(b) *Twin studies.*
- Probandwise concordance UP: monozygotic = 54%, dizygotic = 24%.
- Probandwise concordance BP: monozygotic = 79%, dizygotic = 19%.
(c) *Linkage studies.*
There have been reports of linkage to markers on chromosome 11 and the X chromosome, but these have not been replicated.

*3. Personality.* Twin and adoption studies have shown that monozygotic twins have more similar personalities than dizygotic twins, so that although environment is clearly a major influence, inherited factors are also important.

*4. Neurosis.* There is a tendency for there to be greater rates of obsessional neurosis, anxiety disorder and phobias in first-degree relatives of individuals with these disorders, but there are problems establishing whether these are due to genetic or environmental factors.

*5. Other disorders.* Mental retardation (see Mental handicap – genetic causes, p. 196), addictive behaviour (see Addiction – aetiology, p. 1), eating disorders (see Eating disorders – aetiology, p. 118), delinquency (see Delinquency and antisocial personality, p. 81).

**Ethics and counselling**

Concerns have been raised that genetic research will lead to the practice of eugenics, to the neglect of non-biological research and interventions, and to therapeutic nihilism. Genetic research is actually more likely to lead to clarification of the aetiology of disorders and identification of psychological and environmental interventions.

Genetic counselling in psychiatric disorders is aimed at providing information about familial risks (schizophrenia and bipolar disorder) and advice about avoiding, for example, alcohol (alcoholism) and illicit drugs (schizophrenia). The only current exception to this is Huntington's disease, where closely linked markers on chromosome 4 allow <5% or >95% predictions of risk in individuals because the inheritance is dominant with complete penetrance. However, this is not entirely straightforward, as information from other relatives is required, as is careful pre- and post-test counselling. Pre-natal testing can also be carried out with this marker test but it may only be possible to predict a 50% risk. The pathological mutation has now been identified so it may become possible to be more specific about individual risk.

## Further reading

McGuffin P, Murray R. (eds) *The New Genetics of Mental Illness.* London: Butterworth-Heinemann, 1991.
McGuffin P, Owen MJ, O'Donovan MC, Thapar A, Gottesman II. *Seminars in Psychiatric Genetics.* London: Gaskell, 1994.
Weatherall DJ. *The New Genetics and Clinical Practice,* 3rd Edn. Oxford: Oxford University Press, 1991.

## Related topic of interest

Mental handicap – genetic causes (p. 196)

# PSYCHIATRIC DISORDERS – LIFE EVENTS

Recent studies have examined how life events and chronic difficulties interact with other variables, including the possible genetic vulnerability, personality predisposition and co-morbidity between stress-induced disorders, in predicting illness.

## Specific stressors

**Child sexual abuse**

- Comparison of abused children with normal comparison groups reveals a wide variety of increased psycho-pathology.
- When sexually abused children are compared with other clinical psychiatric samples, however, only two syndromes clearly emerge as more common: post-traumatic stress disorder (PTSD) and sexualized behaviour.
- Variables which increase the likelihood of adverse outcome include a close perpetrator, high frequency of sexual abuse, a long duration of abuse and the use of force and sexual acts that include penetration, and a lack of maternal support at the time of disclosure.

**Other stressors in children**

- Children of depressed mothers are at greater risk of childhood psychiatric disorders.
- Social supports can buffer the effects of stressors causing depression in children.

**Marital breakdown**

- Divorce is a significant life event with substantial psychosocial sequelae.
- Men and women who are divorced are at greater risk of depression.
- There is some evidence that men are at greater risk of depression following marital breakdown than women.

**Unemployment**

- Remains a significant risk factor for psychiatric illness.
- In one study, 12 months after voluntary redundancy depression (but not anxiety) was the major outcome.
- The emotional effects of unemployment on women are as significant as they are for men.

**Single traumatic event**

- Major disaster continues to be a fruitful area for study.
- The relevance of the severity and duration of the life-event stressor as an important variable in generating PTSD has recently been questioned.
- Among 2000 people directly affected by the King's Cross Fire in London, 44% had a GHQ score indicating probable caseness out of 82% of passengers and by-standers who had sought help from a helpline.

- The symptoms of the disorder were not related to the severity of the stressor.
- In the King's Cross study, the symptoms were related to the 16-item Impact of Events score, which is probably a reflection of an underlying personality problem (see Stress reactions, p. 330).

# Specific syndromes

**Schizophrenia**

- There is consistent evidence that the course of schizophrenic illness is affected by stressor life events, but somewhat less evidence that its initial onset is so determined.
- Stressors have a significant impact on non-psychotic symptoms in schizophrenics.

**Affective disorders**

1. *Depression.*
(a) In general, life events close to onset have a significant bearing on affective disorders.
(b) Brown *et al.* (1993) found that severe childhood adversity (sexual or physical abuse or gross parental indifference involving physical or emotional neglect) were associated with both depressive and anxiety disorders.
(c) Similarly, an acute event before onset was commonly found in both anxiety and depressive disorders.
(d) In contrast, longer-term adult adversity (death of a child or spouse, marital separation and divorce, multiple abortions and sexual and physical violence) only affected depression but not anxiety.
(e) Recovery from depression is also related, in part, to life events: lack of negative self-esteem at the first interview with the experience of 'difficulty reduction' and 'fresh-start' events was associated with recovery from chronic depression in one study.
(f) Post (1992) cites evidence that the first episode of affective disorder is more likely to be caused by a stressor than are subsequent episodes, indicating that the stressor (or the occurrence of the affective episode itself) has induced an enhanced biological vulnerability to subsequent depressive episodes.

2. *Mania.*
(a) There is evidence that first or second episodes of mania are associated with severe life events.

(b) This contrasts with patients who have had many episodes; their reduced social networks result in a reduced chance of exposure to life events.

(c) In a prospective study of bipolar patients there was a statistical association with relapse for severe events (4 or 5 on a 5-point scale) but not minor events.

*3. Puerperal psychosis.* Two studies, performed independently, have demonstrated the absence of a relationship between stressful life events and the onset of puerperal psychosis.

*4. Suicide and suicidal behaviour.*

(a) In a recent uncontrolled psychological autopsy study, 85% reported a significant preceding life event in the 3 months before suicide (job problems, family discord and physical illness were common).

(b) In a study comparing completed suicide in substance misusers and those with affective disorders, those with alcohol-related suicide had an increased frequency of and a broader range of interpersonal stressors in the 6 weeks before death.

*5. Post-traumatic stress disorder.*

(a) Recent research has focused on other psychosocial variables influencing PTSD.

(b) Gross childhood stress (e.g. early childhood physical abuse) is a risk factor.

(c) Personality is also an important risk factor, with high rates found in Vietnam veteran PTSD subjects.

(d) In patients presenting with PTSD, many other psychiatric conditions coexist; for example, major depression, substance misuse, anxiety disorders.

(e) Such co-morbidity often persists over time; for example, in Cambodian refugees living in the USA 10 years after migration, 86% had PTSD and 80% had depressive syndromes.

(f) There is increasing evidence of a genetic basis: after adjusting for differences in combat exposure in Vietnam veterans, genetic factors accounted for 13–30% of symptoms in the 're-experiencing' cluster, 30–34% in the 'avoidance' cluster and 28–32% in the 'arousal' cluster.

(g) Psychobiological factors are important, with the possible involvement of brain structures, including the amygdala, locus ceruleus and hippocampus, as well as noradrenergic, dopaminergic, opioid and cortico-trophin-releasing factors.

**Psychosomatic and other disorders**  Patients with non-organic abdominal pain (often leading to the removal of a normal appendix) and parasuicide patients are more likely to experience a threatening event during the 13 weeks prior to the onset of pain or overdose than members of a community comparison group.

# Further reading

Creed F. Life events and disorder. *Current Opinion in Psychiatry,* 1992; **5**: 300–4.
Tennant C. Life event stress and psychiatric illness. *Current Opinion in Psychiatry,* 1994; **7**: 207–12.

# Related topics of interest

Child sexual abuse – assessment and consequences (p. 55)
Schizophrenia – social aspects (p. 303)
Stress reactions (p. 330)

# PSYCHIATRIC DISORDERS – NEUROENDOCRINE CHANGES

**Neuro-endocrine system**

*1. Hypothalamus.* The hypothalamus is involved in the control of eating and sleeping, etc., the autonomic system and in the secretion of hormones. Neurosecretory neurones are:

- *Magnocellular.* Cells in the supraoptic and paraventricular nuclei which release vasopressin (or anti-diuretic hormone (ADH)) and oxytocin from nerve endings in the posterior pituitary.
- *Parvocellular.* Found in the tubero-infundibular system (which connects the hypothalamus to the anterior pituitary) and in the paraventricular nucleus.

| Hypothalamic hormones | Pituitary hormones |
| --- | --- |
| Vasopressin and oxytocin | |
| Thyroid releasing hormone (TRH) | Thyroid stimulating hormone (TSH) |
| Gonadotrophin releasing hormone (GnRH) | Luteinizing hormone (LH)/follicle stimulating hormone (FSH) |
| Growth hormone releasing hormone (GHRH) | Growth hormone (GH) |
| Growth hormone inhibiting hormone (GHIH) | |
| Cortisol relaeasing factor (CRF) and ADH | Adrenocorticotrophic hormone (ACTH) |
| Dopamine | Prolactin (PRL) |

*2. Pituitary.* The pituitary can be divided into:

- Posterior pituitary which contains nerve endings from the hypothalamus.
- Anterior pituitary which contains a variety of secretory cell types which are regulated by hypothalamic hormones.

*3. Anterior pituitary cell types.*

(a) *Chromophils.*
- Acidophils: somatotrophs (GH), lactotrophs (PRL).
- Basophils: corticotrophs (ACTH), thyrotrophs (TSH), gonadotrophs (LH/FSH)

(b) *Chromophobes.*
- Non-secretory.

**Regulation of hormones**

*1. Growth hormone (GH).* Release is stimulated by: exercise and stress; increased activity of the dopamine, $\alpha_2$-adrenergic and 5-hydroxytryptamine (5-HT) systems; thyroid hormones, opioids and oestrogens; in acromegaly, starvation and in anorexia nervosa. Release is inhibited by glucocorticoids, GH, hypothyroidism and reduced activity of the 5-HT, dopamine and $\alpha_2$-adrenergic systems.

*2. Prolactin (PRL).* The control of PRL release from the anterior pituitary is principally by dopamine which is inhibitory and involved in an autoregulatory feedback loop. L-dihydroxyphenylalanine (L-dopa) and bromocriptine (dopamine agonist) inhibit PRL release. Neuroleptics are dopamine antagonists and therefore increase secretion. Gamma-aminobutyric acid (GABA) increases PRL release, as do TRH, 5-HT, vasoactive intestinal peptide (VIP) and opioids.

(a) *Causes of hyperprolactinaemia.*
- Prolactinomas.
- Lesions of hypothalamus and pituitary stalk.
- Primary hypothyroidism.
- Renal failure.
- Drugs: neuroleptics, anti-emetics, reserpine, methyldopa, TRH, opiates, oral contraceptives.
- Idiopathic causes: stress, hypovolaemia.

*3. Hypothalamo–pituitary–adrenal (HPA) axis.* CRF released from the hypothalamus stimulates release of ACTH from the pituitary which leads to release of cortisol from adrenal glands. Particular aspects of release are a circadian rhythm and release in response to stress.

(a) *Changes in the HPA in depression.*
- Cortisol: increased secretion, reduced amplitude of circadian rhythm and relative resistance to dexamethasone.
- ACTH: normal basal concentrations and relative resistance to dexamethasone suppression.
- CRF: increased secretion.

It is also relevant to note the psychiatric effects of cortisol and related steroids. These can cause depression, mania or psychosis, possibly in predisposed individuals.

*4. Hypothalamo–pituitary–gonadal (HPG) axis.* GnRH is released from the hypothalamus, which stimulates LH and FSH release from the pituitary. Abnormalities of this axis are found in eating disorders, post-partum and during the menopause. In anorexia nervosa FSH and LH are reduced at low weight, as well as oestrogens and testosterone. Circulating hormones return to normal with weight gain but restoration of the normal cyclical pattern is delayed. The pattern of LH release resembles that in prepubertal girls, the response of LH to clomiphene is abnormal, and there is a normal response of FSH but not LH to exogenous luteinizing hormone releasing hormone (LHRH).

**Clinical neuroendocrine changes**

*1. Depression.*

- Cortisol: increased activity of HPA axis (see above).
- GH: reduced response to clonidine.
- TSH: TRH response blunted.
- PRL: response to L-tryptophan (LTP) blunted.

*2. Eating disorders.*
(a) *Anorexia nervosa.*
- HPG axis: reduced LH and FSH, prepubertal pattern of release.
- GH: normal or increased GH level.
- HPA: increased cortisol.
- PRL: increased prolactin.
- Lowered thyroxine (T4).

(b) *Bulimia.*
- Menstrual abnormalities despite normal weight.

# Further reading

Morgan G, Butler S. *Seminars in Basic Neurosciences.* London: Gaskell, 1994.

# Related topics of interest

# PSYCHIATRY IN GENERAL PRACTICE

## Five levels and four filters

These were described by Goldberg and Huxley (1992). They used the General Health Questionnaire (GHQ), an instrument designed for community use, and estimated annual period prevalence rates at each level, per 1000, per year as follows

| | |
|---|---|
| The community | 260–315 |
| filter 1 | |
| illness behaviour | |
| Mental morbidity in GP attenders | 230 |
| filter 2 | |
| ability to detect disorder | |
| Mental morbidity identified by GP | 101 |
| filter 3 | |
| referral to psychiatric services | |
| Total morbidity in psychiatric services | 23.5 |
| filter 4 | |
| admission to psychiatric beds | |
| Psychiatric in-patients | 5.7 |

**Psychiatric morbidity in the community**

Psychological symptoms are very common in the community: for example, Srole *et al.* (1962) found neurotic symptoms in 71%, which thus represents an extreme ceiling on rates of psychiatric morbidity.

Estimates of this vary widely, depending to some extent on the population, but mainly on the definition of a case, as illustrated by studies using psychiatric instruments (e.g. Present State Examination (PSE), research diagnostic criteria (RDC)), which have generally found lower rates than GHQ above: 8–15% in females, slightly less in males.

**Illness behaviour and psychiatric morbidity in GP consulters**

Most people have their own coping mechanisms for psychological distress, such as positive thinking, exercise, prayer, etc. and/or confiding in friends or family. Nevertheless, and perhaps surprisingly, it seems that most people with significant psychiatric morbidity do present to the GP, as indicated by the similarity between the prevalence in the community and in GP attenders (see above).

*1. Consultations with the GP.* However, only a minority of these patients complain directly about psychological symptoms. Bridges and Goldberg (1985) assessed in detail 590 new onsets of illness. 195 (33%) could be ascribed to a mental disorder, which they describe as follows:

|  | Percentage |
|---|---|
| 1. Physical illness with secondary mental disorder | 3 |
| 2. Mental disorder and unrelated physical disorder | 24 |
| 3. Somatization, i.e. complained of physical symptoms but no physical cause, and mental disorder present | 57 |
| 4. Entirely mentally ill | 15 |

Thus, in groups 1–3, physical symptoms are prominent, and are often the focus of treatment. These patients are the 'hidden cases' of mental disorders which GPs are sometimes criticized for not detecting. However, as indicated by Goldberg (1994), many of these patients may:

- Know that their disorders are transient.
- Not wish to be seen as mentally ill: they still regard this as stigmatizing.
- Not desire treatment for symptoms even when it is offered.
- Just want serious physical causes of their somatic symptoms to be excluded.

'Failure to detect disorder can therefore be a collusive phenomenon between a reluctant patient and a GP who is unsure what to do about any disorder that is detected.'

However, in 'defence' of the GP, it should be remembered that:

- It is a expecting a lot of the GP to 'sell' a diagnosis of mental illness during a single 6–10 minute consultation to a patient who begins by complaining of a physical symptom.

- Diagnoses may take more than one consultation, so the detection rate is greater in practice.
- Primary care copes alone with 95% or more of psychiatric cases.
- Even a small increase in referral rates would swamp the psychiatric services.

There is a large variation in the proportion of consulters GPs judge to have a mental disorder, a rate of 20% is accepted as a general guide. A further proportion, perhaps 10–15%, would be regarded as 'cases' by psychiatrists.

**Common syndromes in primary care and their classification**

Various classification systems have been used, such as ICD, ICD-10 (PHC), the version for primary care, multiaxial (physical/psychological/social) and Goldberg's above scheme. They agree that organic psychoses, bipolar affective disorder and schizophrenia form a much lower proportion of primary care psychiatry (perhaps 2% each) than in specialist practice.

However, they do not describe well the depression, anxiety, other forms of neurosis and adjustment disorders which form the vast majority of primary care presentations. Clear-cut psychiatric disorders are the exception, not the rule. A typical case would be a mixture of mild anxiety and depressive symptoms occurring after a 'life event': this might form a case of anxiety in one classification, or depression in another. Furthermore, diagnosis does not predict outcome, although there is a link to symptom severity. GPs seem justified in classifying and treating most cases symptomatically.

*1. Depression.* This can be diagnosed in up to 10% of GP attenders, half of whom have 'major depression'. It is recognized much less frequently, as shown above. It has been shown that training in communication skills can improve GPs recognition of depression. However, reviews (see Ormel and Tiemens, 1995) have indicated little evidence that this alone improves the outcome, without attention to management skills.

Treatments for depression proven effective in psychiatric patients cannot automatically be extrapolated to primary care, where comparatively few trials have been done, though there is evidence from GP populations that full doses of tricyclics are effective in major depression. Many GPs use antidepressants, and find them effective, in doses psychiatrists would regard as inadequate. Few treatments have been rigourously shown to be effective in the commoner 'minor depression'.

2. *Defeat depression campaign.* This is a joint Royal College of General Practitioners/Royal College of Psychiatrists initiative aiming to raise awareness of depression and its treatability amongst the general public, and help GPs to recognize and manage it. Further details and educational materials are available from the Colleges.

3. *Anxiety* of all kinds is very common. Many cases show a mixture of anxiety and depressive symptoms. Presentation is often with the physical symptoms of anxiety. Diagnosis, explanation, reassurance and advice as to self-help (i.e. reading materials, relaxation training) are all that is required in most cases.

In severe, acute anxiety, benzodiazepines are very effective. GPs in the past have over-prescribed them for psychological distress of all kinds, but should not be afraid to use them carefully, according to official guidelines (see British National Formulary (BNF)). Sedative antidepressants are sometimes used where minor tranquillizers would formerly have been given, and their sedative, hypnotic and anxiolytic properties are very useful (though they are not licensed for this indication).

4. *'Heartsink' patients.* A term recently coined by O'Dowd for frequent attenders with multiple psychosomatic complaints. Most probably have somatization disorder perhaps together with personality disorder. Management is by contracting, with a view to harm limitation (see Difficult to help patients, p. 110).

5. *Other diagnoses.* It is impossible to mention all diagnoses in a short account. Further information is available in Goldberg (1994).

6. *Referral.* Studies confirm clinical experience that referral often takes place for reasons other than the clinical state of the patient, for example illness in a carer.

There is little evidence that referral influences long-term outcome, for example the important Edinburgh Primary Care Depression Study (Scott and Freeman, 1992): patients diagnosed as depressed by their GP improved just as markedly when randomized to usual GP care as when given specialist care (costing at least twice as much).

7. *Organization of services.* GP fundholding has given GPs budgets to purchase services for their patients, and increasingly, they are choosing to provide more mental health services 'in house', rather than referring. Many employ counsellors, and some even 'purchase' staff such as community psychiatric nurses and occupational therapists. Some psychiatrists feel there is a danger that resources may thus be channelled towards the 'worried well' and away from the severely mentally ill, many of whom, especially in inner cities, find it difficult even to find a GP.

Most mental health professionals remain employed in secondary care, however, even if they work increasingly outside hospital, such as working in clinics in health centres and visiting patients in their homes.

# Further reading

Bridges K, Goldberg D. Somatic presentations of psychiatric illness in primary care settings. *Journal of Psychosomatic Research*, 1985; **32:** 137–44.

Goldberg D. In: Pullen I *et al. Psychiatry and General Practice Today.* London, Royal Colleges of Psychiatry and General Practice, 1994.

O'Dowd TL. Five years of heartsink patients in general practice. *British Medical Journal,* 1988; **297:** 528–30.

Ormel J, Tiemens H. Recognition and treatment of mental illness in primary care. *General Hospital Psychiatry*, 1995; **17,** 160–4.

Scott D, Freeman C. Edinburgh primary care depression study. *British Medical Journal*, 1992; **304:** 883–7.

Srole T *et al. Mental Health in the Metropolis*. New York: McGraw Hill, 1962.

# Related topics of interest

# PSYCHOLOGICAL TREATMENT – BEHAVIOUR THERAPY

This therapy is based on the premise that all behaviour, including abnormal behaviour, can be self-sustaining. Symptoms are improved as a result of changed behaviour, and are based on psychological principles of learning, including classical and operant conditioning. It places less importance on diagnosis and on past (e.g.childhood) experiences. The cornerstone of this approach is observation of the antecedents and consequences of behaviours by means of a 'functional analysis'.

**Assessment**

The initial step is a detailed assessment of behaviour, which includes the following areas:

- Problem situation.
- Problem clarification.
- Motivational analysis.
- Developmental analysis.
- Self-control.
- Social relationships.
- Norms of the patient's environment.

Following assessment, goals for changed behaviour will be set and strategies for measuring outcome put in place. Failure to progress results in re-analysis of behaviour.

Although each case should be treated on the basis of a functional analysis, in practice the following types of procedure tend to be used in the following conditions.

*1. Pad and bell for enuresis.* A child sleeps on a pad which completes an electrical circuit and rings a bell when wetted. The child then gets up, empties bladder and remakes the bed. Effective in >60% of cases.

*2. Systematic desensitization for phobias.* The patient is first trained to relax. Patient and therapist construct a hierarchy of gradually more difficult situations and plan a series of tasks. The tasks involve exposure to the feared situation, either by use of slides, video or audio tapes, imagery or real life (*in vivo*). The patient carries out the agreed tasks, either alone or with the therapist or a friend providing support. At each stage the patient must achieve relaxation and cope with the stimulus before moving on to the next task. Within-session habituation has been shown to be an important factor in success. As therapy proceeds the conditioned response to the feared situation is extinguished. Modifications of this technique have also been applied more recently to rape/assault victims, post-traumatic stress disorder and 'needle freaks' in drug addiction.

*3. Flooding for phobias.* Patients are exposed to the feared object or situation and required to stay there until the fear has abated. Serious side-effects have occurred in only 0.26% of patients in one study, and several studies suggest efficacy comparable to systematic desensitization. Despite this, it is less often used.

*4. Relaxation.* This technique is widely used as a general method for relieving anxiety. It forms part of many other therapies, including systematic desensitization and cognitive behaviour therapy (CBT) and is used in biofeedback strategies for headaches, chronic pain, hypertension and diabetic control. Patients are given education about the physiological processes underlying anxiety and are then trained in techniques of controlled breathing and progressive muscular relaxation.

*5. Response prevention for obsessive-compulsive disorder (OCD).* (See Obsessive-compulsive disorder, p. 219). The success rate is reported to be 70%.

*6. Applied behaviour analysis.* This is an individualized approach utilizing a range of techniques, with emphasis on measurement and modification of a defined range of behaviours. The usual application is in chronic conditions, including learning disability, chronic schizophrenia, chronic physical illness, mutism, self-injury, violence, hyperactivity, lack of self-care, hoarding, stereotyped movements. It includes the concept of the 'token economy', in which a specified desired behaviour is rewarded with tokens which are convertible into privileges.

*7. Self-control for smoking, obesity, alcohol, etc.* Behavioural analysis helps patients to identify mediating triggers for behaviour and thus to change their behaviour by avoiding them or substituting other rewarding behaviour.

*8. Social skills training.* This is suitable for any patient (unless very psychotic) with difficulty in forming/maintaining relationships with others. This uses modelling, social reinforcement, shaping, role playing and modification of expectancies. Evidence exists that in schizophrenia, social skills training reduces the time spent in hospital and reduces the relapse rate.

## Further reading

Kanfer FH, Saslow G. Behavioural diagnosis. In: Franks CM (ed.) *Behaviour Therapy: appraisal and status.* New York: McGraw-Hill, 1969.

Lieberman RP, Mueser KT, Wallace CJ. Social skills training for schizophrenic individuals at risk for relapse. *American Journal of Psychiatry,* 1986; **143:** 523–6.

Marks I. *Fears, Phobias, and Rituals.* Oxford: Oxford University Press, 1987.

Paul GL, Lentz RJ. *Psychosocial Treatment of Chronic Mental Patients.* Cambridge, Mass: Harvard University Press, 1977.

## Related topics of interest

Learning (p. 171)
Psychological treatment – cognitive therapy (p. 261)

# PSYCHOLOGICAL TREATMENT – COGNITIVE THERAPY

**Theory**

This therapy is based on the cognitive model of emotional disorders which assumes that an individual's affect and behaviour are largely determined by the way in which he/she structures the world. It was developed by A.T Beck in the 1970s. The therapy is collaborative, structured, problem oriented and educational. It is time limited and goal oriented and includes elements of:

- Cognitive therapy.
- Behavioural treatment.
- Problem solving.
- Coping strategies.

**Cognitive model of emotional disorders**

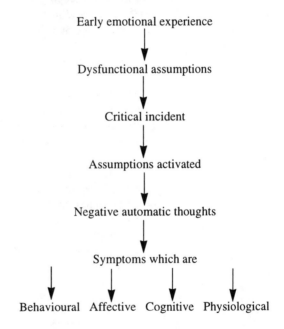

Early emotional experience

Dysfunctional assumptions

Critical incident

Assumptions activated

Negative automatic thoughts

Symptoms which are

Behavioural    Affective    Cognitive    Physiological

*1. Dysfunctional assumptions* tend to be:

- Unreasonable and rigid.
- Excessive.
- Interfere with other goals.
- Associated with powerful emotion.
- Usually unconscious.

For example, if I can't do something very well, there's no point in doing it at all.

*2. Cognitive distortions* are an important concept in the cognitive model and include the following:

- Black and white thinking.
- Overgeneralization.
- Selective abstraction.
- Mind reading.
- Fortune telling.
- Catastrophizing.
- Labelling.
- Personalizing.

**Treatment**

*1. Assessment.* This may be achieved over several sessions and uses history taking, standardized questionnaires, for example, Beck Depression Inventory, and self-assessment with diary keeping and event monitoring by the patient. These can lead to construction of a formulation and include identification of coping resources .

*2. Formulation.* Often using a diagram based on the 'Cognitive model of emotional disorders' above and showing vulnerability factors, precipitants, current situational variables, the current problem in behavioural, affective, cognitive and physiological terms, maintaining factors and hypotheses about targets for change.

*3. Goal setting.* Specific, positive goals, which are measurable and realistic, and often collaboratively planned. Often a hierarchy is used, tackling easiest goals first to create the experience of success with the technique.

*4. Questioning dysfunctional assumptions.* This can be achieved by a variety of methods, including 'Socratic questioning', and leads to the planning of behavioural experiments.

*5. Review.*

**Application**

- Simple phobias.
- Panic disorder and agoraphobia.
- Anxiety.
- Depression.
- Eating disorders.
- Sexual problems.

- Obsessive-compulsive disorder.
- Social phobias.
- Addictions.
- Gambling.
- Functional somatic symptoms.

## Further reading

Greenberger D, Padesky CA. *Mind Over Mood. A Cognitive Therapy Treatment Manual for Clients.* Hove: Guildford Press, 1995.
Hawton K, Salkovskis P, Kirk J, Clark D. *Cognitive Behaviour Therapy for Psychiatric Problems: A Practical Guide.* Oxford: Oxford University Press, 1989.

## Related topics of interest

# PSYCHOLOGICAL TREATMENT – CRISIS INTERVENTION

Crisis occurs:

> *when a person faces an obstacle to important life-goals that is, for a time, insurmountable through the utilisation of customary methods of problem solving. A period of disorganisation ensues, a period of upset, during which many abortive attempts at solution are made.*
>
> (Caplan 1961)

Thus a crisis may be thought of as a situation which one needs to negotiate, and the concept of coping is important. Successful and mature coping usually makes use of some sort of problem-solving ability. When this fails less mature strategies may be used such as regression, denial or even inertia, which is usually accompanied by feelings of hopelessness. Thus a crisis which causes a person to present for help may pass through the following phases:

(a)  Arousal and attempts at problem solving.
(b)  Arousal reaches a level which hinders rather than promotes coping behaviour.
(c)  Emergency resources mobilized and novel methods of coping tried.
(d)  Continuing failure leads to deterioration, exhaustion and decompensation.

**Common problems encountered**

- *Loss.* Feelings of loss may occur in relation to several events, including loss of a loved one (see Bereavement and grief counselling, p. 47), loss of health or physical integrity, loss of resources especially financial, loss of a valued role such as occurs on retirement.
- *Change problems.* Adjustment to a new social role, for example marital status, parenthood, work, identity.
- *Interpersonal problems.*
- *Conflict problems,* where the individual faces a difficult or apparently impossible choice.

**Intervention**

Aims at 'the psychological resolution of the immediate crisis and restoration to at least the level of functioning that existed prior to the crisis' (Aguilera and Messick, 1974). The literature about crisis intervention is diverse, but has some common themes which include:

- Helping the individual to gain cognitive mastery of the situation.
- Dealing with excessive use of the defence of denial.
- Mobilizing and dealing with appropriate affect.

The patient–therapist relationship is vital, and in particular attention should be paid to whether the patient is being offered and accepting the sick role or not – usually not unless decompensation is severe.

*1. Initial assessment.* Detailed enquiry about the events of the last 48 hours. Elicit the:

- Current problems.
- Level of coping ability.
- Degree of support from family and friends.
- Degree to which home situation is helpful or the opposite.
- Mental state.

A decision is made about whether the patient should have responsibility for his/her affairs temporarily taken over by others.

*2. Intensive care.* In this type of crisis intervention there is explicit transfer of responsibility from the patient leading to:

- Organization of immediate practical tasks.
- Removal of patient from stressful environment, which may involve admission to hospital.
- Lowering arousal and distress by psychological support or failing that by drugs. It is especially important to ensure adequate sleep.
- Reinforcing appropriate communication.
- Showing concern and warmth and encouraging hope.

*3. Crisis counselling.* In this type of crisis intervention there is a verbal contract which defines the patient–therapist relationship and extent of intervention. The patient is regarded as an adult seeking help. If the patient is unable to agree or conform to this contract, then brief goal-oriented crisis counselling is precluded. Strategies in crisis counselling include:

- Facilitating the expression of affect.
- Facilitating communication.
- Facilitating the patient's understanding of both his/her problems and feelings.
- Showing concern and empathy and bolstering self-esteem.
- Facilitating problem-solving behaviour by teaching the patient the following procedure, known as problem-solving therapy (see Cognitive function – assessment, p. 66).

*4. Problem-solving therapy.*

- Identify and define problem.
- Identify alternative methods of coping with that problem.
- Cognitively rehearse each alternative and become clear about its implications.
- Choose one alternative to follow.
- Define the behavioural steps required to carry out that alternative.
- Carry out the alternative, step by step.
- Check the effects of this behaviour to ensure that the choice of alternative has been a suitable one.

The choice leading to a good outcome may still be an intuitive process, but the chances of making an appropriate choice are generally enhanced by following the above steps.

The role of the therapist may be to:
- Explain the principles of the technique.
- Help with problem definition.
- Suggest additional coping methods.
- Remind patient where his/her strengths and weaknesses lie.
- Help patient to confront reality if necessary.
- Help patient break down action into manageable behavioural steps.
- Help in evaluation of coping behaviour.

*Note:* The help given to someone in crisis may also involve expert advice; for example, medical, legal, financial.

Prescription of the following medication may be helpful;
- Minor tranquillizer to lower arousal.
- Hypnotic to ensure adequate sleep.
- Antidepressant if depression is inhibiting coping behaviour.

# Further reading

Aguilera DC, Messick JM. *Crisis intervention: theory and methodology.* St Louis, MO: CV Mosby, 1974.

Bancroft J. Crisis intervention. In: Bloch S (ed.) *An Introduction to the Psychotherapies.* Oxford: Oxford University Press, 1979; Chap. 4.

Brandon S. Crisis theory and possibilities of therapeutic intervention. *British Journal of Psychiatry,* 1970; **117:** 627–33.

Caplan G. *An Approach to Community Mental Health.* London: Tavistock, 1961.

# PSYCHOLOGICAL TREATMENT – FAMILY THERAPIES

Family therapy is a generic term for techniques involving working with families. It has an eclectic basis which draws on concepts and techniques from a broad range of fields. These include, in particular, concepts from psychodynamic (especially group) therapy, from systems theory and from learning theory. There are increasing similarities with marital therapy which is considered below.

## Family therapy

**Schools**

1. *Structural family therapy.* This is based on the concept that the family structure is formed by regulating codes and therapy aims to change the structure, communication and function of the family in order to change the symptoms of the presenting individual. The boundaries of and within the family derive from who participates and how, and boundaries can be too rigid (disengaged) or too weak (enmeshed). Family health is measured by a well-defined and elaborated, flexible and cohesive structure. Alignment is the joining or opposition of two family members in carrying out an operation. Techniques include joining, reframing, enactment, marking boundaries, unbalancing. It was originally developed by Minuchin.

2. *Strategic family therapy.* Strategic and systemic family therapy are based on different concepts but they each use principles and techniques from the other.

Strategic family therapy is a problem based therapy, where although understanding the meaning of the problem is important it is not the basis for intervention. It is pragmatic and behaviour-oriented, directives are given and the therapist designs a strategy using: relabelling, unbalancing, prescribing, amplifying, seeding ideas, encouraging relapse, task setting, paradoxical instructions.

There are similarities with structural therapy, as well as using techniques from systemic therapy.

3. *Systemic family therapy.* This is based on the concept that families are systems where (a) individuals are not independent, and (b) in the pursuit of homeostasis changes are often focused on one individual who then presents as the problem. It includes the Milan approach which is

characterized by having a team behind the mirror as well as the therapist(s), with pre-, mid- and post-session discussions. Techniques include hypothesizing, circularity, neutrality, triadic questioning, difference questioning, positive connotations, family rituals, paradox and counter-paradox and invariant prescriptions (although these techniques may also be used in strategic therapy).

**Assessment**

Assessment involves collecting information about the presenting problem, but also about family functioning in general and in response to the perceived problems. Family assessments allow observation of the relationships within the family, and of the perception of the problems from different family members, which is then used to carry out the appropriate management techniques.

**Indications**

- Evidence of a malfunctioning group.
- Evidence that this family dysfunction is related to the problems for which help is being sought.
- The patient is a child or adolescent (or an adult with strong family involvement, for example in eating disorders).
- Availability of appropriately skilled therapist(s).

Family intervention is also used in schizophrenia to reduce high expressed emotion which has a detrimental effect on the prognosis.

**Contraindications**

- All the key members cannot or do not want to be there.
- The problems are too chronic or ingrained (i.e. unlikely to be changed).
- If family therapy might make the problems worse before making them better.
- If there is severe depression or emotional deprivation, because family therapy may not help, may upset the family balance and requires skilled therapist(s).
- Care should be taken if the family has been referred by the school or court, because motivation may be complicated.

# Marital therapy

With the changes in family structure, there is increasing overlap between family and marital therapy, and they have a significant amount in common in terms of techniques. The problems presented reflect the stage of the relationship, people's changing expectations and any associated mental illness.

Marital therapy is often eclectic in approach, using techniques from any of the following forms, but generally with the therapist(s) as arbiter and interpreter.

| | |
|---|---|
| **Behavioural marital therapy** | This identifies problems in terms of the individual's behaviour, and in particular the ability or lack of ability to reward each other. Interventions also involve setting positive behavioural goals for each partner, and progress is monitored and treatment modified as appropriate. |
| **Psychodynamic marital therapy** | The therapist tries to help the couple understand their problems in terms of their early experiences and subsequent unconscious wishes and expectations by interpretation, particularly of the transference between the couple. |
| **Systems family therapy** | This examines patterns of communication and the effects of trying to maintain homeostasis, and aims to change these patterns. |

Marital therapy may be carried out by mental health professionals if the problems present to these services first, or by agencies such as Relate if more appropriate. The therapy aims to help the couple resolve their difficulties and may result in separation and/or divorce. Therapy where one partner has significant mental health problems needs to be carried out by skilled therapists because of this extra dimension and because therapy may exacerbate the problems.

## Further reading

Barker P. *Basic Family Therapy*, 2nd Edn. London: Collins, 1986.
Minuchin S, Fishman H. *Family Therapy Techniques*. Harvard: Harvard University Press, 1981.
Sauber SR, L'Abate L, Weeks GR, Buchanan WL. *The Dictionary of Family Psychology and Family Therapy,* 2nd Edn. Newbury Park, CA: Sage, 1993.
Stagoll B. Aspects of family therapy. *Current Opinion in Psychiatry*, 1993; **6:** 343–7.

## Related topics of interest

# PSYCHOLOGICAL TREATMENT – GENERAL PRINCIPLES

*. . . the informed and planful application of techniques derived from established psychological principles, by persons qualified through training and experience to understand these principles and to apply these techniques with the intention of assisting individuals to modify such personal characteristics as feelings, values, attitudes and behaviours which are judged by the therapist to be maladaptive.*
(Meltzoff and Kornreich, 1970).

Recent interest has focused on the efficacy of the various psychotherapies. This has become increasingly important as purchasers of health services require information about the outcome of psychological treatments in which they have invested tax-payers' money.

The following are generally agreed to be common features of the psychotherapies:

**Common features**
- An intense and confiding relationship.
- A process which occurs in a healing setting.
- A process which is founded on a rationale of therapy.
- A process which involves a defined therapeutic procedure.

**Psychotherapy groups**

The psychotherapies can be grouped in the following way:

*1. Supportive.*
(a) A patient with a chronic and relatively severe mental illness has therapy which is aimed at preventing deterioration and promoting the best possible level of functioning.
(b) A patient who otherwise functions well is helped to negotiate a psychological or social transition (see Psychological treatment – crisis intervention, p. 264).
(c) A patient is in the acute stage of an illness and is given supportive therapy in the interim before a medication has had time to work or in preparation for another type of therapy. Important elements of this type of therapy are:
- The interview itself.
- Reassurance when this is realistic and given after thorough listening to the patient's problem.
- Explanation, for example of illness, treatment and likely outcome.
- Guidance and suggestion.
- Ventilation of feelings.

2. *Re-educative.*
(a) Aims to readjust habits and attitudes.
(b) No direct attempt to understand unconscious motivations.
(c) Remodelling of the patient's attitudes and behaviour.
(d) Techniques may be used to help the patient make change in one significant area of his/her life, based on the theory that this will lead to an increased sense of mastery and then generalize across other areas of life.
(e) Includes:
- Behavioural and cognitive behaviour, therapy (see Psychological treatment – behaviour therapy, p. 258 and Psychological treatment – cognitive therapy, p. 261).
- Rogerian counselling (Carl Rogers) which assumes the self-actualizing quality of the human and concentrates on the notion of personality development. Key features are:
  — genuineness: congruence between how therapist feels and what he/she says and does directly
  — caring: prizing the client, unconditional positive regard
  — empathy: ability to enter into the patient's world.
- Gestalt therapy (Fritz Perls):
  — notion of psychological homeostasis, i.e. human organism is in a self-regulating balance with its social and physical boundaries
  — therapy aims to increase patient's awareness of self and improve relationship with the outside world.
- Primal therapy (Arthur Janov). Physical expression of expressed pain by a systematic attack on the psychological defences of the patient. Intense therapy which includes long sessions with individual therapist, emphasis being on the visceral sensations of the patient.
- Psychodrama (Moreno):
  — group setting in which patients re-enact real-life situations
  — process makes use of emotive release therapies, learning theories and interpretive theories of psycho-analysis.
- Transactional analysis (Eric Berne):
  — ego described in terms of child, adult and parent roles

— problems described as the result of imbalance or inappropriate adoption of roles
— describes a number of 'life games' which people engage in
— describes positive and negative 'strokes' which are the result of humans' interaction. Ideally positive strokes are sought, but a negative stroke may be considered better than none and therefore accepted by an individual.

*3. Reconstructive psychotherapies.* These are the psychotherapies which have developed from the psychoanalytical ideas of Freud. They include therapies practised according to the ideas of Rank, Jung, Adler, Anna Freud, Horney, Sullivan and Klein, as well as Freud himself.

- The unconscious is described in terms of the Id, Ego and Superego.
- Free association is a key technique pioneered by Freud.
- Recognition, working through and verbalization of the transference is a fundamental process of psychoanalysis.

The therapies subsumed under this group range from those labelled 'brief dynamic therapy', in which five to 30 sessions occur at weekly intervals, to much longer therapies of many years in which a patient may be seen up to five times weekly.

There is an interesting recent suggestion that the attachment theory of Bowlby may be a bridge between psychoanalytical principles and biological processes, since detailed study of parent–infant interactions reveals the following parallels with the psychotherapist and patient relationship:

- The provision of a secure base.
- The emergence of a shared narrative.
- The processing of affect.
- Coping with loss.

**Evaluating psychotherapy**

1. In comparison with other forms of psychiatric treatment it is difficult to collect convincing evidence about the efficacy of treatment or suitability of various treatment types in particular situations.

2. Strategies to evaluate psychotherapy:
(a) Symptoms are rated by the doctor and complaints are rated by the patient both before and after therapy. Thus

a change in symptomatology can be assessed and should reflect improvement.

(b) Ability to work improved.

(c) Ability to relate to others improved.

(d) Personality vulnerabilities which could lead to relapse should be lessened.

(e) Improvement should continue after the treatment.

(f) Improvement should be greater than that which may be attributed to the following:
- Spontaneous remission.
- Regression to the mean.
- Response to placebo or non-specific clinical care over the same period.

3. There is good evidence for the efficacy of behavioural and cognitive behaviour therapy in specific conditions.

4. While opinions differ, Andrews makes the case that there is no good evidence to support the efficacy of psychodynamic psychotherapy after the factors noted above have been considered. Most work has been done on brief forms of therapy. Long-term psychotherapy is even more difficult to investigate soundly.

# Further reading

Andrews G. The essential psychotherapies. *British Journal of Psychiatry*, 1993; **162:** 447–51.

Clare AW. Individual psychotherapies. In: Kendell RE, Zealley AK (eds) *Companion to Psychiatric Studies*. Edinburgh: Churchill Livingstone, 1988; Chap.36.

Holmes J. Attachment theory: a biological basis for psychotherapy. *British Journal of Psychiatry*, 1993; **163:** 430–8.

Meltzoff J and Kornreich M. *Research in Psychotherapy*. New York: Atherton, 1970.

# Related topics of interest

# PSYCHOLOGICAL TREATMENT – GROUP THERAPIES

*Man is not an individual, but a social organism* (Trigant Burrow)
*The group is the matrix of individual development* (Foulkes)

The process of treating people in groups, rather than individual therapy, was first developed by Trigant Burrow, and later by Bion and Foulkes, working with 'war neurosis' veterans. The use of group settings has been extended beyond psychodynamic groups into the cognitive and behavioural sphere, but although the methods used vary, the same principles can be applied to the effectiveness of the group.

Therapeutic factors, present to varying degrees in different types of groups, are identified by Yalom:
(a) *Instillation of hope,* is crucial to all psychotherapies, which offer hope of a way out of or through problems.
(b) *Universality* is the process by which patients learn that they are not unique or alone in having problems.
(c) *Imparting of information* consisting of preparatory interviews and briefings for the group, and giving of knowledge by the therapist or others in the group.
(d) *Altruism.* Patients discover that they can be of importance to others, and this boosts self-esteem.
(e) *The corrective recapitulation of the primary family group.* Individuals will play out and recapitulate early family conflicts, and the group provides a setting in which these conflicts can be contained and reworked.
(f) *Development of socializing techniques.* The group provides a mirror to reflect back to the individual on their behaviour, and its effect on others, and to allow them to experiment with other types of interaction in a way which is not possible in outside life. This results in improved empathy and responsiveness, less judgemental attitudes and better conflict resolution.
(g) *Imitative behaviour.* Members of the group identify with other members or the therapist, and take up their behaviours.
(h) *Interpersonal learning:*
  (i) *Importance of interpersonal relationships.*
  (ii) *Corrective emotional experience.* Group support and protection in allowing strong interpersonal emotions to be expressed, and interpersonal beliefs and behaviours tested out, facilitating the person's ability to interact with others more openly and deeply.
  (iii) *The group as a social microcosm* reflecting interpersonal styles of its members, and allowing them to observe, receive feedback and accept personal responsibility. This leads to increasing personal responsibility for change, and an adaptive spiral increasing self-esteem and individual autonomy.
Individual psychotherapy focuses on the dyadic relationship, whereas group therapy extends beyond that allowing 'psychotherapy of the group, by the group'.

(i) *Group cohesiveness.* An important determinant of therapeutic outcome. Cohesive groups are more able to express hostility and criticism of one another and the leader. This allows maximum participation in the therapeutic group tasks of:

(i) *Acceptance of patient role.*

(ii) *Self-disclosure.*

(iii) *Honesty.*

(iv) *Non-defensiveness.*

(v) *Interest in, and acceptance of others.*

(vi) *Support of the group.*

(vii) *Personal improvement.*

(j) *Catharsis.* The free expression of affect is vital in therapeutic gain, but not sufficient in itself.

(k) *Existential factors.* Insights into the way of the world, 'the meaning of life', for example:

(i) *Responsibility* = it's down to you.

(ii) *Basic isolation* = you're on your own.

(iii) *Contingency* = you can only have *this* if you do *that*.

(iv) *Recognition of one's own mortality, and that of others.*

(v) *Capriciousness of existence* = 'Life's a bitch and then you die'.

Different types of groups emphasize different factors, and groups may evolve through stages where different ones become more or less important.

**Levels of communication within groups**

Four levels can be identified, corresponding with different views of the world, and facets of human experience:

- *'Normative':* everyday, current (Social Psychology)
- *'Transference':* relating to past experiences (Freudian)
- *'Projective':* shared and projected (often bodily) experiences (Kleinian)
- *'Primordial':* archetypal and universal images and myths (Jungian)

Groups vary in the degree to which they facilitate or use communications at different levels. Groups run on behavioural or cognitive lines (Stern and Fernandez, 1991), for example, will encourage a focus on the everyday and current, and discourage other levels, whereas dynamic groups, allowing regression to occur, may work at all levels.

**Group formation and functioning**

Described by Tuckman as four phases:

- *Forming:* the group starts to learn how to become a group, and their places within it.
- *Storming:* the group becomes angry and rebellious, testing the boundaries imposed upon it, and challenging the leader.

- *Norming:* the group develops its own rules and structures within which it functions.
- *Performing:* the group is able to work productively in the 'here and now'.

The group may go through these phases more than once, and the resulting group is able to work towards resolution of problems and accomplishment of tasks in the 'here and now'.

*1. Basic assumptions.* This 'working group' may under pressure regress to the 'basic assumption' level of functioning, first described by Bion, which is a retreat into fantasy in order to avoid confronting and solving problems in the 'here and now'. There are three possible basic assumptions:

- *Fight or flight:* the group becomes mobilized against some perceived external threat.
- *Dependency:* the group invests its hopes and expectations in one individual, who is expected to 'save' it. Often this is the group leader, but sometimes a powerful member of the group.
- *Pairing:* a fantasized union or pairing of two people, usually members of the group, comes to dominate the group processes, and is expected to provide a solution for problems.

Bion pointed out that these types of basic assumption also operate within societies, and are reflected in the formation of social institutions (the army, church and monarchy respectively). More malign results of basic assumption groups may be seen in dictatorships and other forms of extreme politics (Skynner and Cleese, 1983).

**Outcomes**

*After successful psychoanalytic treatment, the patient is definitely less neurotic...,
but perhaps not definitely more mature. On the other hand, after group therapy,
the patient is not necessarily less neurotic, but inevitably more mature.* (Bion)

That this can have powerful effects upon both psychological and physical disorders is indicated in studies of the use of group techniques in the treatment of both hypochondriasis (Stern and Fernandez, 1991) and metastatic breast cancer (Spiegel *et al.,* 1989). In the latter study, supportive group therapy plus self-hypnosis increased survival in women with metastatic breast cancer, the effect becoming noticeable and progressively more pronounced from 20 months into the study, 8 months after the active treatment phase had finished.

# Further reading

Skynner R, Cleese J. *Families and How to Survive Them. Afterthought: paranoia and politics.* London: Methuen, 1983; 131–42.

Spiegel D, Bloom JR, Kraemer HC, Gottheil E. Effect of psychosocial treatment on survival of patients with metastatic breast cancer. *Lancet,* 1989(2); 888–91.

Stern R, Fernandez M. Group cognitive and behavioural treatment for hypochondriasis. *British Medical Journal,* 1991; **303:** 1229–31.

With acknowledgement to lecture notes prepared for the Institute of Group Analysis Introductory General Course in Group Work, 1989 by Dr Lionel Kreeger.

# Related topics of interest

# RATING SCALES

Rating scales are used in psychiatry for a variety of purposes both in clinical practice and research. They provide a method of assessing and quantifying psychiatric symptoms and syndromes, and complement the clinical assessment.

**Definitions**

*1. Validity.* This is the extent to which a scale measures what it sets out to measure. Although validity implies that a measure can be compared with a gold standard, in psychiatry it is a relative term.

- Face validity means that the scale appears to measure what it intends to measure.
- Content validity describes the extent to which the test assesses all aspects of the specific subject of interest.
- Criterion validity decribes how well a measure distinguishes between individuals who have been shown to differ on an external measure. The two main sorts of criterion validity are *concurrent validity*, which is how the two measures compare when carried out at the same time, and *predictive validity* means that the scale can predict, for example, an outcome as measured on a different scale.
- Construct validity is related to the concepts underlying the purpose of the measure and includes *convergent validity* which is how well two measures which should be related compare, and *discriminant validity* is how well the measure discriminates from an unrelated measure.
- Incremental validity is the extent to which the new measure adds more information or contributes to more informed decisions.

*2. Reliability.* This is the degree to which tests can be replicated, in various ways.

- Inter-rater reliability (kappa) measures the chance-corrected agreement between different raters.
- Test-retest reliability reflects the measure's stability.
- Split half reliability reflects a measure's internal consistency.

*3. Sensitivity.* This is the ability of a measurement to identify those with a particular condition (i.e. the proportion of those with the disorder who have a positive test).

*4. Specificity.* This is the ability of a measurement to exclude those who do not have a condition (i.e. the proportion of those without the disorder who have a negative test).

*5. Predictive value.*

- Positive predictive value is the proportion of patients with a positive test result who also have the disorder.
- Negative predictive value is the proportion of subjects with a negative test who also do not have the disorder.

Predictive values may be more informative because sensitivity and specificity values (although not the actual figures) vary less predictably with prevalence than do predictive values.

**Completion of scales**

Rating scales can be completed by self-report, observation or interview, and may rate signs and/or symptoms. The questioning may be *closed*, for example, checklist methods (all-or-none), numerical scales or forced-choice methods; or *open,* for example, assessing severity, intensity or frequency.

*1. Types of psychiatric scales.*

- Differential or discriminatory: designed to provide diagnoses or classification.
- Intensity or descriptive: designed to measure severity.
- Prognostic scales: designed to assess course and outcome.
- Selection scales: designed to measure the outcome following a specific treatment

*2. Errors.* These may arise from a variety of sources:

- Error of central tendency where people tend to ignore extremes.
- Halo error where answers are chosen to fit with other answers.
- Response set error where people tend to either agree or disagree with questions.
- Hawthorne effect where researchers alter situation by investigating, in that people behave or respond differently when they know they are being studied.
- Social acceptability errors where individuals give expected answers.

**Specific aspects of established psychiatric rating scales**

*1. Diagnostic instruments.*

- The Present State Examination (PSE) is completed from a semi-structured interview carried out by a trained interviewer, which produces ICD diagnoses using the CATEGO programme.

- The Schedule for Affective Disorders and Schizophrenia (SADS) is scored from a structured interview and leads to current or lifetime Research Diagnostic Criteria (RDC) diagnoses.
- The Clinical Interview Schedule (CIS) is completed from a semi-structured interview and is designed for use in community surveys.
- The National Institute of Mental Health Diagnostic Interview Schedule (DIS). This is a highly structured interview which leads to diagnoses according to DSM, RDC or Feighner criteria.

2. *Defining 'cases'.* The above instruments can be used for this purpose as well as the General Health Questionnaire (GHQ) (a self-administered questionnaire).

3. *Measuring psychiatric symptoms.* These scales are designed to measure severity and/or change in patients already diagnosed. The SADS and CIS can be used as well as the following:

(a) *Global symptom scales.*
- Brief Psychiatric Rating Scale (BPRS): based on verbal report and observation and designed for assessing psychiatric in-patients.
- Symptom Rating Test (SRT): semi-structured interview for measuring change in neurotic symptoms.

(b) *Depression rating scales.*
- Hamilton Rating Scale for Depression (HRSD): an observer-rated scale for measuring changes in severity.
- Beck Depression Inventory (BDI): a self-rating scale, mainly for assessing psychiatric in- and out-patients.
- Montgomery and Asberg Depression Rating Scale (MADRS): completed from a clinical interview measuring the psychological symptoms of depression (therefore especially useful in the presence of physical illness).
- Hospital Anxiety and Depression Scale (HAD) is a self-rated scale for assessing patients in non-psychiatric hospital departments.

(c) *Anxiety rating scales.*
- The State-Trait Anxiety Inventory (STAI): self-rated.
- Hamilton Anxiety Scale (HAS): unstructured interview.

(d) *Mania rating scale.*
- Manic Rating Scale (MS): measures severity by observation.
- Modified Manic Rating Scale (MMS): completed from a structured interview and measures severity.

(e) *Obsessive compulsive rating scales.*
- Leyton obsessional inventory.
- Maudsley obsessive-compulsive inventory.

(f) *Personality disorder scales.*
- Personality assessment schedule (PAS).

*4. Elderly.* CAMDEX: this is a broad assessment designed to provide a psychiatric diagnosis. It consists of an interview, physical, mental state and cognitive (CAMCOG) examinations, and interview with chief carer.

*5. Rating long-term patients.*

- Standardized psychiatric assessment scale.
- Life skills profile.
- Morningside rehabilitation status schedule.

*6. Measures of social adjustment.*

- Social functioning scale.
- Self report social adjustment scale.

*7. Psychometric tests.*

- Personality: Minnesota Multiphasic Personality Inventory, Eysenck Personality Inventory – both self-rater.
- Intelligence: Stanford-Binet, Wechsler Adult Intelligence Scale (WAIS) (verbal and performance scores).
- Neuropsychology: Wisconsin card sorting test, WAIS, mini-mental state examination (MMSE).

**Development of a new rating scale**

It is important first to consider what the scale should measure (for diagnosis, symptoms or severity), how it is to be completed (self-report, observation, interview) and which group of subjects it will be administered to. If there are no current criteria, then these may have to be created and these should be discussed with colleagues for clinical validity. The scale should be validated against psychiatrists' judgement/diagnosis and particularly predictive and incremental validity. Reliability, particularly split-half and test-retest reliability should be measured. A pilot study including an appropriate control group should be carried out, and the sensitivity and specificity measured using a random sample from the appropriate population.

Measures may be assessed by numerical scales or graphic/visual analogue scales; attitudes can be measured on Likert scales (5-point scale from strongly agree to strongly disagree) or Thurstone scales where the questions used are those which give the most agreement in attitudes by a group of judges. Concepts should be carefully and operationally defined.

## Further reading

Freeman C, Tyrer P. *Research Methods in Psychiatry*, 2nd Edn. London: Royal College of Psychiatrists/Gaskell, 1992.

Weller M, Eysenck M. (eds). *The Scientific Basis of Psychiatry*, 2nd Edn. Philadelphia: WB.Saunders, 1992.

## Related topics of interest

# RECURRENT BRIEF PSYCHIATRIC SYNDROMES

People with these syndromes do not play a major part in psychiatric practice, but may present more often to general practitioners, or not present at all. Most psychiatric syndromes have built into their definition criteria for duration. These vary, being up to 6 months for DSM-IV schizophrenia. For depression and anxiety disorders, the qualifying period is 2–4 weeks.

Recurrent brief psychiatric syndromes are those which do not meet these duration criteria. They have been most studied by Angst, in the context of the Zurich study, in which a cohort of men from the canton of Zurich is being followed up over time. Angst describes recurrent brief depression, mania, neurasthenia, anxiety and also sporadic panic.

**Recurrent brief depression**

Recurrent brief depression (RBD) is included under the section of syndromes for further study in DSM-IV. The characteristics are:

- Criteria, except duration, for major depressive disorder are met.
- Depressive periods last at least 2 days but less than 2 weeks.
- Depressive periods occur at least once a month for 12 consecutive months, and are not associated with the menstrual cycle.
- There is significant impairment to some aspect of daily living.
- Not due to pharmacological or medical conditions.
- Never depressive episode, dysthmia, manic episode.

Recurrent brief depression may be more common than major depressive disorder, though it is often co-morbid with other conditions, including major depression ('combined depression'). In particular, the suicide rate is reported to be as high as in major depression, and 30% of individuals with 'combined depression' have attempted suicide by the age of 30. The disorder seems to be equally prevalent in men and women. There is also an association with migraine, in marked contrast to major depressions, and onset is most often in adolescence.

RBD is more common in individuals with childhood histories suggestive of personality disorder, and shares some features of borderline personality.

*1. Treatment.* There is not very much data on the treatment of RBD, but a mixture of biological and social approaches is suggested by Montgomery (1991). The following lifestyle advice can be given:

(a) Recognize the intermittent nature of the illness.
(b) Retreat emotionally and possibly physically during episodes.
(c) Choose an appropriate occupation:
  • With low emotional content.
  • Which will allow unpredictable days off.
(d) Avoid family conflicts when ill, require that family be tolerant and non-intrusive.

*2. Drug treatment.*
(a) Treat over long- not short-term.
(b) Use safe drugs preferentially:
  • Low dose neuroleptic, e.g. flupenthixol.
  • Lithium.
  • Monoamine-oxidase inhibitors.
(c) Avoid toxic tricyclic antidepressants which may lead to suicide.
(d) Avoid benzodiazepines or alcohol.

**Recurrent brief hypomania**

One-year prevalence of hypomania (diagnosed by DSM-IIIR criteria) was found to be 4% in the Zurich cohort (Wicki and Angst, 1991). Frequently recurring episodes lasting for a week or less were the pattern in 80% of cases. There was an excess family history (six times) of psychiatric illness, RBD and major depression were common (40% were treated for depression within the year being studied), and the rate of attempted suicide was as high as other affective disorder groups (3.8 times the control group).

**Recurrent brief anxiety**

Diagnosis is made by Angst and Wicki (1992) on the basis of:

(a) Anxiety.
(b) 3/4 DSM-III categories of symptoms of generalized anxiety disorder:
  • Motor tension.
  • Autonomic hyperactivity.
  • Apprehensive expectation.
  • Vigilance and scanning.
(c) Anxious mood present 1–13 days, with recurrence at least once a month in past year.
(d) Subjective work impairment.

On these criteria, the 30-year-old cohort being studied had prevalence rates of 3.3% for males and 2.1% for females (the opposite of the sex ratio for generalized anxiety). Co-morbidity with panic disorder and depression (particularly RBD) was very high, with 75% of the patients already having a lifetime history of treatment for these conditions. There is also frequently a family history of anxiety or depression. Unlike RBD, there is no association with migraine. There is no data available on treatment but, given the overlap with RBD and panic disorder, treatments aimed at these might be expected to be effective.

**Sporadic panic**

This is defined (Vollrath *et al.*, 1990) as the presence of symptoms of PD, occurring less frequently than needed for this diagnosis. Unlike RBD, there is no sharp delineation between the groups with panic disorder and sporadic panic. The symptomatology in the two groups is similar and both show a very high degree of overlap with depression (major and RBD), isolated depressive symptoms, tension and somatic anxiety.

**Neurasthenia**

Merikangas and Angst (1994) found that reducing the duration criterion from 3 months to 1 month resulted in a tenfold increase in the prevalence of neurasthenia (to 12% in 1 year). Significant subjective distress, occupational and social impairment was reported by most subjects. The longitudinal course is as stable as any other neurotic illness, with 50% continuing to exhibit the disorder at follow-up. There is considerable overlap with both depression and anxiety disorders, and neurasthenia may be an early symptom, or a consequence of these disorders.

**Conclusions**

Recurrent brief psychiatric syndromes, or syndromes not meeting normal duration and frequency criteria, are very common, and probably reflect as much as anything the continuous spectrum between normality and neurotic illness. There is considerable impairment in people with such 'subthreshold' psychiatric syndromes.

# Further reading

Angst J, Wicki W. The Zurich Study XIII. Recurrent brief anxiety. *European Archives of Psychiatry and Clinical Neuroscience,* 1992; **241:** 296–300.

Merikangas K, Angst J. Neurasthenia in a longitudinal cohort study of young adults. *Psychological Medicine,* 1994; **24:** 1013–24.

Montgomery SA. Recurrent brief depression. In: Feighner JP, Boyer WF (eds) *The Diagnosis of Depression.* Chichester: John Wiley & Sons, 1991; 119–34.

Vollrath M, Kick R, Angst J. The Zurich Study IX. Panic disorder and sporadic panic: symptoms, diagnosis, prevalence, and overlap with depression. *European Archives of Psychiatry and Clinical Neuroscience,* 1990; **239:** 221–30.

Wicki W, Angst J. The Zurich Study X. Hypomania in a 28 to 30-year old cohort. *European Archives of Psychiatry and Clinical Neuroscience,* 1991; **240:** 339–48.

## Related topics of interest

Affective disorders – classifications and epidemiology (p. 15)
Chronic fatigue syndrome (p. 59)
Neurosis divisible? (p. 206)

# RESEARCH METHODS

In psychiatry as in any medical discipline, the way in which information is collected and the reasons for collecting it are crucial to the answers which can be inferred from the results.

*Epidemiology* can be defined as the study of disease in populations. It aims to establish the nature of illnesses and, in particular, what risk factors there are and their effects on the frequency and nature of illnesses. This can be extended to study the effect of interventions and therefore be used in healthcare planning.

**Definitions**

- *Incidence/inception rates* describe the rate of first episodes of illness.
- *Prevalence* is the number of people suffering from a disorder at a particular point in time (point prevalence) or over an interval (period prevalence). The figures depend on the course of an illness and its incidence.
- Rates can be divided into *true rates* (when numerator and denominator (top and bottom of a fraction) are in the same units, e.g. people, and those in the numerator also come from the population of the denominator), and *ratios* (when numerator and denominator are in different units, e.g. admissions/population).
- *Cases* are those which reach the required criteria for a disorder or level of morbidity. The inferences that are made depend on how cases are defined and measured.

  Some studies analyse information which has been collected for another reason, e.g. official mortality, morbidity, suicide and first admission statistics and so the definition of a case has been defined beforehand and not for the purpose of the study. This can therefore lead to methodological flaws because the information has not been collected with the specific hypothesis in mind, but has the advantage that the information is already available. For example, case registers record and collate all contacts with the psychiatric services. This can then form a record linkage system which can be used to follow a cohort over time. National registers exist in Sweden and Denmark, and regional ones in USA, UK and one for Scotland. However they are expensive and have not been set up to test a specific hypothesis.
- In *population surveys* cases can be defined using interviews, questionnaires or observation depending on the proposed hypothesis, how the results will be analysed, and what the information is to be used for (see below).
- Similarly, the method of *sampling* dictates the relevance and conclusions of a study. Sampling (studying part of

the population of interest) can be random, systematic (e.g. every tenth admission), stratified (e.g. random samples from different groups according to age, sex, or severity of illness), multistage sampling (e.g. by area and then by age) and non-random (e.g. identifying other subjects through known subjects). The sample size needs to be carefully considered before starting measurements in order to ensure that there is sufficient power to measure a difference.

**Studies**

Studies that provide epidemiological information can be:

- Observational or intervention.
- Descriptive or analytical.
- Prospective or retrospective.

*1. Cross-sectional studies.* These are observational and descriptive and measure the prevalence of disorders or morbidity.

*2. Case-control studies.* These compare affected and unaffected individuals in order to identify factors which may contribute to the disorder. They are retrospective in nature. The control group can be matched individually or (more easily) as a group. Matching is often by, for example, age, sex, social class. It is important to avoid 'overmatching', that is matching so much that this hides the variable(s) of interest.

*3. Cohort studies.* These are observational and analytical, and are usually prospective (although may be retrospective if the outcome of interest has already occurred). A group is followed over time (longitudinal) and they are therefore particularly useful for investigating causal associations, but are expensive. In interpreting the results it is important to take into account the possible effects of developing illness, effects of age (e.g. alcohol intake decreases and suicide increases with increasing age) and period effects (e.g. war, economic recession, new treatments). As measurements are only made at the beginning and the end of the study, the results are an average of change over that time and should be interpreted as such.

*4. Controlled clinical trials.* These investigate the outcome of treatments in affected and unaffected individuals, compared with established treatments and placebo. The design is important in order to be able to conclude that the difference reflects a real difference rather than chance or bias in the study. In designing trials, important considerations include:

- Pilot studies.
- The time interval.
- Washout periods for previous drug treatments.
- Randomized and double-blind designs.
- The relative advantages and disadvantages of a cross-over design.
- Inclusion of appropriate control groups (placebo, no treatment, established treatment) which are matched.
- Appropriate (blind) follow-up.

*5. Risk.* The information from epidemiological studies can be expressed in terms of risk which reflects the effect of a risk factor on those exposed to it. *Relative risk* is the ratio of the incidence in those exposed to a factor to the incidence in those not exposed. *Standardized risks* are calculated by taking into account confounding variables such as age, sex and social class (e.g. standardized mortality rates (SMRs)).

*6. Meta-analysis.* This describes various methods of combining results from multiple randomized trials in order to draw conclusions about a particular treatment. Meta-analyses are most informative when the studies use similar methods so the likelihood of differences between trials being due to chance or spurious factors is reduced.

**Classification**

Diagnoses are concepts which in psychiatry are principally based on symptoms because as yet aetiology is rarely known. Diagnosis is usually based on a group of symptoms rather than on a single pathognomonic symptom.

Classification systems can be categorical or dimensional. Categorical systems are familiar, easy to understand, remember and use, do not require numeracy, and lead easily on to treatment decisions. However, clinical validity may be sacrificed for these advantages. Dimensional classifications produce finer distinctions, are more flexible and can be converted into categories. They do not imply unproven qualitative differences and do not impose what may be false boundaries. ICD-10 and DSM-III-R/IV are both categorical classifications, but ICD-10 is descriptive and DSM-III-R/IV uses operational criteria which need to be satisfied to make a diagnosis. DSM-III-R/IV is multi-axial, and ICD-10 now also has provision for description on different axes.

In psychiatry there is also a diagnostic hierarchy whereby the highest appropriate diagnosis is used. The hierarchy starts with organic diagnoses at the top, followed by schizophrenia, affective disorders, stress-related, neurotic and somatoform disorders.

## Further reading

Freeman C, Tyrer P. *Research Methods in Psychiatry*, 2nd Edn. London: Gaskell (Royal College of Psychiatrists), 1992.

## Related topics of interest

Drug development (p. 115)
Rating scales (p. 278)
Statistics (p. 327)

# SCHIZOAFFECTIVE DISORDERS

*...An uninterrupted period of illness during which at some time there is a [major affective] episode concurrent with symptoms (of) schizophrenia... (at least 2 weeks of) delusions or hallucinations in the absence of mood disturbance, (and) mood disturbance for a significant proportion of the total illness (DSM-IV)*

The diagnosis has been seen as one of exclusion, only to be used if neither a diagnosis of schizophrenia or major affective psychosis adequately describes the symptomatology. Two forms are described: a depressed form and a manic or mixed form.

**Cycloid psychoses**

Described particularly by Kleist, Leonhard and Perris, cycloid psychoses have sudden onset with a bipolar fluctuation in mood and a good short-term prognosis but a high rate of recurrence. Clinically, in addition to mood fluctuations, they are also characterized by at least two of the following:

- Confusion (from slight perplexity to gross disorientation).
- Paranoid delusions or mood-incongruent hallucinations.
- Motility disturbances: hypo- or hyperkinesia.
- Ecstasy.
- Pananxiety (overwhelming fear of some catastrophe).

This symptomatology is common in puerperal psychosis, and various studies have shown 8-12% of psychotics to have cycloid psychoses. Sufferers are predominantly female. Similar psychoses are found in first degree relatives. Three types are described (Hamilton, 1984):

*1. Anxiety-elation psychosis.* Either pronounced anxiety, with depressive delusions, or enthusiastic euphoria, with grandiosity. Rapid oscillations between these states are common.

*2. Confusion psychosis.* Disorder of thinking, rather than affectivity or psychomotor activity. Pressure of speech is marked.

*3. Motility psychosis.* Hyperkinetic states with motor restlessness, inarticulate screaming; lasting a few weeks, alternating with hypokinetic states, including catatonic motor disorders and incoherent speech.

Although Kendell (1993) is of the opinion that these are in fact forms of bipolar disorder with unusually acute onset, he states that the concept is worthy of further investigation. This group of disorders is sufficiently different in course, prognosis and family history to be considered separately, and in many ways they resemble the affective form of schizoaffective disorder.

**Differential diagnosis**

A degree of affective symptomatology is common in schizophrenia, and depression is common in its aftermath (post-schizophrenic depression). Distinction also needs to be made from true bipolar disorder. Drug-induced psychoses are often schizoaffective in form, as are puerperal psychoses.

**Demographic factors**

These are exactly what would be expected of a disorder intermediate between schizophrenia and affective disorder. The female:male ratio in schizoaffective disorder is higher than in schizophrenia, but lower than in affective disorders. Incidence and prevalence are not accurately known, but DSM-IV states that it is probably less common than schizophrenia. Peak age of onset is in early adulthood, rather later than in schizophrenia. There is some evidence that bipolar types of schizoaffective disorder are more common earlier, and depressed types later in life. There is a raised incidence of both schizophrenia and affective psychoses in first degree relatives.

**Course and prognosis**

There is a tendency to recurrence, with full recovery between episodes, although the depressed type has more tendency to develop a chronic defect state typical of schizophrenia, and recurrent episodes are often typically schizophrenic in nature.

The prognosis is better than schizophrenia (as might be expected, given that an affective component within schizophrenia is a good prognostic sign). The prognosis of the manic form is similar to that of bipolar disorder, whereas that of the depressed form is considerably worse than in affective disorder.

**Is schizoaffective disorder a separate diagnostic category?**

A number of hypotheses have been advanced to explain the nature of schizoaffective disorder (Kendell, 1993). They depend, to some extent, upon theoretical notions of whether or not schizophrenia and bipolar disorder are separate entities, as first postulated by Kraeplin, or are part of a spectrum of psychotic disorders '*Einheitpsychosen*'.

*1. Misdiagnosis.* Schizoaffectives are in fact just people with schizophrenia or affective psychosis who have incidental symptoms of the other disorder.

*2. Co-morbidity.* One simple explanation is that schizoaffective disorder is simply a conjunction, in the same patient, of separate schizophrenia and affective psychosis. The main problem with this hypothesis is that the disorder is far too common for this to be the case.

*3. Continuum.* There is no real separation of schizophrenia from affective psychoses: inheritance is polygenic, and schizoaffective disorder is one of the expected variety of intermediate forms between the two 'pure' illnesses. A strong exponent of this hypothesis is Crow, who musters considerable evidence in its support (Crow and Harrington, 1994), and it is gaining in acceptability (Kendell, 1993).

*4. Unrelated disorder.* Schizoaffective disorder is unrelated to schizophrenia or affective disorder. The familial association with both disorders, as opposed to the 'breeding true' which would be expected of a separate disorder, renders this unlikely.

**Treatment**

Symptoms of psychosis should be treated with antipsychotic drugs, and those of affective disorder with lithium. Antidepressants are not said to be helpful in the depressed form, although electroconvulsive therapy (ECT) is effective. Maintenance treatment with antipsychotics is more effective than with lithium (Crow and Harrington, 1994).

# Further reading

Crow TJ, Harrington CA. Aetiopathogenesis and treatment of psychosis. *Annual Review of Medicine*, 1994; **45:** 219–34.
Hamilton M. Fish's Schizophrenia. In: *Special Varieties of Schizophrenia*, 3rd Edn. London: John Wright and Sons, 1984, Chap. 6.
Kendell RE. Paranoid and other psychoses. In: Kendell RE, Zealley AK (eds), *Companion to Psychiatric Studies*, 5th Edn. London: Churchill Livingstone, 1993; 459–71.

# Related topics of interest

Affective disorders – classification and epidemiology (p. 15)
Schizophrenia – natural history and prognostic features (p. 299)

# SCHIZOPHRENIA – BIOLOGICAL AND PSYCHOLOGICAL ASPECTS

Schizophrenia is being seen increasingly as a brain disorder with a physical basis, and this is reflected in the categories of markers that are associated with the disease, and in current theories of aetiology. Family, twin and adoption studies have shown a strong genetic (and therefore biological) component in the aetiology of schizophrenia, and recent theories of the causation of schizophrenia have tried to relate biological and psychological abnormalities to underlying cerebral abnormalities.

**Biological abnormalities**

*1. Dopamine hypothesis.* This has developed from a range of observations about the connection between the dopamine system and schizophrenia. Firstly, neuroleptic drugs principally act by blocking dopamine receptors, particularly $D_2$ receptors, and for most neuroleptics (except clozapine) $D_2$ postsynaptic receptor blockade potency is directly related to their clinical efficacy. Secondly, amphetamine, which increases dopamine transmission, can produce a schizophrenic-type psychotic illness. Thirdly, an increased density of postsynaptic $D_2$ receptors has been shown in the caudate nucleus and nucleus accumbens in post-mortem studies. But these findings could merely be a consequence of neuroleptic administration. With the recent advances in imaging techniques it has been possible to study the dopamine system in drug-free and drug-naïve patients but the results of studies of drug-free schizophrenics using positron electron tomography (PET) scans have been ambiguous. One study showed an increase in $D_2$ receptor density in the basal ganglia, but two other studies failed to show this. Other dopamine receptors, particularly $D_4$, may be involved in schizophrenia and the action of anti-psychotics because clozapine has a high affinity for these receptors.

It is therefore becoming more likely that dopamine blockade is not the primary change or site of action of neuroleptics. This would also be consistent with the fact that neuroleptics are not specific for schizophrenia alone (cf. mania, other psychoses), and that the time course for changes in dopamine transmission is generally in terms of hours, whereas that for a clinical response is several weeks.

*2. Ventricular size changes.* Enlargement of the third and lateral ventricles was initially seen by air encephalography, but more recently by computerized tomography (CT). The majority of studies have shown an increase in the ratio of ventricle to brain size, but the increase is not generally that large. The greatest increases tend to be seen in males with poor premorbid functioning, early onset, cognitive decline and a poor prognosis. Magnetic resonance imaging (MRI), because of its greater resolution, is confirming and extending these findings. Ventricular enlargement is not progressive.

As well as ventricular enlargement, studies have shown volume reductions in medial temporal lobe structures such as the amygdala and hippocampus. In studies of discordant twins the lateral and third ventricles were larger, and the hippocampi were smaller, almost always in the schizophrenic twin.

*3. Neuroanatomical changes.* Direct studies of the sizes of various anatomical structures from treatment-free post-mortem brains have shown a decrease in the size of the amygdala, hippocampus, parahippocampal gyrus and globus pallidus, and an increase in the size of the lateral ventricles, especially in the temporal lobes and particularly on the left. Cellular abnormalities include a reduction in the number of cells in various structures, and disordered orientation of pyramidal cells of the hippocampi suggesting migrational abnormalities during neurodevelopment. A significant finding is the absence of gliosis. So overall the evidence is of gross and cellular abnormalities which may be due to neurodevelopmental abnormalities or a pathological process occurring before birth. This may reflect genetic influences, a perinatal insult, such as obstetric complications (which may be more common in patients with schizophrenia), or a prenatal factor such as influenza infection in the third trimester. There is evidence for an excess of schizophrenic winter births and an association with influenza epidemics, but the proportion of patients with schizophrenia where influenza contributes to the aetiology is unclear.

*4. Cerebral activity.* Functional studies of brain activity using PET and single photon emission tomography (SPECT) have shown reductions in regional cerebral blood flow (RCBF), both resting and with psychological activation in the frontal lobes. Similar changes in oxygen and glucose metabolism have been shown. However, hypofrontality is also seen in affective disorders so the significance is unclear.

Overactivity in the hippocampus and other temporal areas has been shown. It has been suggested that hypofrontality is related to negative symptoms and overactivity in temporolimbic structures is related to positive symptoms.

5. *Other neurotransmitters.* Abnormalities of glutamate transmission have been identified in schizophrenia, particularly loss of non-$N$-methyl-D-aspartate (NMDA) receptors in the hippocampus and entorhinal cortex. These changes may link in with changes in cytoarchitecture because excitatory amino acids are involved in trophic changes in the brain during development. The serotonin (5-$HT_2$) system may be involved in the aetiology of schizophrenia, and the therapeutic effects of drugs as clozapine and risperidone may be through binding 5-$HT_2$ receptors. There has also been interest in cholecystokinin and opiate receptors.

6. *Other abnormalities.* Changes in platelet monoamine oxidase (MAO) activity have been shown in schizophrenia but not consistently. They are not necessarily specific to schizophrenia, and may not relate to changes in brain activity. Abnormal eye tracking movements have been shown in patients with schizophrenia and in their relatives. Abnormal sensory evoked potentials have been found in schizophrenic patients, particularly in terms of latency in the auditory evoked P300 potential, and although similar abnormalities may be found in affective disorders the evidence suggests a possible trait abnormality of auditory processing.

7. *A current integrated theory* proposes a genetic pre-disposition or prenatal insult which contributes to neuro-developmental changes. These changes then lead to or reflect the anatomical and neurotransmitter changes seen in schizophrenia.

**Psychological aspects**

The psychological abnormalities in schizophrenia range from global impairment to specific defects on neuro-psychological testing, and may contribute to symp-tomatology, particularly thought disorder, and also may reflect underlying pathological brain changes (e.g. anatomical, biochemical and functional).

1. *Cognitive function.* Extensive studies have shown, overall, a general decline in cognitive function which is not

necessarily explained by thought disorder, negative symptoms or medication. Although there is some evidence that this is related to the structural brain changes in schizophrenia, this is conflicting. Cross-sectional studies indicate that this impairment of cognitive function is static, which is consistent with evidence from neuroanatomical studies which show lack of progression of cellular abnormalities.

*2. Executive skills.* The majority of patients, however, do not have global impairment, but some do have specific problems particularly in executive skills which reflect frontal function (Wisconsin Card Sorting Test). These deficits may contribute to symptoms such as apathy and poor motivation, and changes in affect, but may also reflect the hypofrontality seen on functional imaging.

*3. Memory impairment.* This has also been shown in schizophrenia which is out of proportion to any general impairment and unlikely to be explained by negative symptoms or medication. Problems with memory, especially semantic memory, could explain some schizophrenic symptoms, most particularly the wide range of abnormalities included in schizophrenic thought disorder, but this is currently at the level of speculation. Memory problems may be related to changes in brain activity in the medial temporal areas.

*4. Psychological models.* Several psychological models have been suggested but remain to be tested. Frith postulates that abnormalities of volition, namely a failure to turn intentions into actions, contribute to negative symptoms, and that abnormalities of central monitoring of intentions and actions contribute to positive symptoms. Schizophrenic patients show abnormalities of latent inhibition (blocking of subsequent conditioning by previous association without reward), which may be useful as an animal model (because it can be influenced by the dopamine system), and may explain some symptoms by suggesting a defective filter against irrelevant information.

*5. Lateralization.* The debate continues as to whether the cognitive defects in schizophrenia are lateralized (to the left side).

*6. Rehabilitation.* With the identification of cognitive abnormalities in schizophrenia, interest is developing in cognitive rehabilitation to attempt to ameliorate some of the symptoms of schizophrenia and subsequent disabilities. Psychological methods are also used in general rehabilitation and family interventions.

## Further reading

Chua SE, McKenna PJ. Schizophrenia - a brain disease? *British Journal of Psychiatry*, 1995; **166**: 563–82.

Frith C. Functional imaging and cognitive abnormalities. *Lancet,* 1995; **346**: 615–20.

Jones P, Murray RM. The genetics of schizophrenia is the genetics of neurodevelopment. *British Journal of Psychiatry*, 1991; **158**: 615–23.

Mortimer AM, McKenna PJ. Levels of explanation - symptoms, neuropsychological deficit and morphological abnormalities in schizophrenia. *Psychological Medicine,* 1994; **24**: 541–5.

Sedvall G, Farde L. Chemical brain anatomy in schizophrenia. *Lancet,* 1995; **346**: 743–9.

Weinberger DR. From neuropathology to neurodevelopment. *Lancet,* 1995; **346**: 552–7.

## Related topics of interest

# SCHIZOPHRENIA – NATURAL HISTORY AND PROGNOSTIC FEATURES

*Schizophrenia does not have a natural history that unfolds independently of its cultural and social milieu* (Harrison *et al.*, 1994)

**Natural history**

When discussing the natural history of schizophrenia, it is important to be clear exactly which syndrome is being discussed. DSM-IV schizophrenia, which excludes illnesses of less than 6 months' duration, has a much poorer prognosis than more loosely (or less exclusively) defined syndromes. There is some evidence that schizophrenia in the early decades of this century had a poorer prognosis than latterly: Kraeplin's 10-year follow-up in 1913 shows 83% with bad outcome, with more recent studies showing only about 30%. The improvement in outcome precedes neuroleptics, so is not due to the use of these.

One of the most detailed descriptions is that of Manfred Bleuler, who followed his patients for well over 20 years in some cases. The long-term prognosis in these subjects was as follows:

- 20% had a single episode with full recovery and no recurrence.
- 35% suffered from repeated episodes, with full recovery between episodes.
- 35% suffered mild chronic psychosis, with severe exacerbations.
- 10% showed severe deterioration to the extent that they needed continuous care.

Prognosis on first admission is that roughly a quarter will never be re-admitted, a quarter will become chronically psychotic, and half will have a relapsing-remitting course with some degree of continuing impairment. Fifteen per cent will be deluded or hallucinated at any one time, and up to 70% may have neurotic (usually depressive) symptoms.

Whilst the lifetime incidence of schizophrenia is similar throughout the world, at about 1%, the prognosis tends to be better in less developed countries. This may be due to greater acceptance of mental illness by families, or to higher death rates in more severe cases.

**Does schizophrenia 'get better'?**

Other studies have looked at the very long-term outcome in discharged patients. The Vermont study investigated a cohort discharged from detention as a result of a planned deinstitutionalization programme in the 1950s. At 10 and 20 years, the outcome was poor, with many patients having persistent social and occupational difficulties. At 25 years, however, a surprising change had occurred, and over 60% of this sample of 'chronic back ward' patients showed full recovery, or only mild impairment (Harding et al., 1987a,b). This is similar to the results obtained by Ciompi and Bleuler (for discussion see Hamilton, 1984).

**Prognostic features**

There is increasingly compelling evidence that schizophrenia is a neuropsychological disorder (Pilowsky, 1992), with evidence of behavioural disturbance in pre-schizophrenic children 15 years before the development of frank psychosis (Done et al., 1994). Perhaps not surprisingly, premorbid abnormalities of social, motor and language development are more pronounced in those with juvenile-onset schizophrenia (Hollis, 1995).

A poor prognosis is associated with the following clinical features in the first episode:

- Insidious rather than acute onset.
- Long episode before treatment.
- No clear precipitating factors.
- Poor premorbid adjustment or personality (especially schizoid).
- Childhood behavioural problems.
- Early onset.
- Male sex.

Of these, poor premorbid social and sexual adjustment is the most powerful single predictor, but only about a third of the variance in outcome can be accounted for by any measurable predictors. The current form of the illness has little, if any, predictive value.

The role of negative symptoms is of interest. It has become clear in recent years that they are not simply a long-term outcome of institutionalization, but may be present right from the onset of the illness in 25% of patients. In follow-up, the proportion of patients with negative symptoms does not vary, but the extent to which individuals suffer from them does.

**Can treatment improve outcome?**

*1. Drug treatment.* Given the evidence of neuropsychological studies which suggest important developmental origins of schizophrenia, there is no possibility of curing the underlying abnormality. This does not mean, however, that treatment will not affect long-term outcome. Neuroleptics are a valuable symptomatic treatment for positive symptoms of schizophrenia, and their use probably explains the extreme rarity in developed countries of severe catatonic schizophrenia, and possibly the extreme rarity of the progressive malignant course described by Kraepelin. Their role in shortening periods of hospitalization, and the severity of positive symptoms, should be expected to contribute to better long-term adjustment. However, the major long-term disabilities of the illness are mainly due to negative symptoms, which are far less amenable to drug treatment. Atypical antipsychotics, which act through mechanisms other than, or in addition to, dopamine blockade, may have more effect on negative symptoms. Trials of clozapine in treatment-resistant schizophrenia indicate that it is more effective than chlorpromazine, and has the potential, in about 50% of these patients, to move them one step up the rehabilitation ladder (institutionalized to group home, supported accommodation to independent living). Other less toxic drugs, such as risperidone, which has a similar pharmacological profile to clozapine, seem to show similar promising effects against both positive and negative symptoms (Marder and Meibach, 1994).

*2. Rehabilitation.* It should be the case that vigorous, early, appropriate and sustained rehabilitation, aimed at minimizing the development and impact of negative symptoms, should improve long-term functioning. The possibility that this may be true is indicated by a recent 13-year follow-up of the Nottingham cohort of first-episode psychosis (Harrison *et al.,* 1994). This revealed high levels of employment and independent living, no homelessness or institutionalization, and nearly half having (and needing) no contact with psychiatric services in the previous 2 years. The authors point out that Nottingham has an extensive spread of community-based acute and rehabilitation services, and attribute the good outcome at least in part to this.

# Further reading

Done OJ, Crow TJ, Johnstone EC, Sacker A. Childhood antecedents of schizophrenia and affective illness: social adjustment at ages 7 and 11. *British Medical Journal,* 1994; **309:** 699–703.

Hamilton M. *Fish's Schizophrenia*, 3rd Edn. Bristol: PSG Wright, 1984, Chap. 7.

Harding CM, Brooks GW, Ashikaga T, Strauss JS, Brier A. The Vermont longitudinal study of persons with severe mental illness. I: methodology, study sample, and overall status 32 years later. *American Journal of Psychiatry,* 1987a; **144:** 718–26.

Harding CM, Brooks GW, Ashikaga T, Strauss JS, Brier A. The Vermont longitudinal study of persons with severe mental illness. II: Long-term outcome of subjects who retrospectively met DSM-III criteria for schizophrenia. *American Journal of Psychiatry,* 1987b; **144:** 727–35.

Harrison G, Mason P, Glazebrook C, Medley I, Croudace T, Docherty S. Residence of incident cohort of psychotic patients after 13 years of follow up. *British Medical Journal,* 1994; **308:** 813–19.

Hollis C. Child and adolescent (juvenile onset) schizophrenia: a case study of premorbid developmental impairments. *British Journal of Psychiatry,* 1995; **166:** 489–95.

Marder SR, Meibach RC. Risperidone in the treatment of schizophrenia. *American Journal of Psychiatry,* 1994; **151:** 825–39.

Pilowsky LS. Understanding schizophrenia. *British Medical Journal,* 1992; **305:** 327–8.

## Related topics of interest

# SCHIZOPHRENIA – SOCIAL ASPECTS

Although schizophrenia is now increasingly being seen as a brain disease, social factors are important, particularly in terms of precipitating relapse (life events and expressed emotion), predicting reponse to medication (expressed emotion) and in reducing the disabilities associated with schizophrenia (institutionalization and rehabilitation).

**Aetiology**

Social factors have been implicated in aetiology, but it now seems that these associations are due to the illness rather than contributing to it.

*1. Socioeconomic class (SEC).* First-admission rates are greater in urban as opposed to rural settings, and there is a gradient from low SEC (higher rates) to higher SEC (lower rates). But rather than contributing to schizophrenia these factors seem to be a consequence of social drift due to the illness. The distribution of SEC of the parents does not differ from the general population, and those with a history of schizophrenia, or those in the early stages of the illness, tend to move into urban areas.

*2. Race and migration.* The incidence of schizophrenia appears to be relatively constant in a wide range of countries and cultures, but the incidence of schizophrenia in immigrants is raised. Interpretation of these findings is difficult. It is most likely to be a spurious artefact resulting from an increased likelihood of admission (rather than of developing illness) if the person is from a foreign culture, rather than the migration of vulnerable individuals or the stresses of migration.

*3. Marriage/fertility.* The incidence of schizophrenia is increased in the unmarried compared to the married and their fertility is low. This again is most likely to be a consequence rather than a cause of the illness.

*4. Family factors.* Theories about contribution of family behaviour to aetiology of schizophrenia include, for example, schizophrenogenic mothers, double-bind theory, marital schism and marital skew. The studies which suggested these theories had major methodological flaws, and although abnormalities may be observed they do not contribute to the aetiology of schizophrenia. These abnormalities are that parents of schizophrenic patients are more often psychiatrically disturbed, more mothers show schizoid traits, there is more parental conflict and mothers are more often overprotective (see expressed emotion). These could all be explained, however, by genetic influences.

5. *Life events.* The evidence that life events contribute to the incidence of schizophrenia is equivocal at best. Although a study of US army recruits showed a greater incidence of first episodes of schizophrenia in the first month compared with the subsequent two years, and a UK study showed a significantly higher rate of independent life events in the three weeks before the first episode of schizophrenia, compared to normal controls, these studies are methodologically flawed. However, the evidence for contribution to relapse is much more robust (see Psychiatric disorders – life events, p. 246). There is a raised frequency of independent life events (both major and minor) in the three weeks before relapse of florid symptoms.

**Relapse**

1. *Life events* (see above).

2. *High expressed emotion.* This is characterized by critical comments, hostility and emotional overinvolvement. It is a better predictor of risk of relapse (>35 h exposure/week) than compliance with medication, but medication, reduced exposure and family intervention mitigate the effects of high expressed emotion.

|  |  |  | % Relapse within nine months |
| --- | --- | --- | --- |
| Low expressed emotion (drugs and no drugs) |  |  | 13 |
| +drugs | 12 |  |  |
| -drugs | 15 |  |  |
| High expressed emotion (all categories) |  |  | 51 |
| <35 hours per week (+/- drugs) |  | 28 |  |
| +drugs | 15 |  |  |
| -drugs | 42 |  |  |
| >35 hours per week (+/- drugs) |  | 69 |  |
| +drugs | 53 |  |  |
| -drugs | 92 |  |  |

Exposure can be reduced by a job, day hospital or sheltered workshop. Family intervention by a psychoeducational approach (Falloon *et al.*, 1985) has also been shown to improve the relapse rates, and this improvement continued on follow-up (two years). The intervention involves education about the effects of illness on the patient's functioning, the opportunity to talk about problems, and a problem-solving and behavioural approach to dealing with these difficulties.

**Institutionalization and rehabilitation**

The Three Hospitals study (Wing and Brown, 1961) identified some common characteristics of long-stay patients with schizophrenia as being the result of their environment rather than the illness alone. In particular, social withdrawal and socially embarassing behaviour were greater in individuals from the hospital with the most rigid routine, and on follow-up, when the hospital routine had become more personalized, these behaviours had declined as a result. These principles have been incorporated into the management of chronic patients and in particular their rehabilitation. So a balance has to be struck between the understimulation of an institutional environment and overstimulation, which can lead to excessive expressed emotion and to eventual relapse. With the changes to community care and the consequent move of patients from hospitals to more independent accommodation one might expect institutionalization to become less of a problem, but in fact living in bed-and-breakfast accomodation can be just as devoid of stimulation.

# Further reading

Falloon IRH, *et al.* Family management in the prevention of morbidity of schizophrenia. *Archives of General Psychiatry*, 1985; **42**: 887–96.
Vaughan CE, Leff JP. Influence of family and social factors on the course of psychiatric illness. *British Journal of Psychiatry,* 1976; **129**: 125–37.
Wing JK, Brown GW. Social treatment of chronic schizophrenia: a comparative survey of three mental hospitals. *Journal of Mental Science*, 1961; **107**: 847–61.

# Related topics of interest

# SELF MUTILATION

Self-mutilation may take a number of forms, varying from the infliction of minor scratches or cuts to serious injuries. Any form of self-harm causes a great deal of concern to both health professionals and others. The important differential diagnosis is between the following groups of patients:

- Those with severe psychotic illnesses, who may perform bizarre self-mutilations, usually as a response to delusional ideas or command hallucinations.
- Failed violent suicide attempts in those with severe mental illness.
- Single episodes of deliberate self-harm.
- 'Multiple self-cutters'.

As with all patients after deliberate self-harm, a careful history should be taken, with particular reference to suicidal intent, and to reasoning behind self-mutilation in order to distinguish to which group the patient belongs. The following deals with the treatment of self cutters. Treatment of the other groups is described in the appropriate sections.

**'Cutters'**

The final group of 'cutters' causes great anxiety, and their correct diagnosis and management is important, both for mental health services and for their own correct management. The characteristics of multiple self-cutters are:

- Young.
- Single.
- Female.
- Often with a medical or nursing background or family.
- Personality problems or personality disorder.
- Background social problems are common.
- Concurrent eating disorders or dysorexia.
- Sexual problems.

The attempt is made in response to threats of loss, and the following clinical features are evident:

- Increasingly intolerable feelings of depersonalization and escalating tension precede the attempt.
- Multiple superficial cuts are made on wrists or arms.
- No pain is felt during the act, and there is often none for several hours afterwards.
- The drawing of blood is important, and the sight of it is described as giving relief from tension.

The complete anaesthesia accompanying the cutting is one index of an extremely unusual alteration of consciousness, another sign of which is the complete flattening of polygraph traces taken during the episode of derealization.

Self-cutters are rarely suicidal, and it has been noted that the cutting is in many ways the obverse of suicide, attempting as it does to bring the sufferer back to a connection with reality from which they have found themselves uncomfortably removed. However, serious injury is possible.

**Management**

Management involves careful briefing of involved professionals that the cutting is not a sign of suicidal attempt, and concerted action to encourage other more adaptive forms of help-seeking.

A behavioural approach is adopted towards cutting, with attention viewed as a reinforcer, if cutting occurs, it should be ignored as much as possible, and treated as not significant. Cuts should be checked to ensure no deep structures are damaged and, if possible, the patient should then be given dressings to apply themselves.

It is important to explore the events leading up to an episode of cutting, and the affects associated. The patient should be encouraged to ask for attention as early as possible in the prodromal period, and immediate attention be given when requested. Other stress-relieving activities, such as progressive muscular relaxation, should be taught, and their use encouraged as an alternative form of coping. Regular, scheduled sessions ensure that attention is not contingent upon illness behaviour, and should be used to explore the psychosocial background which is often an important factor in cutting. In particular, attention should be given to reactions to loss, which can be seen by these patients as potentially overwhelming. The therapeutic contract should contain specific plans for the duration of treatment, review dates, and specific assurance of further treatment if necessary or desirable. Termination of therapy should be a specific issue discussed, and worked through. Treatment of underlying personality disorder can be planned and in some studies has been shown to be of benefit (Linehan *et al.*, 1991).

# Further reading

Hawton K. Self cutting: can it be prevented? In: Hawton K, Cowen P. (eds) *Dilemmas and Difficulties in the Management of Psychiatric Patients.* Oxford: Oxford University Press, 1990; 91–104.

Linehan MM, Armstrong HE, Suarez A, Allmon D, Heard HL. Cognitive treatment of chronically parasuicidal borderline patients. *Archives of General Psychiatry*, 1991; **48**: 1060–4.

# Related topics of interest

# SEXUAL DISORDERS

Sexual disorders can be divided into dysfunctions of the normal sexual response cycle, and variations or deviations from normal sexual attitudes and behaviour. These categories are defined and influenced by social and cultural factors.

**Normal response cycle**
(Kaplan, 1974; Masters and Johnson, 1966)

- Desire: affected by cultural, social, personal and hormonal influences.
- Excitement: consists of subjective excitement and physiological changes. Genital vasodilation (parasympathetic) leads to erection; vaginal swelling and lubrication occur in females.
- Plateau: physiological changes include increases in blood pressure, heart rate and respiratory rate; skin flushing; elevation of testes, elevation of cervix and ballooning of upper vagina.
- Orgasm: increasing sympathetic activity with emission, ejaculation and orgasm in men, and contraction of the perineal muscles in women.
- Resolution: reversal of above changes followed by a refractory period. This is shorter in women than men, and in men it increases with age. Resolution is slower if there is no orgasm.

**Dysfunctions**

*1. Classification.* Sexual disorders can be described as primary or secondary, as psychological or organic, as acute or insidious, total or partial, or specific or global. Another useful system is to classify according to stage.

| Stage | Men | Women |
|---|---|---|
| Desire/initiation | Low sexual drive, avoidance | |
| Excitement/arousal | Erectile impotence<br>Premature ejaculation | Unresponsiveness/lubricative failure |
| Penetration | Failure to sustain erection | Vaginismus (involuntary spasm of perineal muscles on penetration) |
| Orgasm | Premature ejaculation, ejaculatory disorders (delayed or absent, partial incompetence, retrograde, anejaculatory orgasm) | Orgasmic dysfunction |
| Resolution | Priapism (sustained and painful erection) | Pelvic engorgement |
| Other | Low sexual enjoyment, dyspareunia (especially women) | |

2. *Epidemiology.*
(a) General population.
- Erectile impotence    0.1% under 20 years
                                  7% 40–50 years
                                    30% by 70 years
                                    75% over 75 years

(b) Presenting to sexual dysfunction clinics.

| | | |
|---|---|---|
| Men: | erectile impotence | 50% |
| | premature ejaculation | 13% |
| Women: | low interest | 50% |
| | dyspareunia | 11% |
| | vaginismus | 13% |
| Problems in both partners | | 30% |
| Organic cause | | 10% |

3. *Aetiology.*
(a) *Psychological.*

Predisposing factors may include difficult family relationships, traumatic sexual experiences and negative family attitudes.

Precipitating and maintaining factors include performance anxiety, ignorance, relationship problems, guilty or negative attitudes towards sex, fear of consequences, for example, pain, pregnancy, low self-esteem (short or long term), an adverse life situation, for example, redundancy.

(b) *Psychiatric.*

Depressive illness can lead to reduced libido. Alcohol problems can reduce sexual drive and cause impotence. Mania can result in hypersexuality and disinhibition.

(c) *Organic.*
- Genital: congenital abnormalities, pelvic inflammatory disease, episiotomy, prostatectomy, endometriosis.
- Cardiovascular: myocardial infarction, peripheral vascular disease.
- Neurological: epilepsy, peripheral nerve damage, spinal cord damage.
- Endocrine: diabetes, hypogonadism, hyperprolactinaemia.
- Musculoskeletal: arthritis.
- Drugs: tricyclic antidepressants, selective serotonin reuptake inhibitors (SSRIs), monoamine-oxidase inhibitors (MAOIs), anxiolytics, antipsychotics, antihypertensives, diuretics, steroids and the oral

contraceptive, alcohol and other drugs of abuse, cimetidine.
- Pregnancy: reduced interest in first trimester and up to one year post-natally.
- Ageing.

*4. Assessment.* Assessment should focus on presenting problem and consequences, sexual history and current and past relationships; psychiatric, medical and drug history; sexual knowledge, understanding of problem and attitudes to treatment. The mental state in particular, and physical examination as appropriate, should be examined, as well as observation of the patient's relationship. Investigations may be indicated, for example, glucose, liver function tests, hormone levels. The problem(s) is then presented as a formulation which is used as the basis for management.

*5. Management.* Treat any underlying disorder, for example if there is evidence of an organic or psychiatric cause. Explanation of the problem and further information can often make a significant difference.

If further intervention is required, this generally takes the form of couple therapy (Masters and Johnson, 1966), which involves a graded programme of exercises from non-genital to genital sensate focus to reduce anxiety. Additional treatment techniques depend on the dysfunction, as follows.

- Erectile impotence may require medical intervention with intercavernosal papaverine injections.
- Premature ejaculation can be managed with the squeeze technique to delay orgasm.
- Vaginismus is improved by relaxation techniques, graded vaginal dilatation and education.
- Orgasmic dysfunction can be helped with a masturbation training programme.
- Difficulties relating to pregnancy need education about, for example, the safety of intercourse during pregnancy, and alternatives to intercourse.
- Similar approaches apply to post-myocardial infarction, for example, issues such as when an individual is fit to restart a physical relationship, the role of medication, and how to approach this level of activity.

*6. Prognosis.* This depends on the disorder, the development and duration of the disorder as well as individual and situational factors. The best outcome is for premature ejaculation and vaginismus, particularly if the problem is acute and in the context of a good relationship with good premorbid adjustment. The prognosis for erectile and orgasmic dysfunction depends on the cause and is generally moderate. Overall approximately one-third of individuals attending a sexual dysfunction clinic show a very significant improvement, in one-third this is moderate, and one-third show no improvement or drop out of treatment.

**Sexual variations/deviations**

*1. Exhibitionism* (indecent exposure describes the criminal offence). This can be divided into type 1 and type 2.

- In type 1 (80% of cases) there is a compulsion for the individual to expose himself, the penis is flaccid, he does not masturbate and he feels guilty afterwards. It generally occurs in inhibited, emotionally immature young men. The prognosis is good.
- In type 2 (20%) the individual has an erect penis and masturbates, he feels little guilt and may even experience sadistic pleasure. This tends to be associated with sociopathic personality traits and has a worse prognosis.

Indecent exposure is the commonest sexual offence, and the incidence is increasing in young men. The peak age of onset is 15–25 years. 5% are psychotic or have learning disabilities, but other factors include personality traits (immature or enjoy risk taking), poor family relationships, sexual problems, stress or depression. In terms of management the court appearance is often a deterrent and 80% do not re-offend. Psychiatric intervention is indicated if the offence is repeated and this may involve aversion techniques individually or in groups. Favourable prognostic factors include type 1 behaviour, stable personality, good work record and relationships. Unfavourable factors include type 2 behaviour, exposure to young children, previous convictions for other offences and late onset which is linked to brain damage or psychosis. In the longer term 12% of people convicted of rape, arson, or robbery with murder have a previous conviction for indecent exposure. Individuals are more likely to show future violence if physically or verbally aggressive towards the victim.

*2. Paedophilia.* This can occur in men of all backgrounds; intercourse is rare. There is a preferred gender of victim.

10% are bisexual, and homosexual paedophiles are more likely to re-offend. This behaviour is often associated with alcoholism and occurs in vulnerable individuals; it is particularly related to stress and loneliness in older men with paedophiliac tendencies. The victims can be either accidental, or are vulnerable to being selected because of social problems or sexual precociousness.

*3. Incest.* This is most commonly brother–sister or father–daughter. Related factors include learning disabilities, adoption of the surrogate mother role, overcrowding, isolation, alcoholism and marital disharmony. Most victims subsequently lead normal lives.

*4. Sex killing.* This may occur in sadistic or psychopathic individuals, to hide evidence of an assault or to obtain a corpse for necrophilia.

*5. Rapists.* They may have aggressive or inhibited personalities, may be sadistic, paedophiliac or mentally ill or suffer from learning disabilities or alcohol problems. The behaviour may be stress-related or circumstantial. A small proportion re-offend and this is more likely in younger individuals with previous offences, social difficulties, mental illness, abnormal fantasies and available victims. Treating any underlying disorder and improving social functioning can help.

*6. Necrophilia.* Many individuals who practice necrophilia are psychotic or have learning difficulties.

*7. Sexual assault.* Assault can be a result of underlying mental disorder, for example, personality disorder or learning difficulties.

*8. Transvestitism and transsexualism.* (See Gender identity disorders, p. 148).

*9. Homosexuality.* This occurs in approximately 4% of men and 1% of women. It is not an illness but may lead to psychiatric ill-health due to stigma.

- Aetiological factors include genetic, other biological and social influences.
- Twin studies have suggested a genetic contribution.

- Anatomical differences have been suggested in the hypothalamus, the suprachiasmatic nucleus and the anterior commissure.
- Social factors are more difficult to investigate but it has been suggested that family relationships, and attitudes to homosexuality in society can contribute to homosexual behaviour.

*10. Fetishism and sadomasochism.* These present less often as problems and do so generally because they place strain on a relationship.

## Further reading

Bancroft J. Sexual disorders. In: Kendell RE, Zealley AK (eds) *Companion to Psychiatric Studies*, 5th Edn. Edinburgh: Churchill Livingstone, 1993; 553–75.
Hawton K. *Sex Therapy: A Practical Guide.* Oxford: Oxford University Press, 1985.
Kaplan HS. *The New Sex Therapy.* Bailliere Tindall, 1974.
Masters WH, Johnson VE. *Human Sexual Response.* London: Churchill Livingstone, 1966.

## Related topic of interest

Gender identity problems (p. 148)

# SLEEP DISORDERS – ASSESSMENT AND MANAGEMENT

Poor sleep is a major cause of serious morbidity including accidents, psychiatric sequelae and reduced quality of life, and has a major economic impact.

**Insomnia**

Insomnia can present as lack of sleep, poor quality of sleep or reduced daytime performance. It is probably the commonest complaint presented to general practitioners; for example, a Los Angeles population survey showed a 42.5% prevalence of insomnia. Hypnotic use is still common despite recent changes in prescribing (in Sweden over a 15 year period one in five men and one in three women used hypnotics regularly). Primary insomnia is rare. Causes of insomnia include (with estimated rates): psychiatric disorders (36%), psychophysiological insomnia (sleeplessness phobia) (16%), drugs and alcohol (12%), periodic limb movement disorder (12%); and sleep apnoea, pseudo-insomnia, sleep–wake schedule disorder (e.g. related to shift work) and medical disorders which account for 6% each. However, social and personal factors are also very important in determining who presents, for example women report insomnia twice as often as men, and rates are higher in the unemployed.

**Assessment**

- Patient's description of the problem, including the onset, length and quality of sleep, and any daytime drowsiness or reduced performance.
- Objective observations by patient and spouse/partner/relative.
- Possible general medical, psychiatric or drug problems.
- Details of the sleep environment and hygiene.
- Drug history, both prescribed and recreational.
- Current circumstances and stresses.
- Sleep diary including caffeine, alcohol and drugs.

People often overestimate the length of time to get to sleep, even to the extent that good and poor sleepers can have similar sleep patterns. However the quantity of sleep can be relied on in assessing the presence of insomnia. Pathophysiological changes which affect the quality of sleep include reduced growth hormone release in slow wave sleep (SWS), raised body temperature during sleep, increased metabolism (and greater oxygen consumption) during sleep, failure of normal nocturnal release of prolactin and an alpha electroencephalogram (EEG) pattern during sleep, and circadian dysrhythmia.

Excluding psychiatric causes, *psychophysiological insomnia* is the most likely cause of sleep disturbance. Features of this include: the complaint of insomnia and reduced performance when awake, trying too hard to get to sleep, evidence of increased tension with physical symptoms, increased sleep latency, reduced sleep efficiency and increased number and duration of awakenings on EEG. In particular it is not accounted for by medical psychiatric conditions. Other sleep disorders, for example, poor sleep hygiene and obstructive sleep apnoea, can coexist.

**Management**

Any underlying causes should be treated, for example, medical or psychiatric disorders.

Having done this, symptomatic treatment would include:

- Education and advice on sleep hygiene, for example, avoiding caffeine and alcohol.
- Optimizing the temperature of bedroom.
- Encouraging a regular routine.
- Exercising late in the afternoon or in the evening.
- Small food intake in the evening.
- Relaxation techniques can also be very helpful.
- Advice about problem-solving and dealing with intrusive thoughts can reduce difficulties with getting off to sleep and arousals.

1. *Psychotropic drugs and sleep.*
(a) *Drugs used to improve sleep.* Particularly benzodiazepines, which can be used in short-term treatment for poor sleep associated with acute stress. Benzodiazepines reduce rapid eye movement (REM) sleep and SWS, and increase stage 2 sleep. Tolerance and REM sleep rebound occur on discontinuation. Zopiclone increases SWS, and is reported to cause less tolerance and dependence.
(b) *Drugs used to reduce sleepiness.* These are, for example, amphetamines, pemoline and selegiline. These reduce total sleep, REM sleep and SWS, delay sleep onset and cause fragmented sleep.
(c) *Drugs used to treat psychiatric disorders.*
   - Antidepressants. Some are alerting, for example, fluoxetine and some monoamine-oxidase inhibitors (MAOIs); some are sedative, which is generally related to their anticholinergic properties (most

tricyclics). In general, antidepressants suppress REM sleep. MAOIs are used for atypical depression which is characterized by hypersomnia and hyperphagia.
- Mood-stabilizers. Lithium reduces REM sleep and delays onset. Carbamazepine reduces REM sleep and increases SWS, and can cause initial drowsiness.
- Anti-psychotics. These reduce periods of wakefulness, increase SWS. They can increase or decrease REM sleep, depending on the dose. Total and REM sleep are reduced on stopping.

*2. Non-psychotropic drugs.*
Non-psychotropic drugs can affect sleep by crossing the blood–brain barrier (especially if they affect the noradrenergic or cholinergic system), or by causing or exacerbating a disorder which disrupts sleep (e.g. sleep apnoea). Common causes of sleep disturbance include appetite suppressants, anti-emetics, antihistamines, corticosteroids, cardiovascular drugs and hormones.

*3. Recreational drugs.*

- Alcohol promotes sleep in small amounts but in larger amounts causes insomnia later in the night due to rebound and withdrawal effects. Its soporific effect depends on level of sleep deprivation, and interactions with other drugs.
- Nicotine can disrupt sleep.
- Caffeine causes an increased number of arousals and decreased REM sleep. It has a half-life of five hours. Withdrawal symptoms also occur which disrupt sleep.

*4. Illicit drugs.*

- Cannabinoids reduce REM sleep, and increase SWS initially but decrease it after several days. Habitual use leads to excessive sleeping and lassitude, with sleep disturbance on withdrawal.
- Narcotic analgesics cause a drowsy state followed by reduced REM and SWS. Sleep disturbance occurs on withdrawal.
- Cocaine reduces total sleep, SWS and REM sleep. Excessive sleeping occurs on withdrawal (rebound).
- Hallucinogens do not affect sleep directly except by 'bad trips'.

- Benzodiazepines, psychostimulants and appetite suppressants, see above.

5. *Withdrawal.*
Sedatives and hypnotics cause rebound insomnia usually for seven days but it can be for up to two months. Insomnia is more severe but less prolonged for drugs with a shorter half-life. Chloral hydrate gives fewer problems with withdrawal but is less efficacious.

Abrupt withdrawal from antidepressants can lead to short-lived rebound insomnia and panic.

Antipsychotics rarely cause dependence or withdrawal.

# Further reading

Lewis SA. Sleep disorders. *Current Opinion in Psychiatry,* 1994; **7:** 106–9.
Shapiro C. *ABC of Sleep Disorders.* London: BMJ Publishing Group, 1993.

# Related topics of interest

Electroencephalogram (EEG) (p. 134)
Sleep disorders – syndromes (p. 319)

# SLEEP DISORDERS – SYNDROMES

**Sleep**

*1. Stages of sleep and the electroencephalogram (EEG).*

- Stage 1: mixed frequency, low voltage. $\alpha$(8–12 Hz) and $\theta$(4–6 Hz).
- Stage 2: low voltage, slower frequencies. Contains sleep spindles (12–14 Hz) and high amplitude 'k' complexes.
- Stages 3 and 4: high amplitude, low frequency (2 Hz) $\delta$ waves. Stage 3 characterized by <50% $\delta$ waves with sleep spindles. Stage 4 is characterized by >50% $\delta$ waves but no sleep spindles. Stages 3 and 4 comprise slow wave sleep (SWS). As sleep progresses through stages 1 to 4 low frequencies increase at the expense of the higher frequencies which are characteristic of waking.

*2. Rapid eye movement (REM) (desynchronized or paradoxical sleep).* The EEG shows a low voltage, mixed frequency spectrum with characteristics of cortical activation. It is associated with rapid eye movements, signs of autonomic arousal and paradoxical low muscle tonus, and this is when dreams occur.

*3. Sleep architecture.* From waking, individuals pass through stages 1 to 4, then into REM sleep. REM sleep then alternates with non-REM. REM sleep comprises approximately 20% of total sleep time, and occurs at 80 to 90 minute intervals. Stages 3 and 4 comprise 15–20% of total sleep time. The majority of time is spent in stage 2. SWS occurs mainly early on in sleep with REM sleep later. SWS and REM sleep are highest in neonates, and decrease in amount with increasing age.

*4. Functions of sleep.* Theories about the function of sleep include conservation of energy versus brain or body restoration. REM sleep has been proposed to reflect brain functions, and SWS to be associated with bodily functions (as the amount of SWS is related to the amount of energy expended, it is increased with exercise and decreased in hyperthyroidism). It has been suggested that sleep can be divided into core and optional sleep based on observations that:

- Only 30% of total sleep lost is regained after sleep deprivation, especially SWS and REM.

- Short sleepers have similar early sleep patterns to longer sleepers.
- Gradual sleep reduction down to five hours is well tolerated.

*5. Sleep, arousal and performance.* The reticular activating system is involved in arousal, and the induction of sleep is an active rather than passive process. The Yerkes–Dodson curve describes the phenomena of increasing then decreasing performance with increasing arousal. The peak is reached and exceeded more quickly for difficult than for easy tasks. Poor sleep affects the ability to perform simple, mundane tasks but not more complex ones which require more attention. Drugs can affect both performance (via drowsiness) and sleep, for example, antidepressants, antipsychotics, benzodiazepines, antihistamines and alcohol (see Sleep disorders – assessment and management, p. 315).

**Clinical syndromes**

*1. Epidemiology.*

- Narcolepsy: 0.15% (i.e. rare).
- Sleep apnoea: 4–8% of men; 2–4% of women.
- Nightmares: occasional in 50% of adults, regular in 1%.
- Insomnia: 30% in one year.

*2. Classification.*

- Dysomnias: poor sleep (see Sleep disorders – assessment and management, p. 315).
- Medical/psychiatric sleep disorders: i.e. secondary.
- Parasomnias: abnormalities during sleep.
- Specific sleep disorders.

(a) *Parasomnias.* These are acute, undesirable, episodic physical phenomena which usually occur during, or are exacerbated by sleep. There is an interaction between psychological (especially stress) and biological factors. Generally treat with reassurance, education and practical advice. These occur in different stages of sleep:
- SWS: disorders of arousal; sleepwalking and night terrors. Sleepwalking is often exacerbated by excessive sleepiness. Night terrors occur early in sleep, the individual is difficult to rouse and generally has no recall.
- REM sleep: patients rouse easily. These are usually nightmares or dream anxiety attacks which are

frightening, with clear recall. They may be related to psychological precipitants, fever or drug withdrawal (amphetamines, anti-depressants, benzodiazepines, alcohol). Other disorders are sleep-related cluster headaches and sleep-related asthma; the REM sleep behavioural disorder which involves loss of the usual atonia in REM sleep so the individual acts out dreams which are often violent.

- Other parasomnias. Enuresis (patients may have different sleep patterns and therefore not be able to sense the need to urinate); bruxism (teeth-grinding); head banging; familial sleep paralysis.

(b) *Specific sleep disorders.*

- Narcolepsy: characterized by hypersomnolence, cataplexy, sleep paralysis and hypnogogic hallucinations (tetrad is Gelineau's syndrome). 50% also have major affective disorders and/or personality problems. Aetiology unknown; family history is common but there is often a precipitant; HLA-DR2 found in 99%. Onset is generally in the teens or early twenties. Sleep attacks are irresistible in boring situations, and cataplexy is often related to emotion. There is a short REM latency. Narcolepsy can be treated with psychostimulants, and support groups are helpful.
- Periodic limb movement disorder: there are repetitive and stereotyped movements during sleep, and the patient is often unaware. It may lead to poor sleep and daytime fatigue, also depression and anxiety. Found in narcolepsy, obstructive sleep apnoea, Parkinson's disease and metabolic disorders. It can be aggravated by tricyclics and phenothiazines and withdrawal from benzodiazepines.
- Kline–Levin syndrome: this occurs generally in adolescent boys, and is characterized by periods of hypersomnia and overeating, often with changes in libido.

3. *Other sleep-related problems.*
(a) *Circadian rhythm disorders.* This describes changes in the timing of sleep, for example in people on shifts and with jetlag.
(b) *Daytime sleepiness.* Narcolepsy, obstructive sleep apnoea, sleep-related motor disorders, depression, postviral fatigue, head injury, metabolic, toxic and drug-

related factors, essential hyper-somnolence, and older age can all cause daytime sleepiness.

4. *Legal aspects.*
(a) *Alertness.* Doctors have a duty to inform patients about the effects of illness and medication (and interaction with alcohol) on driving and occupation. There are clear guidelines about an individual's duty to inform the driving authorities but doctors should only breach confidentiality if there is a significant hazard and the patient cannot be persuaded to give details themselves.
(b) *Violence.* Insane and non-insane automatism (i.e. internal or external aetiology) allows treatment or acquittal following violent crime (see Legal process, p. 175).

# Further reading

Culebras A. Update on disorders of sleep and the sleep-wake cycle. *Psychiatric Clinics of North America*, 1992; **15**: 467–89.
Lewis SA. Sleep Disorders. *Current Opinion in Psychiatry,* 1994; **7**: 106–9.
Shapiro C. *ABC of Sleep Disorders*. London: BMJ Publishing Group, 1993.

# Related topics of interest

# SOCIAL ASPECTS OF PSYCHIATRY

Knowledge of the social context and aspects of society that contribute to psychiatric disorders and to their presentation and course is vital in making specific management plans and in planning services. This area of psychiatry reflects the changing society we live in and the developing ideas about the management of, and services for, the mentally ill.

**Socio-economic class**

This is one of the strongest predictors of morbidity, including psychiatric disorders. There is an inverse relationship, with those in the lower socioeconomic classes (SECs) being significantly more likely to experience psychiatric disorders or psychological ill-health. The possible reasons for this can be divided into the social causation theory, and the social selection (and drift) theory. The social causation theory says that the increased adversity experienced by those in a lower SEC contributes to the psychiatric disorder, whereas the social selection theory says that people with psychiatric disorders either stay in lower SECs or drift down into them.

**Life events**

Life events can predispose an individual to psychiatric disorder, can precipitate the disorder, or can precipitate relapse (see Psychiatric disorders – life events, p. 246).

**Unemployment and work**

Unemployment is associated with increased mortality, but in particular with depression, anxiety, parasuicide and suicide. This has been found in prospective as well as cross-sectional studies. The mechanisms are not clear but are likely to include economic stresses, stigma, loss of status, isolation and inactivity. Conversely, work itself can also be a major source of stress contributing to psychiatric disorders, but, in general, occupation is protective and is a major focus of rehabilitation programmes.

**Other social factors**

Marital status, as well as affecting overall mortality, affects the rates of psychiatric morbidity. Marriage is protective for men, but for women, those who are single fare better than those who are married. A supportive social network is protective in a variety of psychiatric disorders, as well as other environmental factors such as housing.

**Social consequences of psychiatric disorder**

Patients with psychiatric disorders suffer social disadvantages because of (a) the primary clinical symptoms, (b) secondary handicaps such as withdrawal, and (c) tertiary social disabilities such as isolation, poverty, unemployment and stigma. These aspects are the principal targets of rehabilitation programmes.

**Institutions and institutionalization**
(see also 'Schizophrenia – social aspects', p. 303)

General features of institutions relate to isolation and the fact that they contain a selected population, as well as specific aspects such as understimulation, loss of independence, depersonalization and loss of status, and loss of skills. These are due to rigid rules, all activities being carried out in the same place with the same people, and social distance between patients and staff. These aspects lead to lack of motivation, social withdrawal and apathy. Rehabilitation and the moves towards community care aim to avoid or ameliorate these effects.

**Social interventions and rehabilitation**

Rehabilitation aims to help the individual use their remaining skills to function at the best possible level, and overcome or ameliorate the disabilities caused by their illness, including any aspects of institutionalization. Apart from improving their quality of life it has been shown that this reduces admission rates. The problems of individuals requiring rehabilitation stem either directly from their illness (psychiatric and physical disabilities), from social factors such as isolation and expressed emotion, or from poor skills (social and occupational). Assessment therefore concentrates on psychiatric (and physical) symptoms and treatment, potential skills (self-care and domestic, work, social), short- and long-term objectives, what help is available (professional, voluntary, family), and what progress is being made. Regular monitoring and modification is important. Local psychiatric rehabilitation services make use of and liaise with services offering employment, accomodation, and other specific interventions. For employment this includes the Disablement Resettlement Officer, employment rehabilitation centres, sheltered employment and government training schemes. Day centres and day hospitals can offer specific assessments and behavioural interventions. Accommodation ranges from group homes to sheltered housing to independent housing.

**Community psychiatry**

Community psychiatry reflects the recent changes in the organization of psychiatric services in the move away from large institutions. It aims to manage patients in their own environment as much as possible, according to their individual needs, and therefore avoid at least some of the problems of institutionalization (although the community can be just as isolating and unstimulating). The key piece of legislation for this change was the White Paper: *Better Services for the Mentally Ill (1975)*. The changes in psychiatric services include reducing the number of psychiatric beds, moving to acute units attached to general hospitals and developing day hospitals and day centres. The services have also been developed in primary care according to various models (see Psychiatry in general practice, p. 253), and in the community with community psychiatric nurses, crisis intervention teams and mental health advice centres. These are supported by employment services and social services and aim to provide a coordinated and accessible network of help which is responsive to individuals' needs.

There have been several areas of debate associated with these organizational changes, namely coordination, the issues of responsibility and power, and the particular problems of the homeless.

*1. Coordination of care.* One of the potential problems of moving away from the traditional asylum-based service is that care can become fragmented. Two models of specific coordination that have been assessed are case management (assessment, brokerage and monitoring; low staff to patient ratio) and assertive community treatment (direct care as well as coordination; high staff to patient ratio). Studies in patients with schizophrenia have suggested (although there are methodological problems) that assertive community treatment is more effective in improving various outcome measures, particularly use of hospital services, than case management.

*2. Responsibility of care.* A further consequence of the changes is the increased difficulty in maintaining information on, and contact with, patients, which is particularly important for those at risk of self-neglect or danger to others. The Care Programme Approach has been introduced to plan and coordinate care, and supervision registers have been introduced to identify those who pose the most risk. These measures follow several well publicized incidents (Christopher Clunis and Ben Silcock), and are designed to target services appropriately. The debate continues as to whether these will be effective, or whether they lead to more bureaucracy, to responsibility without power or resources, and increased stigma for patients. Another aspect is the debate about how the changes affect the use of the Mental Health Act and whether it should be reviewed accordingly.

*3. Homelessness.* Homelessness is an increasing problem, but the evidence that this is due to deinstitutionalization (rather than to the reduction in available, affordable housing) is not strong. It also seems likely that psychiatric disorders are not often a major cause of homelessness, especially as living on the streets requires resourcefulness, and indeed has major stresses which may contribute to the prevalence of morbidity. Estimates of the rates of morbidity vary: 40–90% of the homeless population have mental health problems, and the majority are related to alcohol or chronic mental and physical problems with 10–13% suffering from active psychotic illness. As well as the higher rates of morbidity the homeless are often isolated, poor and not in contact with psychiatric services, and because of this and their mobility this population is particularly difficult to help through traditional services. The most effective services are those which concentrate on engaging individuals, and offer a range of psychiatric and social services.

## Further reading

Cohen CI, Thompson KC. Psychiatry and the homeless, *Biological Psychiatry*, 1992; **32:** 383–6.

Fisher K, Collins J. (eds) *Homelessness, Health Care and Welfare Provision.* London: Routledge, 1993.

McCarthy A, Roy D, Holloway F, Atakan Z, Goss T. Supervision registers and the care programme approach: a practical solution. *Psychiatric Bulletin*, 1995; **19:** 195–9.

Muijen M. Rehabilitation and care of the mentally ill, *Current Opinion in Psychiatry*, 1994; **7:** 202–6.

Tyrer P, Kennedy P. Supervision registers: a necessary component of good psychiatric practice. *Psychiatric Bulletin*, 1995; **19:** 193–4.

## Related topics of interest

# STATISTICS

In psychiatry, the important concepts to understand include: concepts of measurement and scale (see also 'Rating scales', p. 278), sampling methods (see also Research methods, p. 287), frequency distributions, applications of probability theory to testing the significance of differences, including non-parametric methods, and some likely sources of error or difficulties in interpretation.

**Measurement**

- *Qualitative scales* are either categorical or nominal, for example scales rating depression and anxiety, where there is no numerical relationship between groups.
- *Ordinal scales* measure, for example, severity where the points lie on a spectrum but the intervals are not significant (eg. mild, moderate and severe depression).
- *Quantitative scales* are either interval where the intervals are equal but there is no significance to the ratio and zero is meaningless (e.g. temperature); or ratio where zero is meaningful, and the points on the scale can be related by interval and ratio (e.g. mass in kg).

**Purpose of measurement and statistics**

Statistics can be descriptive or inferential. They can be used for hypothesis testing, especially of the null hypothesis. The null hypothesis is that there is no difference between samples. Statistical significance is a measure of the probability that a difference between samples is a true difference rather than occurring by chance. The usual value (p) is 0.05, that is 95% probability that the observed difference reflects a real difference (and that the null hypothesis is therefore rejected).

A type I error reflects the probability of finding a difference when the null hypothesis is true, that is a false positive. A type II error reflects the probability of accepting the null hypothesis when a difference exists, that is a false negative. If the false negative rate is $\beta$ then the power of a test is 1-$\beta$. The power is a measure of the likelihood that a real difference will be detected and depends on the size of the sample and the size of the difference in the whole population. The power of the test is particularly important if the expected difference is much smaller than the standard error (a measure of range of values in the population).

*1. Descriptive statistics.* Figures can be expressed in the form of tables, graphs (histograms, comparing two variables) or frequency distributions. The latter can be described by figures which reflect features such as central tendency, symmetry, shape and variability. Distributions may be normal (parametric statistics apply), skewed, Poisson or binomial.

Descriptive statistics include the mode (commonest occurring value), median (middle value when ranked) and mean (average – measure of central position); range (highest and lowest values), variance, standard deviation, standard error (all measures of spread).

*2. Inferential statistics.* These allow interpretation of the information, particularly the degree of sampling error, and therefore how much information about the population can be inferred from the sample information.

Confidence intervals describe the range of values which will include the true population value in 95% of samples taken from Gaussian distributions. In other words, 95% of the time the true value of the mean will fall within the 95% confidence intervals. Confidence intervals are calculated using the standard error and can also be calculated for differences between samples.

*3. Tests/measures.* Parametric statistics assume Gaussian or normal distribution and have greater statistical power than non-parametric tests.

Univariate statistics test the sample distribution of one variable in relation to certain theoretical specifications including a null hypothesis. Samples may be independent, paired or repeated. Bivariate statistics analyse the relationship between two variables, and multivariate between many variables. The *chi square test* is used for categorical data, to look for differences between observed and expected frequencies.

|  | Ordinal data | Quantative data (parametric) | Quantative data (non-parametric) |
| --- | --- | --- | --- |
| 2 independent groups | Wilcoxon | Unpaired t test | Mann-Whitney U test |
| Paired data | Wilcoxon | Paired t test | Wilcoxon |
| Repeated measures three or more groups | | ANOVA (analysis of variance) ANOVA (analysis of variance) | |
| Bivariate data | Spearman's | Pearson's (correlation coefficients) | |

Correlation is the association between two variables. Correlation coefficients can range from -1 (inverse relationship) through 0 (no association) to +1. For parametric statistics use Pearson's correlation coefficient, for non-parametric statistics use Spearman's correlation coefficient. Regression statistics allow the value of one variable to be predicted from the known value of the associated variable.

Multiple regression and two-way analysis of variance enable several variables to be studied at once. Factor analysis and cluster analysis are used to study the influences of multiple variables.

*4. Interpretation.* An association can be explained by: direct causality; chance; reverse causality (i.e. disease causes factors, e.g. social drift in schizophrenia); a confounding variable (i.e. associated with both factor and disease so association is spurious); or there may be another intermediate variable. Other common errors are to use poorly defined criteria for those contributing to the numerator, and to use prevalence instead of incidence to study causality.

# Further reading

McGuire RJ. Statistics and Research Design. In: Kendell RE, Zealley AK (eds) *Companion to Psychiatric Studies*, 5th Edn. London: Churchill Livingstone, 1993.
Swinscow TDW. *Statistics at Square One,* 7th Edn. London: British Medical Association, 1980.

# Related topics of interest

Rating scales (p. 278)
Research methods (p. 287)

# STRESS REACTIONS

Stress in one form or another is ubiquitous within society. A certain level is tolerable, and may even be desirable, as a motivator and to provide 'spice' to life. As a term within medicine, it is 'clearly overstretched and should be used sparingly' (Wilkinson, 1991).

Exposure to stressful events, either acutely or chronically, may produce a variety of responses, which occur over a number of time frames:

| | | |
|---|---|---|
| *Acute* | Hours or days | Acute stress reaction |
| *Subacute* | Days or weeks | Adjustment disorders, dissociative disorders |
| *Chronic* | Months or years | Post-traumatic stress disorder |

All share as common diagnostic features the close and apparently causal association with a stressful event, either acute or long-lasting, and which is viewed as threatening. Although *acute and transient psychotic disorders* (F23 in ICD-10) may also occur in association with stress (within 2 weeks), an obvious stressor is not necessary for the diagnosis. Treatment is with antipsychotics.

**Functions of stress reactions**

It is possible to view acute or subacute reactions to stress as to some extent adaptive, in that they allow an individual to continue activities vital in daily living. The fact that post-traumatic stress symptoms such as intrusive flashbacks occur in over 90% of people within days of a serious event, but persist in only a few, suggests that the syndrome is simply an abnormal extension of the normal processing of traumatic memories, perhaps as a consequence of the interaction between the stressor and the underlying personality structure (McFarlane, 1988).

**Clinical features**

*1. Acute stress reaction*
*A transient disorder of significant severity which develops (in the absence of other mental disorder) in response to exceptional physical / mental stress, and which usually subsides within hours or days...* (ICD-10).

*Treatment.* In acute stress reactions, short-term prescription of sedatives and hypnotics may be justified, to normalize sleep and reduce overwhelming anxiety. The cause of the stress should be dealt with if possible. Supportive counselling should focus on supporting and augmenting the coping mechanisms already in use by the individual, on relating the event to previous episodes, and reactivating any coping mechanisms available for use at the time of stress.

2. *Adjustment disorders.* These occur in the context of an acute or continuing stress, with onset within 1 month of the stressful event. Clinical subgroups are:

- Depressed.
- Anxious.
- Depressed and anxious.
- With disturbance of conduct.
- With disturbance of emotions and conduct.

The disturbance should be over and above that to be expected from exposure to the stressor. Adjustment disorder is common, between 5 and 20% of psychiatric out-patients are assigned this diagnosis at presentation. Symptoms usually resolve within a few months, but may be persistent if the source of the stress cannot be removed.

*Treatment* is by psychological methods, of a supportive nature, designed to deal with any continuing stressors, and to mobilize support networks (both professional and personal).

3. *Post-traumatic stress disorder.* This diagnosis has gone through a variety of forms over time. Although other terms such as 'soldier's heart', 'shell shock', 'war neurosis' and 'battle fatigue' have been used, DSM-III introduced the term post-traumatic stress disorder (PTSD) in 1980, and it is only more recently that the same syndrome has been recognized as occurring outside wartime. Lifetime prevalence estimates vary from 1 to 14%.

The qualifying level for the stressor is difficult to determine, but the stress must be of a nature or degree which almost anyone would find extremely disturbing. Definitions involving the specifier 'outside the range of normal human experience' are difficult to interpret, as symptoms of PTSD occur in 10% of victims of road traffic accidents (Mayou *et al.*, 1993), which are relatively common experiences. Rather illogically, DSM-IV advises that people with symptoms of PTSD in response to a lesser stress be diagnosed as having adjustment disorder. This would seem to ignore the probability that onset of symptoms must be determined by a subjective threshold level of stress, determined by interaction of the environment with individual vulnerabilities, and many studies of at-risk groups have shown that the development of symptoms is related to premorbid personality and psychopathology (McFarlane, 1988). The sequelae may be lifelong and serious, particularly in those whose trauma is prolonged or inflicted by other human beings, such as survivors of concentration camps, torture or rape. The effects may extend to the children of these survivors (Garland, 1993). Patients with PTSD have high rates of psychiatric comorbidity.

The cardinal symptoms are:

- Repeated, intrusive *recollections* of the experience, as flashbacks, images, thoughts or nightmares.
- Phobic *avoidance* of objects or situations reminiscent of the experience, or amnesia for aspects of it.
- *Numbing* of responsiveness.
- Increased *arousal* and hypervigilance.

Onset is usually within 3 months of the trauma, but may rarely be delayed 6 months or longer.

Survivors of childhood sexual abuse may exhibit many of the features of PTSD, and borderline personality disorder has been hypothesized to be a form of chronic PTSD.

*Treatment* should be begun promptly, as the prognosis is worse with longer-established PTSD. Both pharmacological and psychological treatments may be of benefit (Adshead, 1995). Almost every pharmacological agent has been tried, and reported at some point to be successful in the treatment of PTSD, and this is perhaps the best indication of the lack of consistent usefulness of any one of them. Pharmacological treatment alone is never sufficient to alleviate the symptomatology of PTSD. However, drugs such as tricyclics, monoamine-oxidase inhibitors, benzodiazepines and, particularly, selective serotonin reuptake inhibitors may provide sufficient symptom relief to allow psychological work to take place.

Psychological treatments focus on the premise that the principal symptom is the repeated re-experiencing of the event, with the avoidance and arousal being secondary elaborations of this. Flashbacks are thought to be a disorder of memory processing, whereby traumatic memories are laid down in iconic form (i.e. in the form of the initial visual images prior to cognitive processing), outside the usual temporally ordered narrative flow of memory. Treatment involves exposure, usually in imagination, to break the cycle of intrusion and avoidance. Repeated working through of the events in narrative form acts as both a form of desensitization (Vaughan and Tarrier, 1992) and to facilitate the linguistic encoding of unverbalized sensations, which are then amenable to normal 'forgetting'.

# Further reading

Adshead G. Treatment of victims of trauma. *Advances in Psychiatric Treatment,* 1995; **1:** 161–9.

Garland C. The lasting trauma of the concentration camps. *British Medical Journal,* 1993; **307:** 77–8.

Mayou R, Bryant B, Duthie R. Psychiatric consequences of road traffic accidents. *British Medical Journal,* 1993; **307:** 457–61.

McFarlane AC. The longitudinal course of posttraumatic morbidity: the range of outcomes and their predictors. *Journal of Nervous and Mental Disease,* 1988; **176:** 30–9.

Vaughan K, Tarrier N. The use of image habituation training with post-traumatic stress disorders. *British Journal of Psychiatry,* 1992; **161:** 658–64.

Wilkinson G. Stress: another chimera. *British Medical Journal,* 1991; **302:** 191–2.

# Related topics of interest

Defence mechanisms (p. 76)
Memory (p. 185)
Personality – borderline disorders (p. 219)
Psychiatric disorders – life events (p. 246)
Psychological treatment – crisis intervention (p. 264)

# STUPOROSE PATIENTS

The assessment of a patient who lies motionless for long periods of time can be difficult, and occasionally the diagnosis is only clear in retrospect. Such a patient may be described as stuporose. The term stupor refers to both organic and non-organic conditions.

## Definitions

- ICD 10:
  *Profound diminution or absence of voluntary movement and normal responsiveness to external stimuli such as light, noise and touch. The individual lies or sits largely motionless for long periods of time. Speech and spontaneous and purposeful movement are completely or almost completely absent. Although some degree of disturbance of consciousness may be present, muscle tone, posture, breathing and sometimes eye opening and coordinated eye movements are such that it is clear that the individual is neither asleep nor unconscious.*
- The term may also be used to describe an organic condition which intervenes between delirium and coma.

**Clinical settings**

*1. Organic conditions.*
(a) *Cerebral*
- Head injury.
- Epilepsy.
- Tumour.

(b) *General*
- Drugs: lithium, neuroleptics, barbiturates, opiates.
- Hypoglycaemia.

*2. Affective disorders.*
(a) *Manic stupor* has a gradual onset following a period of excitement.
(b) *Depressive stupor* has a gradual onset following a period of psychomotor retardation.

*3. Schizophrenia.* Other general features of schizophrenia are likely to be present, in particular other catatonic features such as hyperkinesis, echolalia and echopraxia, automatic obedience, negativism, waxy flexibility, ambitendence and an oneiroid state with vivid scenic hallucinations. However catatonic symptoms can also be caused by organic brain disease, metabolic disturbance, mood disorders, and alcohol or drugs (see above).

*4. Conversion disorder (dissociative stupor).* This has a sudden onset in response to a stressful event, prominent interpersonal or social problems.

5. *Malingering (Z76.5).* Conscious simulation of stupor by a person attempting a favourable outcome.

**Assessment**

*1. Collection* of data from informants, to describe the onset and nature of the presentation.

*2. Information* gathering about:
(a)   Previous mental illness (especially affective disorder).
(b)   Recent life events and difficulties.

*3. Examination,* paying attention to:
(a)   Facial expression.
(b)   General level of self-care.
(c)   Neurological findings.
(d)   Level of consciousness.
(e)   Muscle tone? waxy flexibility.
(f)   Respiratory state.
(g)   Pupillary responses.
(h)   Purposive eye movements are evidence of a conscious state.
(i)   Papilloedema.
(j)   Evidence of drug misuse.
(k)   Evidence of responding to delusions or hallucinations.
(l)   Response to speech.
(m)  Consistency of presentation.

*4. Investigations:*
(a)   Full blood count.
(b)   Urea and electrolytes.
(c)   BM stix and blood glucose.
(d)   Electroencephalogram may be necessary to determine level of cerebral depression.
(e)   Computer assisted tomography or nuclear magnetic resonance imaging may be indicated.

5. *Psychogenic causes.* When psychogenic causes are suspected, an interview under sodium amytal may confirm the situation, while in schizophrenic and depressive stupors the response to ECT can be dramatic.

6. *On recovery,* patients with 'functional' stupors often prove to have retained awareness of what transpired during the episode, whereas in organic stupor the level of awareness as well as the level of responsiveness is usually grossly diminished.

# Further reading

Gelenberg A. The catatonic syndrome. *Lancet,* 1976; **i**: 1339–41.
Johnson J. Stupor: its diagnosis and management. *British Journal of Hospital Medicine,* 1982; **27**: 530–2.

# Related topic of interest

Electroencephalogram (EEG) (p. 134)

# SUICIDAL PATIENTS

Suicide is a common outcome of mental disorder, with a lifetime incidence of 10–15% in major depression or schizophrenia. The assessment and subsequent management of suicidal patients is thus a common problem in psychiatry.

**Detection**

Failure to detect suicidal ideation or intent is almost always due to failure to ask the correct questions. Few patients dissimulate, but many will be reluctant to volunteer information regarding ideas or plans for suicide. Part of the standard psychiatric interview should be to ask about (in order):

- Feelings of depression, worthlessness or hopelessness.
- Feeling that life is not worth living.
- Thoughts about harming oneself.
- Wanting to die.
- Specific plans or preparations.
- Acts of self-harm.

Details should also be sought of any self-harm in previous episodes of illness or stress.

**Parasuicide**

All patients who have self-harmed should be interviewed by someone trained in the assessment of suicidal risk. It is important to take an open, non-judgmental attitude, and encourage the patient to talk freely about the attempt and its circumstances. It is important to understand the history of the attempt, particularly the people involved and their social relationships, and to have a reasonably detailed understanding of the events in the 24 hours leading up to the attempt. Formal psychiatric illness should be specifically enquired after. With regard to the circumstances of the attempt, the following are indicators of seriousness:

- Violent methods.
- Detailed *planning,* as opposed to impulsive action.
- High *subjective* impression of lethality (the patient may be wrong, in either direction).
- Precautions taken to avoid being found.
- Leaving a note, or other explanation, indicating an expectation not to be there to explain.
- Putting affairs in order (e.g. writing a will).
- Regret on first realizing they are still alive.

Continuing high suicidal risk is indicated by:

- Continuing expressed wish to die (or interviewer feeling that this is the case, though not expressed).

- No change in circumstances as a result of the attempt.
- Continuing regret at having survived.
- Hopelessness about the future.
- Alienation.

**'Manipulative' patients**

Whilst the vast majority of patients should have their statements taken at face value, there are a few who may seem to be persistently using the threat of suicide to produce some change in their environment (e.g. to gain admission to hospital, or control relatives' behaviour). Dealing with these patients is difficult, because they may well self-harm, even if the risk of completed suicide is probably low. It is important to understand 'manipulation' as a form of behaviour indulged in by those who feel powerless, in an attempt to gain some control over their lives. With this in mind, it is often possible to negotiate with the patient some acceptable compromise, by accepting that there is a genuine distress underlying the behaviour, and collaboratively working to find ways of reducing this. With some who repeatedly attempt or threaten suicide, it may be necessary to set firm boundaries, for example by stating (and documenting in the notes, and at local accident and emergency departments) that self-harm, or threats thereof, will not result in their being seen or admitted, but that regular appointments in out-patient departments, or with the GP, might be negotiable.

**Home or hospital?**

There is no accurate way of predicting which patients will actually commit suicide, as this is ultimately an individual decision, and frequently an ambivalent and impulsive one. The corollary of this is that 'wrong' decisions are inevitable, and this is what makes the assessment of suicidal risk so difficult and stressful. The presence of psychiatric disorder, a history of past attempts, a serious current attempt, or thoughts and actual plans, should all increase the assessed risk. Although there may be a very few people in whom a decision to end their lives seems rational and ought to be respected as an inalienable right, actively suicidal patients should probably always be admitted to hospital, at least for observation, if necessary on a compulsory order for assessment of mental disorder. The key issue relating to admission or discharge of a suicidal patient should be based on:

(a) The degree of support available at home: either friends, relatives, or community psychiatric services.

(b) The perception of the likelihood of further attempts: there are a significant number who, having made one attempt, are adamant that they will not make another, and statements to this effect are generally to be believed.

(c) The patient's ability and willingness to make other contingency plans for a recurrence of suicidal thoughts (e.g. call a friend or their GP, visit someone, etc.).

(d) If in doubt, admit to hospital, even if the reasons are uncertain.

**Hospital treatment**

Severely suicidal patients in hospital should be placed on close observation, and all reasonable steps taken to remove from them any potentially harmful objects. Vigorous treatment for mental disorder should be instituted, and severe suicidality is one indication for emergency electroconvulsive therapy.

**Services for suicidal patients**

Each general hospital (or provider unit) should have in place a Self Harm Services Planning Group, which sets out to ensure that patients with deliberate self harm are adequately assessed by a designated self harm specialist team. The service should work closely with the Accident and Emergency staff and be audited regularly. (The General Hospital Management of Adult Deliberate Self Harm, 1994).

# Further reading

Hackett TP, Stern TA. Suicide and other disruptive states. In: Cassem NH (ed.) *Massachusetts General Hospital Handbook of General Hospital Psychiatry,* 3rd Edn. New York: Mosby-Year Book, 1991; 281–308.

*The General Hospital Management of Adult Deliberate Self Harm.* A consensus statement on standards for service provision. Council Report CR32. London: Royal College of Psychiatrists, 1994.

# Related topics of interest

Suicide – epidemiology and risk factors (p. 340)
Suicide – prevention (p. 343)

# SUICIDE – EPIDEMIOLOGY AND RISK FACTORS

It is worth noting the distinction made by coroners between suicide, where there is definite evidence that the deceased intended to take their life, and open verdicts, where there is not. Although most of the latter are probably suicides, some may be accidental death during risk-taking behaviour.

**Epidemiology and trends**

*1. Suicide.* Compared with many other countries, the UK has a relatively low incidence of suicide (but a high incidence of parasuicide and deliberate self-harm). The rate in men in 1990 (Platt 1992) was 11.2 per 100 000 (with 5.1/100 000 open verdicts), and in women it was 3.7 per 100 000 (2.8/100 000). It is in the top ten causes of death in every country in Europe, but is second only to road traffic accidents in 15–34-year-old men. Because of the age profile of those affected, it is second only to heart disease in terms of years of life lost.

The commonest methods of suicide are vehicle exhaust poisoning in men, and self-poisoning with drugs in women. In both sexes, hanging is the second commonest method. In the UK over the past 20 years, the rate in women has halved, while that in men has increased by over 50% (Hawton, 1992). Virtually all of the increase in men is in the under-35 age group, where rates have more than doubled, whereas the decrease in women has been in the older age groups. Because of this there is now only a slight increase in rates with age. Marital status shows up to a 16-fold difference in risk, with married people lowest, followed by single, widowed and divorced as the highest. Other risk factors are social class V (2.1 times social class I), especially young unskilled, and unemployment (1.7 times employed).

*2. Parasuicide.* Parasuicide, or deliberate self-harm, is over ten times as common, with rates of 200 per 100 000 in males, and 400 per 100 000 in females recorded in Oxford. The UK has relatively high rates of parasuicide.

**Risk factors**

Retrospective diagnosis in 1974 showed up to 90% of completed suicides to have been suffering from mental disorder, and 15–30% of these to have seen a psychiatrist at some point. It is possible that if a similar 'psychological autopsy' study were to be carried out in the mid 1990s, as many as 50% of completed suicides would not have a formal mental illness. The major risk factors are as follows:

*1. Previous attempt.* This increases risk 100-fold over the general population. The risk is 2.6% in the 2 years following a single attempt, and 3.6% in the 2 years following subsequent attempts. Death rates from all causes seem to be raised in suicide attempters, confirming that they are atypical of the general population (Nordentoft *et al.,* 1993).

*2. Family history.* This is an independent risk factor for completed suicide. What is probably inherited is an abnormality of 5-hydroxytryptamine (5-HT) systems, as low cerebrospinal fluid 5-hydroxyindoleacetic acid (5-HIAA) is found as a trait marker in survivors of suicide attempts, and low brain 5-HT levels in completed suicides is one of the most robust findings in biological psychiatry.

*3. Affective disorder.* This increases risk by a factor of 30, and lifetime risk of suicide in major affective disorder is of the order of 15% (up to 1% per annum early in the history of the illness). Between 30 and 60% of all suicides may be suffering from affective disorder, and most are untreated or inadequately treated at the time of death. Specific factors increasing risk within affective disorder are childhood bereavement, broken home and recent losses, and prominent feelings of worthlessness and hopelessness. Suicide tends to occur at the onset, peak or early in recovery of the illness. Recurrent brief depression (see Recurrent brief psychiatric syndromes, p. 283) may confer particularly high risk.

*4. Schizophrenia.* Schizophrenia confers a 10–15% lifetime risk. Superadded depression, hopelessness and akathisia all increase risk, and suicide is particularly common in young, intelligent, newly diagnosed males with good insight.

*5. Neuroses.* Appleby (1994), reviewing the sometimes contradictory findings with regard to panic, concludes that:

- Mortality, including that from suicide, is raised in patients with severe neuroses, including panic disorder.
- Panic attacks increase short-term risk of suicide in major affective disorder.
- Patients with a history of panic attacks have a high parasuicide rate, though most of this is due to the high co-morbidity of depression or substance (including alcohol) misuse, and personality disorder.

Similar results have been found in a large cohort with 'pure' anxiety neurosis (Allgulander and Lavori, 1991), where the suicide rate over 14 years was as high as for those with depression. Obsessive-compulsive disorder (see p. 209), which is generally atypical of the neuroses, has a low suicide rate.

6. *Substance misuse.* Twenty per cent of suicides are alcoholic, and alcohol is often involved in attempts. 'Dual diagnosis' is common in alcoholism, and depression primary or secondary to alcoholism is probably a significant factor.

7. *Physical illness.* All types increase risk, especially if chronic, neurological disease or cancer. For example, people with multiple sclerosis have twice the population suicide rate.

8. *Interaction of individual and environment.* One powerful short-term predictor of suicide, particularly of psychiatric patients, seems to be that termed 'Malignant Alienation' by Morgan (Watts and Morgan, 1994). This term is used to describe a progressive deterioration of relationships with others, especially staff, who lose sympathy, and come to regard the patient's behaviour as unreasonable. Up to half of all deaths of psychiatric patients may involve alienation to some degree.

# Further reading

Allgulander C, Lavori PW. Excess mortality among 3302 patients with 'pure' anxiety neurosis. *Archives of General Psychiatry,* 1991; **48:** 599–602.

Appleby L. Panic and suicidal behaviour. *British Journal of Psychiatry,* 1994; **164:** 719–21.

Hawton K. By their own young hand: suicide is increasing rapidly in young men. *British Medical Journal,* 1992; **304:** 1000.

Nordentoft M, Breun L, Munck LK, Nordestgaard AG, Hunting A, Bjoeldager PAL. High mortality by natural and unnatural causes: a 10-year follow-up study of patients admitted to a poisoning treatment centre after suicide attempts. *British Medical Journal,* 1993; **306:** 1637–44.

Platt S. Epidemiology of suicide and parasuicide. *Journal of Psychopharmacology,* 1992; **6:** 291–9.

Watts D. Morgan G. Malignant alienation: dangers for patients who are hard to like. *British Journal of Psychiatry,* 1994; **164:** 11–5.

# Related topics of interest

# SUICIDE – PREVENTION

This topic has been included because it is not only 'topical' in 1995 (Health of the Nation, 1993) but also clinically important.

**Introduction**

- According to official statistics, suicide is the cause of approximately 4000 deaths per year in England and Wales, although the true extent is greatly in excess of this figure.
- Rates of attempted suicide (parasuicide or deliberate self-harm (DSH)) in the UK are among the highest in Europe.
- 1% of hospital-referred attempters die by suicide within a year of an attempt (a rate 100 times that of the general population).
- 40–50% of suicides have a history of attempted suicide.
- Most suicides are psychiatrically ill at the time of death (depression 47–70%; alcohol dependence 15–27%; schizophrenia 2–12%).

**Psychiatric disorders**

*1. Depression.*
(a) In depressed patients with a clear tendency to become hopeless, there is a high risk of suicidal behaviour, so attention should be given to prevention and early detection and treatment of future episodes of depression.
(b) Appropriate use of antidepressant drugs in correct dosage.
(c) Possible use of less dangerous preparations; for example, selective serotonin reuptake inhibitors (SSRIs).
(d) Limiting the amount of medication available.
(e) Prophylactic lithium or carbamazepine is effective in reducing episodes of affective disorder and possibly episodes of suicidal behaviour.

*2. Substance misuse.*
(a) Prevention of alcohol misuse and early detection and adequate treatment are important.
(b) Need for close links between general hospital services for suicide attempters and substance misuse services.

*3. Schizophrenia.*
(a) At least 10% of schizophrenics kill themselves.
(b) High-risk group includes young males with a chronic relapsing disorder in which depressive features are common.

(c) Many are unemployed and aware of the effects of their illness and its implications for their future functioning.

(d) Suicide usually occurs during a non-psychotic phase, but when there are depressive features.

(e) The period immediately following discharge from psychiatric in-patient care is a time of very high risk for suicide.

**Physical ill health**

- Chronic physical illness is common among suicides, especially in elderly males.
- Specific conditions that often occur in suicide include peptic ulcer, cardiovascular disease, malignancies and epilepsy.
- Suicide risk is also greatly increased in people with AIDS or HIV infection, so supportive networks are important for this group.

**Social problems**

*1. Unemployment and poverty.*
(a) Both suicide and attempted suicide are closely associated with unemployment.
(b) Poverty is likely to be another linking factor.

*2. Family problems and marital breakdown.*
(a) Increased family breakdown, related to the rapid rise in the divorce rate which occurred among parents of young people in the 1960s and 1970s, might be one reason for the recent increase in young male suicides.
(b) Marital and family counselling agencies such as Relate should therefore be supported.

**Control of measures used for suicide**

- A 34% reduction in suicide rate occurred between 1963 and 1974, in parallel with the change in domestic gas supply from coal gas to non-toxic North Sea gas.
- Reducing the toxicity of car exhausts by means of catalytic converters is likely to prevent some suicides.
- Reducing the number of analgesic tablets (especially Paracetamol) available over the counter and greater use of blister packs might help prevent potentially fatal self-poisoning.
- 'Suicide barriers' should be erected on all high bridges and other such sites strongly associated with suicide.

**Media reporting of suicide**

- There is evidence that media reporting of suicide can be associated with further suicides.
- Straightforward, undramatic, factual reporting of suicide by the media should be encouraged.
- Any presentation of suicide in the context of a drama

should be followed by advertisements for help-lines and encouragement for distressed people to seek help through these or other means.

**Educational measures**

*1. Public.*

(a) Education of the public about the facts of mental illness, including suicide, is important.

(b) Relatives of at-risk mentally ill patients should be provided with appropriate support.

*2. Schools.*

(a) Education and training of young people in 'life skills' for coping with stress, conflicts and crises awaits further evaluation.

(b) Specific education for teachers concerning the early recognition of children and adolescents with psychiatric disorders and the risk factors for suicidal behaviour (not evaluated).

*3. Clinicians.*

(a) Should be trained and encouraged to detect affective disorder and signs of hopelessness in patients with physical ill health.

(b) GPs need to be skilled in the detection and treatment of depression.

(c) A special postgraduate training programme for GPs on the Swedish Island of Gotland was followed by a reduction in the local suicide rate. After the study period, however, suicide rates rose again. Thus the accurate diagnosis and effective treatment of depression, especially in primary care, may have a major bearing on suicide rates. This is recognized by the World Health Organization (WHO) in its guidelines for treatment of recurrent depression (WHO, 1989).

*4. Samaritans.*

(a) Offer confidential telephone counselling with the goal of suicide prevention.

(b) There is no evidence of a significant impact of the Samaritans on suicide rates.

*5. General hospital services for suicide attempters.* A quarter of all suicides have attended hospital in the previous year as a result of a non-fatal act of deliberate self-harm. It follows, therefore, that provision of first-class services for cases of deliberate self-harm represents a potential means of meeting the Health of the Nation target for prevention of suicide (Royal College of Psychiatrists, 1994).

6. *Limitations of suicide prevention.*
(a) Total eradication of suicide will never be feasible.
(b) Even when at-risk groups are identified, prevention is not easy.
(c) Economic and social factors, as well as clinical factors, have an impact on suicide.
(d) No single means of prevention by itself is likely to have a major lasting impact on the problems of suicide and attempted suicide.

# Further reading

Gunnell D, Frankel S. Prevention of suicide. Aspirations and evidence. *British Medical Journal*, 1994; **308**: 1227–32.
Hawton KE. Suicide. In: Paykel ES, Jenkins R (eds) *Prevention in Psychiatry.* Gaskell, 1994; 67–79.
Royal College of Psychiatrists. The General Hospital Management of Adult Deliberate Self Harm. A Consensus Statement on Standards for Service Provision. Council Report CR32. London: Royal College of Psychiatrists, 1994.
Rutz W, von Knorring L, Walinder J. Frequency of suicide on Gotland after systematic postgraduate education of general practitioners. *Acta Psychiatrica Scandinavica*, 1989; **80**: 151–4.
World Health Organization. Pharmacotherapy of depressive disorders. A consensus statement. WHO mental health collaborating centres. *Journal of Affective Disorders*, 1989; **17**: 197–8.

# Related topics of interest

# TOURETTES AND RELATED CONDITIONS

**Tourettes syndrome**

Tourettes syndrome is a rare disorder, with a prevalence of 4–5/1000, characterized by multiple motor and vocal tics. A tic is defined as a sudden, rapid, recurrent, non-rhythmic, stereotyped motor movement or vocalization. The vocalizations are of enormous variety: barking, grunting, sneezing, as well as fully formed words.

The tics are increased by:

- Anxiety.
- Stimulant drugs

and reduced by:

- Absorbing situations.
- Relaxation and sleep.

Although involuntary, the tics can be controlled for a short time by efforts of will.

Accompanying symptoms include:

- *Coprolalia*. Inappropriate foul language.
- *Echolalia*. Compulsive repetition of things said by others (as opposed to mimicry, which is voluntary, playful repetition).
- *Echopraxia*. Compulsively copying actions or gestures of others.

Severe occupational and social impairment may result, as may self-injury.

The disorder typically begins in childhood or adolescence, and the prognosis is poor, with at least 50% continuing to have symptoms into adulthood, although these may be controlled by medication. In some patients, tics may be used to advantage (Sacks, 1986).

**Treatment of Tourettes**

Treatment is pharmacological, usually with drugs which block dopamine receptors. Low doses of haloperidol and pimozide are the most commonly used. Clonidine, a presynaptic alpha$_2$, receptor blocker, may be useful in resistant cases, but treatment is often only partially successful.

**Tourettes and OCD**

Evidence for a link between the two syndromes is of two types.

*1. Genetics.* A significant proportion of Touretteurs have obsessional disorder, and about 20% of obsessive-compulsive disorder (OCD) patients have tics. A number of pedigrees show an association of Tourettes and OCD in the same families, with suggestions of an autosomal dominant mode of transmission.

*2. Organic features.* Positron emission tomography (PET) scanning shows metabolic abnormalities in the orbital frontal cortex and caudate nucleus of OCD patients, in areas with high serotonergic innervation. This is in keeping with the finding of low CSF 5-hydroxyindoleacetic acid (5-HIAA) in untreated patients, and the marked anti-obsessional effects of drugs blocking the reuptake of serotonin, which probably act by downregulating transmission at synapses in these areas. Similar abnormalities in frontal lobes, corpus striatum and caudate nucleus occur in Tourettes syndrome. However, treatment is usually with drugs blockading dopamine: haloperidol or pimozide.

At a fundamental level, both diseases can be viewed as disorders of impulse control, involving irresistible impulses to think or act in certain ways. Impulsivity as a behavioural trait is related to central serotonergic activity, but the initiation of motor activity is controlled by the extrapyramidal motor system. Thus, the two disorders are acting at different levels: Tourettes at the level of motor behaviour, OCD more at the cognitive and affective level.

## Further reading

Kendell RE, Zealley AK (eds) *Companion to Psychiatric Studies* (5th Edn). Churchill Livingstone.
Pigott TA, L'Heureux F, Dubbert B, Bernstein S, Murphy DL. Obsessive-compulsive disorder: Comorbid conditions. Journal of Clinical Psychiatry, 1994; **55**(10, suppl): 15–27.
Sacks O. "Witty, Ticky Ray" In: *The Man Who Mistook His Wife for a Hat*. Pan Books, 1986.

## Related topic of interest

Obsessive-compulsive disorder (OCD) (p. 209)

# TREATMENT-RESISTANT DEPRESSION

The treatment of depression is one of the success stories of modern psychiatry. Well-conducted trials of biological and psychological treatments consistently show response rates of 70%, compared to placebo response rates of around 30% (BMJ, 1965). However, even this level implies that nearly one-third of patients are not successfully treated, and it is of note that using the more rigorous 'intention to treat' as opposed to 'completion of treatment' reduces the success rate to around 50%. In those patients unwilling or unable to comply with medication, or in those who cannot tolerate antidepressants, a trial of cognitive therapy or interpersonal therapy may be worthwhile, particularly if there are obvious cognitive or social precipitating or maintaining factors (Gelder, 1990).

**Adequate dosage**

In practice, results do not always match those cited, because the consistent finding in both hospital and community studies is that the commonest cause of failure to respond is failure to treat with adequate dosage for an adequate time. An adequate dose of an antidepressant is at least 150 mg of imipramine or the equivalent, and dosage should be increased stepwise, 50 mg per week up to 200 mg, then 25–50 mg per week to 300 mg or more, or until a response is observed, or side-effects become limiting. Selective serotonin reuptake inhibitors (SSRIs) show less of a dose-response relationship, but dose should be increased to 40 mg of fluoxetine or the equivalent, and some patients respond only to doses of 60 mg or more. Adequate time is at least 8 weeks, because, although most responses are observed within 2–4 weeks, there is a group of patients who respond late.

**Psychotic depression**

This should be treated from the outset with a combination of antidepressant and antipsychotic medication, which works better than either of these alone. Alternatively, ECT is extremely effective, although the risk of relapse after stopping it is very high, so it should be used concurrently with drug treatment.

**Change of antidepressant**

If there is no response to a full therapeutic trial of one antidepressant, it is worth considering switching to one of a different class (monoamine reuptake inhibitor (MARI) such as imipramine, to SSRI or monoamine-oxidase inhibitor (MAOI)).
MAOIs should be considered in those with:

- Retained mood reactivity.
- Reversal of usual biological features (i.e. hypersomnia, hyperphagia and weight gain, hypersexuality).

- Panic symptoms.
- Premorbid rejection sensitive personality traits ('hysteroid dysphoria').

In this sort of 'neurotic' picture, they have been demonstrated to be superior to imipramine (Liebowitz *et al.*, 1988). Tranylcypramine, which has a combination of MAOI, noradrenaline reuptake inhibitor, and amphetamine-like action is occasionally successful where all other drugs have failed. However, it is both the most dangerous of the MAOIs and the only addictive antidepressant (and therefore has a withdrawal syndrome), so it should be used with circumspection! Alternatively augmentation of an antidepressant of one class with one from another may be effective (see below), but great care must be taken when combining MAOIs with tricyclics. Adding the tricyclic to the MAOI may cause a rise in blood pressure, so it is important to start cautiously, with a low dose. The combination of clomipramine or SSRIs with MAOIs is absolutely contraindicated: a fatal serotonin syndrome has been reported. The serotonin syndrome has also been reported with combinations of 5-HT reuptake inhibitors with lithium, L-tryptophan and pethidine. The symptoms are caused by $5\text{-HT}_{1A}$ receptor hyperstimulation in the brainstem and spinal cord, and are of 3 types:

- *Mental state* changes (confusion, hypomania).
- *Autonomic* (diaphoresis, diarrhoea).
- *Motor* (restlessness, hypertonia, myoclonus, hyper-reflexia, incoordination).

It is important to allow a washout period when switching between SSRIs and MAOIs: the exact time needed varies from 1–4 weeks, so manufacturers instructions should always be consulted.

**ECT**

If a patient fails to respond, it is worth considering whether the diagnosis is correct, and drug compliance. Then consider whether electroconvulsive therapy (ECT) would be appropriate. ECT is most effective in moderate or severe depressions with biological features, psychotic depression, or in those with a history of responding to ECT. It should be considered early where there is a significant suicidal risk, as it is the most rapid and effective treatment known. Evidence from studies of suicide suggests that it is usually considered rather late, even in those with a previous history of responding to ECT. An initial course of 6–8 treatments is given, and extended to 12 treatments if necessary. After recovery, drug treatment must be continued, or the risk of relapse is unacceptably high.

**Augmentation**

A combination of drugs may have a synergistic effect. Most commonly, a MARI or SSRI is augmented by adding lithium, in normal therapeutic doses (Katona *et al.*, 1995). The effect is often dramatic, and is usually seen within a week, sometimes as soon as 24–48 hours after treatment. The addition of L-tryptophan 2–3 g nocte to the combination may further enhance its efficacy. In recurrent depression carbamazepine may be used instead of lithium, or in combination with it. The ultimate serotonergic drug cocktail is said to be clomipramine (or an MAOI), lithium, and L-tryptophan. There are some patients who remain well only when on all three of these, in whom withdrawal of any causes relapse. An alternative noradrenergic cocktail uses maprotiline plus lithium.

There is some data to suggest that combining noradrenaline reuptake inhibitors (most tricyclics) with SSRIs may be as effective as the combination with lithium. A few patients respond to augmentation with small doses of thyroxine, 20–50 µg daily (Targum *et al.*, 1984), or to the use of clonazepam 0.5–2 mg b.d.

**Psychosurgery**

This is a treatment of last resort, for patients who remain severely depressed for over a year despite maximal combination chemotherapy, and at least 2 courses of ECT. In this group, a referral for stereotactic subcaudate tractotomy may be considered. The operation may be successful in abolishing symptoms in up to 50%, with some improvement in another 20% (Bridges, 1990).

# Further reading

Bridges PK. Treatment of Resistant Depression. Hospital Update: April, 1990; 346–52.

Clinical Trial of the Treatment of Depressive Illness: Report to the Medical Research Council by its Clinical Psychiatry Committee. *British Medical Journal,* 1965; **1:** 881–6, (1965).

Gelder MG. Psychological treatment for depressive disorder. *British Medical Journal*, 1990; **300:** 1087–8.

Katona RLE, Alou-Saleh MT, Harrison DA, Nairac BA, Edwards DRL, Lock T, Burns RA, Robertson MM. Placebo-controlled trial of Lithium augmentation of Fluoxetine and Lofepramine. *British Journal of Psychiatry*, 1995; **166:** 80–6.

Liebowitz MD, Qutikin FM, Stewart JW *et al.*, Antidepressant specificity in Atypical Depression. *Archives of General Psychiatry,* 1988; **45:** 129–37.

Targum SD, Greenberg RD, Harman RL *et al.* Thyroid hormone and the TR4 test in refractory depression. *Journal of Clinical Psychiatry,* 1984; **45:** 345–6.

## Related topics of interest

# VIOLENT PATIENTS

**Violence: classification**

- Actual or threatened.
- Directed toward self or others.

**Violence: epidemiology**

- Most episodes are non-psychiatric: typically minor, unreported and between adolescent or young adult males.
- This may be becoming generally more common: but perception could be real or due to increased media coverage.
- However, it does seem to be occurring in situations where it was once rare: for example, assaults on health-care staff.
- There is no evidence that psychiatric patients are more likely to be violent than the general population, but see below for particular conditions.

**Violence towards the self**

Suicide and attempted suicide are covered elsewhere (see Suicidal patients, p. 337). Relevant here are:

*1. Habitual self-harmers* (see Self mutilation, p. 306). The 'cutter' may assault the carer who is trying to remove a sharp object during a cutting episode, rather than waiting until it is over, when the patient is often calm.

*2. Suicide-homicide.* In rare cases when a person, often with a mental disorder, kills another, usually a relative, and then kills himself/herself. Associated disorders include:
(a) Postnatal psychosis/depression.
(b) Psychotic depression.
(c) Pathological jealousy.
(d) Substance misuse.

**Threats of violence to others**

- May be a criminal offence.
- In certain cultural backgrounds are not entirely untoward.
- Must always be taken seriously in psychiatric settings.
- Even if not acted on or apparently meant seriously, can cause great distress to staff or other patients.
- A full assessment is essential.

**Management of threats of violence to others**

- If the risk appears real, the main treatment should be geographical: for example, the child abuser/violent husband leaves the family home.
- If the risk remains, consider informing person(s) at risk and the police: balance duty of confidentiality against duty to others. In the USA, many States impose a 'duty to warn' on psychiatrists. (Tarasoff doctrine: in therapy, a

male student said that he intended to kill female student Tatiana Tarasoff and later did so. Her family then sued.)

Psychiatrists routinely assess a patient's risk of self-harm, but frequently fail to assess the risk to others.

**Warning signs of impending violence**

*See also Dangerousness assessment, p. 73.*

Defusing a potentially violent situation, for example by briefly postponing a psychiatric interview, is much better than dealing with actual violence. Although a precise prediction of risk is impossible as it varies according to the situation, recognized warning signs include:

- A history of violence.
- Angry, impulsive, emotional, demanding or threatening demeanour.
- Substance misuse, especially present intoxication or withdrawal.
- Patient with grievance.
- Never ignore the interviewer's own anxiety or fear.

For example, a person with brain damage, who has been drinking, and who has waited a long time in casualty to see a doctor, could fit into this category.

**Safe interviewing**

If one or more of the above signs apply, and the interview really is immediately necessary, the interviewer should routinely take the following precautions:

- Be in an open space, not a claustrophobic room.
- There should be an accompanying colleague, with others nearby.
- Staff should be nearest door.
- Have a panic button to hand.
- Staff should be trained in breakaway techniques (but avoid getting into that situation).
- Adopt a non-confrontational approach.

**Interviewing the potentially violent patient**

Much can and should be done before the interview:

- Review all the notes.
- Discuss the case with present and previous carers.
- Seek advice from senior colleagues.

The more fraught the situation, the greater the dividend from pausing briefly to think and confer.

The assessment attempts to avoid violence by the following procedures:

- Take a non-confrontational approach.
- Remain polite, calm and unhurried.
- Stay focused and problem-oriented.
- Indefatigable efforts at complete assessment should be made, but although laudable in other situations, certain aspects (e.g. family history), may seem interfering or aggressive to the disturbed patient.

**Calming the violent patient**

Sometimes the above approach is ineffective, and actual violence occurs:

- Do not attempt to tackle the person singlehandedly.
- Leave the interview room.
- Damage to property is of no immediate importance.
- Summon assistance.

**Control and restraint then becomes necessary**

- Restraint techniques must be safe for staff and patient.
- Specially trained three-person teams should be used, more if available. The presence of large numbers of staff may cause a patient to 'think twice' about continuing violence, and they may submit meekly.
- Doctors are usually not directly involved.
- Even psychotic patients often settle without physical restraint when they observe the control and restraints (C and R) team.
- In extreme cases, shields and/or helmets may be needed to protect staff.
- Summon the police if the violence is clearly not psychiatric in origin.

**Medication**

- Indicated where the violence is clearly psychiatric in origin or if it is uncontrollable by other means.
- Choice of antipsychotics versus combinations.
- Royal College Consensus Report disfavours traditional mega-dose antipsychotic regimes (there have been well-publicized cases of unexplained sudden death in violent, restrained patients).
- If antipsychotic treatment is ineffective (e.g. chlorpromazine 100–200 mg x 2), consider adding a second class of drug, for example, lorazepam 1–2 mg.
- Route orally if possible, otherwise IM.

**After the acute incident**

1. *Clopixol acuphase* (2–4 day acting depot antipsychotic). This drug is very useful for maintaining sedation.

2. *Seclusion or 'time out'.* A side room with minimal furniture can help to calm some patients. It must be used briefly and judiciously, not as a punishment.

3. *Physical restraints.* Their use is rare, and they are probably under-used in the UK. It could be queried whether ethical objections are intrinsically greater than for other involuntary treatments.

4. *Review placement.*
(a) Most restrained patients are cared for in the same institution.
(b) Patients probably need increased care, e.g. day patients become in-patients.
(c) Review diagnosis and care plan.
(d) Consider increasing staffing to 'special' the patient.
(e) Consider transferring to more secure care if the patient appears uncontainable.

5. *Legal aspects.*
(a) Common law: allows involuntary emergency treatment such as C and R, medication.
(b) Section under the Mental Health Act: not always needed; some incidents are 'one-offs', but usually consider formal assessment if there is likely to be a continuing need for compulsory assessment or treatment.

6. *Case notes.* A full account is needed.

7. *Staff needs.*
(a) Most staff receive their support informally.
(b) Staff-support groups are often advised, but are often problematical in practice.
(c) 'Critical incident debriefing' is fashionable in an effort to prevent post-traumatic stress disorder, but is unevaluated and can re-traumatize.
(d) Identify needs for further training.

8. *Audit of violent incidents.*
(a) Identifies problems; for example, an excess in one ward.
(b) Necessary to satisfy interested bodies; for example, Mental Health Act Commission.
(c) Allows appropriate representations to purchasers and managers.

# Further reading

Brown TM. *Handbook of Emergency Psychiatry.* Edinburgh: Churchill Livingstone, 1990.

# Related topics of interest

# INDEX

Head injury, 51, 99, 151, 334
Heartsink patient, 110, 256
Hepatic coma, 136
Herpes simplex, 51
Homelessness, 326
Homosexuality, 313
Hormones, 131
Hospital Anxiety Scale, 64
Hospital order, 178
HRT, 240
Human Immunodeficiency Virus (HIV), 99, 137, **155**
Huntington's disease, 89, 99, 136
Hydrocephalus normal pressue, 90
Hyperkinetic syndrome, 43, 334
Hyperventilation, 40, **159**
Hypochondriasis, 48, 160, 182
Hypoglycaemia, 334
Hypothalmo-pituitary-adrenal (HPA) axis, 251
Hypothalmo-pituitary-gonadal (HPG) axis, 251

ICD-10, 96
Id, 234
Illness behaviour, **162**
Illness worry, 180
Imaging, 30, 90, 92, 295, 335
Impulse control, 348
Incest, 313
Incidence, 287
Infanticide, 177
Informed consent, 145
Insomnia, 315, 320
Institutionalization, 303, 324
Intelligence test, 67
Intensive care, 265
Interpersonal therapy, 128
Intoxication, 167, 178
Involuntary hospitalization, 146
Irritable bowel syndrome, 63

Jung, 227, 234

Kleinfelter's syndrome, 149, 197
Kline-Levin syndrome, 321
Kluver-Bucy syndrome, 99
Kohlberg, 106
Koro, 70

Korsakoff's psychosis, 51, 187

Latah, 70
Learning disabilities, 50, 66
Leukoencephalopathy, 155
Lewy body dementia, 89, 98
Life events, 19, 303, 323
    affective disorders, 247
    depressive disorders, 247
    schizophrenia, 247
Life review therapy, 21
Life stresses, 162, 246
Linkage, 242
Lithium, 22, 90, 195, 334, 351

Malingering, 141, 180, 335
Mania, 15, 48, 283
Marital therapy, 268
Maslow, 224
Maternity blues, 205
Memory, 66
Meningitis, 155
Menopause, 238
Mental Deficiency Act (1913), 200
Mental handicap, **200**
Mental Health Act, 132, 145, 175, 201, 325, 356
Methadone, 13
Migration, 71, 303
Mini Mental State Examination, 66
Moral philosophy, 144
Multi-infarct dementia, 89, 97, 137
Multiple personalities, 181
Multiple sclerosis, 89
Munchhausen's syndrome, 183
Myalgic encephalomyelitis, 59, 163
Myxoedema, 51

Naltrexone, 13
Narcolepsy, 320
Negativism, 334
Neurasthenia, 59, 180, 285
Neurofibrillary tangles, 30
Neuroleptic malignant syndrome, 36
Neuropathology, 100, 155
Neurosis,157, **206**
Neuroticism
    extravert, 215
    introvert, 215

# Key Topics in Accident & Emergency Medicine

**P. Howarth & R. Evans**
*respectively Royal Cornwall Hospital, Truro, UK; and Cardiff Royal Infirmary, UK*

An ideal reference and revision aid for postgraduate examinations, providing the key information on acute injuries and sudden illness which commonly present at Accident and Emergency Departments.

"Within a logical and attractive layout it covers 91 topics... All are relevant to everyday practice as well as being likely topics to be covered at some stage during the accident and emergency fellowship examination... readable and up-to-date... especially useful for candidates working for the fellowship examination." *BMJ*

## Contents

100 key topics in current accident and emergency medicine presented in alphabetical order.

## Of interest to:

Medical and nursing staff working in Emergency and Surgical Departments, particularly candidates for Fellowship or other postgraduate qualifications (such as the FRCS examination in Accident and Emergency Medicine). Also useful as a reference for paramedics; nurses and practitioners.

1872748678; 1994; Paperback; 332 pages

# Key Topics in Anaesthesia 2/e

**T.M. Craft & P.M. Upton**
*respectively Royal United Hospital, Bath; and Treliske Hospital, Truro, UK*

The ideal reference and revision aid for trainee anaesthetists with essential information on 100 major subjects pertinent to modern clinical practice in anaesthesia. The text is presented in a uniform, systematic format to encourage a problem-based approach to clinical scenarios.

"I think this book is a winner. What about those to whom it is aimed? I have not yet found a member of our junior staff who, prior to taking the test [FRCA part III], has not already purchased a copy. May I also recommend it to their teachers?" *Today's Anaesthetist*

## Contents

Each topic includes (wherever the subject allows): introduction; essential problems; anaesthetic management - assessment and premedication, conduct of anaesthesia, and postoperative care; further reading; and related topics of interest.

## Of interest to:

Trainee anaesthetists studying for postgraduate examinations (e.g. FRCA, European Academy of Anaesthesiology examination, etc.); qualified anaesthetists, anaesthetic assistants, nurse anaesthetists and surgeons.

1859960758; 1995; Paperback; 360 pages

ALSO AVAILABLE FROM BIOS SCIENTIFIC PUBLISHERS LTD

# Key Topics in Obstetrics and Gynaecology

**R.J. Slade, E. Laird & G. Beynon**
*respectively University Hospital of Wales, Cardiff, UK; Northampton General Hospital, UK; and Queen Elizabeth II Hospital, Gateshead, UK*

The ideal reference and revision aid for postgraduate examinations in obstetrics and gynaecology. Contains essential information on 100 major subjects presented in a uniform, systematic style.

"Whilst one hesitates to recommend such volumes as a basis for learning, this particular publication will be found by many to be a useful guide to preparation for examinations from final MB to the MRCOG." *Br.J.Obstetrics & Gynaecology*

**Contents**

**Of interest to:**

Trainee obstetricians and gynaecologists studying for a postgraduate examination, such as the MRCOG part II; also general practitioners and medical students.

1872748074; 1993; Paperback; 296 pages

# Key Topics in Ophthalmology

**R. Taylor\*, P. Shah, P.I. Murray & A. Fielder**
*respectively Royal Hallamshire Hospital, Sheffield, UK\*; and Birmingham and Midland Eye Hospital, UK*

Essential information on approximately 100 major subjects, chosen for their importance and their incidence in examinations. The book is an ideal reference and revision aid for ophthalmology postgraduate examinations.

## Contents

Approximately 100 key topics presented in alphabetical order; ranging from AIDS, Allergy and Anisocoria to Scleritis, Uveitis and Watery eye.

## Of interest to:

Postgraduate examination candidates, e.g. FRCOphth or MRCOphth; also useful for qualified ophthalmologists and general practitioners with a special interest in ophthalmology.

1872748384; 1995; Paperback; 304 pages

# Key Topics in Orthopaedic Surgery

**I. Nugent, J. Ivory & A. Ross***
*respectively Royal United Hospital, Bath, UK; and *Royal United Hospital and Royal National Hospital for Rheumatic Diseases, Bath, UK*

An excellent revision and reference aid for surgeons intending to specialize in orthopaedics, covering 100 of the most common problems and areas encountered in orthopaedics.

## Contents

## Of interest to:

Postgraduate examination candidates, e.g. the FRCS (Orth) Part III examination, or its equivalent; orthopaedic trainees and consultants.

1872748333; 1995; Paperback; 364 pages

ALSO AVAILABLE FROM BIOS SCIENTIFIC PUBLISHERS LTD

# Key Topics in Otolaryngology

**N.J. Roland, R.D.R. McRae & A.W. McCombe**
*respectively Royal Liverpool University Hospital, UK; Royal Liverpool University Hospital, UK; and Bristol Royal Infirmary, UK*

Essential information on 100 major subjects pertinent to modern clinical practice in otolaryngology. The ideal reference and revision aid for postgraduate examinations.

## Contents

100 key topics in current ENT practice presented in alphabetical order.

## Of interest to:

Postgraduate examination candidates, e.g. the FRCS Clinical Surgery in General with Otolaryngology Part II and DLO (Otolaryngology) examinations and their equivalent. Also ideal as a reference source for general practitioners.

1872748686; 1995; Paperback; 368 pages

# Key Topics in Paediatrics

**A.E.M. Davies & A.L. Billson**
*respectively Bristol Royal Hospital for Sick Children, UK; and University of Nottingham, UK*

The ideal reference and revision aid for a postgraduate qualification in paediatrics or child health. Systematically describes the important issues and the identification and management of problems.

"recommended to trainees aiming at taking the MRCP and DCH examinations ... would also be of use to any member of the ward team for quick reference." BMJ

## Contents

100 key topics in current paediatrics presented in alphabetical order.

## Of interest to:

Candidates studying for a postgraduate examination in paediatrics, such as the MRCP (Paed) Parts I and II or the Diploma of Child Health. Also useful as a reference source for all general practitioners, paediatricians, students and nurses.

1872748589; 1994; Paperback; 348 pages

# ORDERING DETAILS

**Main address for orders**

**BIOS Scientific Publishers Ltd**
**9 Newtec Place, Magdalen Road,**
**Oxford OX4 1RE, UK**
**Tel: +44 1865 726286**
**Fax: +44 1865 246823**

**Australia and New Zealand**
DA Information Services
648 Whitehorse Road, Mitcham, Victoria 3132, Australia
Tel: (03) 873 4411
Fax: (03) 873 5679

**India**
Viva Books Private Ltd
4325/3 Ansari Road, Daryaganj, New Delhi 110 002, India
Tel: 11 3283121
Fax: 11 3267224

**Singapore and South East Asia**
(Brunei, Hong Kong, Indonesia, Korea, Malaysia, the Philippines,
Singapore, Taiwan, and Thailand)
Toppan Company (S) PTE Ltd
38 Liu Fang Road, Jurong, Singapore 2262
Tel: (265) 6666
Fax: (261) 7875

**USA and Canada**
Books International Inc
PO Box 605, Herndon, VA 22070, USA
Tel: (703) 435 7064
Fax: (703) 689 0660

Payment can be made by cheque or credit card (Visa/Mastercard, quoting number and expiry date). Alternatively, a *pro forma* invoice can be sent.

Prepaid orders must include £2.50/US$5.00 to cover postage and packing
(two or more books sent post free)